PHANTOMS IN THE BRAIN

V.S. RAMACHANDRAN MD, PHD is one of the world's leading brain researchers. He is Professor and Director of The Center for Brain and Cognition, University of California, San Diego and adjunct Professor at the Salk Institute, La Jolla. He is the recipient of many scientific honours including a gold medal from the Australian National University and a visiting fellowship at All Souls College, Oxford. He also gave the 'Decade of the Brain' lecture at the Silver Jubilee meeting of the Society for Neuroscience. He lives in Del Mar, San Diego.

SANDRA BLAKESLEE is an award-winning *New York Times* science writer and co-author of the bestselling *Second Chance.*

Other books by Sandra Blakeslee

Second Chances
with Judith Wallerstein, PhD

The Good Marriage
with Judith Wallerstein, PhD

V.S. RAMACHANDRAN
and SANDRA BLAKESLEE

Phantoms in the Brain

Human Nature and the
Architecture of the Mind

HarperCollins*Publishers*

HarperCollins*Publishers*
1 London Bridge Street,
London, SE1 9GF, United Kingdom

www.harpercollins.co.uk

First Published in Great Britain by Fourth Estate 1998

10th impression 2016

The name of people and distinctive characteristics referred
To in the case histories in this book have been changed to
Protect the identities of the individuals concerned

ISBN-13: 978-0-00-725389-0

SCIENCE

HarperCollins *Publishers*
A-75, Sector 57, NOIDA, Uttar Pradesh – 201301, India
1 London Bridge Street, London, SE1 9GF, United Kingdom
Hazelton Lanes, 55 Avenue Road, Suite 2900, Toronto, Ontario M5R 3L2
and 1995 Markham Road, Scarborough, Ontario M1B 5M8, Canada
25 Ryde Road, Pymble, Sydney, NSW 2073, Australia
195 Broadway, New York, NY 10007, USA

Printed and bound at
Replika Press Pvt. Ltd.

To my mother, Meenakshi
To my father, Subramanian
To my brother, Ravi
To Diane, Mani and Jayakrishna
To all my former teachers in India and England
To Saraswathy, the goddess of learning, music and wisdom

Foreword

The great neurologists and psychiatrists of the nineteenth and early twentieth centuries were masters of description, and some of their case histories provided an almost novelistic richness of detail. Silas Weir Mitchell—who was a novelist as well as a neurologist—provided unforgettable descriptions of the phantom limbs (or "sensory ghosts," as he first called them) in soldiers who had been injured on the battlefields of the Civil War. Joseph Babinski, the great French neurologist, described an even more extraordinary syndrome—anosognosia, the inability to perceive that one side of one's own body is paralyzed and the often-bizarre attribution of the paralyzed side to ***another person.*** (Such a patient might say of his or her own left side, "It's my brother's" or "It's yours.")

Dr. V.S. Ramachandran, one of the most interesting neuroscientists of our time, has done seminal work on the nature and treatment of phantom limbs—those obdurate and sometimes tormenting ghosts of arms and legs lost years or decades before but not forgotten by the brain. A phantom may at first feel like a normal limb, a part of the normal body image; but, cut off from normal sensation or action, it may assume a pathological character, becoming intrusive, "paralyzed," deformed, or excruciatingly painful—phantom fingers may dig into a phantom palm with an unspeakable, unstoppable intensity. The fact that the pain and the phantom are "unreal" is of no help, and may indeed make them more difficult to treat, for one may be unable to unclench the seemingly paralyzed phantom. In an attempt to alleviate such phantoms, physicians and their patients have been driven to extreme and desperate measures: making the amputation stump shorter and shorter, cutting pain or sensory tracts in the spinal cord, destroying pain centers in the brain itself. But all too frequently, none of these work; the phantom, and the phantom pain, almost invariably return.

To these seemingly intractable problems, Ramachandran brings a fresh and different approach, which stems from his inquiries as to what phantoms ***are,*** and how and where they are generated in the nervous system. It has been classically considered that representations in the brain, including those of body image and phantoms, are fixed. But Ramachandran (and now others) has shown that striking reorganizations in body image occur very rapidly—within forty-eight hours, and possibly much less—following the amputation of a limb. Phantoms, in his view, are generated by such reorganizations of body image in the sensory cortex and may then be maintained by what he terms a "learned" paralysis. But if there are such rapid changes underlying the genesis of a phantom, if there is such plasticity in the cortex, can the process be reversed? Can the brain be tricked into *unlearning* a phantom?

By using an ingenious "virtual reality" device, a simple box with a transposing mirror, Ramachandran has found that a patient may be helped by merely being given the sight of a normal limb—the patient's own normal right arm, for example, now seen on the left side of the body, in place of the phantom. The result of this may be instantaneous and magical: The normal look of the arm competes with the feel of the phantom. The first effect of this is that a deformed phantom may straighten out, a paralyzed phantom may move; eventually, there may be no more phantom at all. Ramachandran speaks here, with characteristic humor, of "the first successful amputation of a phantom limb," and of how, if the phantom is extinguished, its pain must also go—for if there is nothing to embody it, then it can no longer survive. (Mrs. Gradgrind, in *Hard Times*, asked if she had a pain, replied, "There is a pain somewhere in the room, but I cannot be sure that I have got it." But this was her confusion, or Dickens's joke, for one cannot have a pain except in oneself.)

Can equally simple "tricks" assist patients with anosognosia, patients who cannot recognize one of their sides as their own? Here too, Ramachandran finds, mirrors may be of great use in enabling such patients to reclaim the previously denied side as their own; though in other patients, the loss of "leftness," the bisection of one's body and world, is so profound that mirrors may induce an even deeper, through-the-looking-glass confusion, a groping to see if there is not someone lurking "behind" or "in" the mirror. (Ramachandran is the first to describe this "mirror agnosia.") It is a measure not only of Ramachandran's tenacity of mind but of his delicate and supportive relationship with patients that he has been able to pursue these syndromes to their depths.

The deeply strange business of mirror agnosia, and that of misattributing one's own limbs to others, are often dismissed by physicians as irrational. But these problems are also considered carefully by Ramachandran, who sees them not as groundless or crazy, but as emergency defense measures constructed by the unconscious to deal with sudden overwhelming bewilderments about one's body and the space around it. They are, he feels, quite normal defense mechanisms (denial, repression, projection, confabulation, and so on) such as Freud delineated as universal strategies of the unconscious when forced to accommodate the intolerable or unintelligible. Such an understanding removes such patients from the realm of the mad or freakish and restores them to the realm of discourse and reason—albeit the discourse and reason of the unconscious.

Another syndrome of misidentification that Ramachandran considers is Capgras' syndrome, where the patient sees familiar and loved figures as impostors. Here too, he is able to delineate a clear neurological basis for the syndrome—the removal of the usual and crucial affective cues to recognition, coupled with a not unnatural interpretation of the now affectless perceptions ("He can't be my father, because I *feel* nothing—he must be a sort of simulacrum").

Dr. Ramachandran has countless other interests too: in the nature of religious experience and the remarkable "mystical" syndromes associated with dysfunction in the temporal lobes, in the neurology of laughter and tickling, and—a vast realm—in the neurology of suggestion and placebos. Like the perceptual psychologist Richard Gregory (with whom he has published fascinating work on a range of subjects, from the filling-in of the blind spot to visual illusions and protective colorations), Ramachandran has a flair for seeing what is fundamentally important and is prepared to turn his hand, his freshness, his inventiveness, to almost anything. All of these subjects, in his hands, become windows into the way our nervous systems, our worlds, and our very selves are constituted, so that his work becomes, as he likes to say, a form of "experimental epistemology." He is, in this way, a natural philosopher in the eighteenth-century sense, though with all the knowledge and know-how of the late twentieth century behind him.

In his Preface, Ramachandran tells us of the nineteenth-century science books he especially enjoyed as a boy: Michael Faraday's *Chemical History of a Candle,* works by Charles Darwin, Humphry Davy and Thomas Huxley. There was no distinction at this time between academic and popular writing, but rather the notion that one could be deep and serious but completely accessible, all at once. Later, Ramachandran tells us, he enjoyed the books of George Gamow, Lewis Thomas, Peter Medawar, and then Carl Sagan and Stephen Jay Gould. Ramachandran has now joined these grand science writers with his closely observed and deeply serious but beautifully readable book *Phantoms in the Brain*. It is one of the most original and accessible neurology books of our generation.

—Oliver Sacks, M.D.

Preface

In any field, find the strangest thing and then explore it.

—John Archibald Wheeler

This book has been incubating in my head for many years, but I never quite got around to writing it. Then, about three years ago, I gave the Decade of the Brain lecture at the annual meeting of the Society for Neuroscience to an audience of over four thousand scientists, discussing many of my findings, including my studies on phantom limbs, body image and the illusory nature of the self. Soon after the lecture, I was barraged with questions from the audience: How does the mind influence the body in health and sickness? How can I stimulate my right brain to be more creative? Can your mental attitude really help cure asthma and cancer? Is hypnosis a real phenomenon? Does your work suggest new ways to treat paralysis after strokes? I also got a number of requests from students, colleagues and even a few publishers to undertake writing a textbook. Textbook writing is not my cup of tea, but I thought a popular book on the brain dealing mainly with my own experiences working with neurological patients might be fun to write. During the last decade or so, I have gleaned many new insights into the workings of the human brain by studying such cases, and the urge to communicate these ideas is strong. When you are involved in an enterprise as exciting as this, it's a natural human tendency to want to share your ideas with others. Moreover, I feel that I owe it to taxpayers, who ultimately support my work through grants from the National Institutes of Health.

Popular science books have a rich, venerable tradition going as far back as Galileo in the seventeenth century. Indeed, this was Galileo's main method of disseminating his ideas, and in his books he often aimed barbs at an imaginary protagonist, Simplicio—an amalgam of his professors. Almost all of Charles Darwin's famous books, including *The Origin of Species, The Descent of Man, The Expression of Emotions in Animals and Men, The Habits of Insectivorous Plants*—but not his two-volume monograph on barnacles!—were written for the lay reader at the request of his publisher, John Murray. The same can be said of the many works of Thomas Huxley, Michael Faraday, Humphry Davy and many other Victorian scientists. Faraday's *Chemical History of a Candle*, based on Christmas lectures that he gave to children, remains a classic to this day.

I must confess that I haven't read all these books, but I do owe a heavy intellectual debt to popular science books, a sentiment that is echoed by many of my colleagues. Dr. Francis Crick of the Salk Institute tells me that Erwin Schrödinger's popular book *What Is Life?* contained a few speculative remarks on how heredity might be based on a chemical and that this had a profound impact on his intellectual development, culminating in his unraveling the genetic code together with James Watson. Many a Nobel Prize–winning physician embarked on a research career after reading Paul de Kruif's *The Microbe Hunters,* which was published in 1926. My own interest in scientific research dates back to my early teens, when I read books by George Gamow, Lewis Thomas, and Peter Medawar, and the flame is being kept alive by a new generation of writers—Oliver Sacks, Stephen Jay Gould, Carl Sagan, Dan Dennett, Richard Gregory, Richard Dawkins, Paul Davies, Colin Blakemore and Steven Pinker.

About six years ago I received a phone call from Francis Crick, the codiscoverer of the structure of deoxyribonucleic acid (DNA), in which he said that he was writing a popular book on the brain called *The Astonishing Hypothesis.* In his crisp British accent, Crick said that he had completed a first draft and had sent it to his editor, who felt that it was extremely well written but that the manuscript still contained jargon that would be intelligible only to a specialist. She suggested that he pass it around to some lay people. "I say, Rama," Crick said with exasperation, "the trouble is, I don't *know* any lay people. Do you know any lay people I could show the book to?" At first I thought he was joking, but then realized he was perfectly serious. I can't personally claim not to know any lay people, but I could nevertheless sympathize with Crick's plight. When writing a popular book, professional scientists always have to walk a tightrope between making the book intelligible to the general reader, on the one hand, and avoiding oversimplification, on the other, so that experts are not annoyed. My solution has been to make elaborate use of end notes, which serve three distinct functions: First, whenever it was necessary to simplify an idea, my cowriter, Sandra Blakeslee, and I resorted to notes to qualify these remarks, to point out exceptions and to make it clear that in some cases the results are preliminary or controversial. Second, we have used notes to amplify a point that is made only briefly in the main text—so that the reader can explore a topic in greater depth. The notes also point the reader to original references and credit those who have worked on similar topics. I apologize to those whose works are not cited; my only excuse is that such omission is inevitable in a book such as this (for a while the notes threatened to exceed the main text in length). But I've tried to include as many pertinent references as possible in the bibliography at the end, even though not all of them are specifically mentioned in the text.

This book is based on the true-life stories of many neurological patients. To protect their identity, I have followed the usual tradition of changing names, circumstances and defining characteristics throughout each chapter. Some of the "cases" I describe are really composites of several patients, including classics in the medical literature, as my purpose has been to illustrate salient aspects of the disorder, such as the neglect syndrome or temporal lobe epilepsy. When I describe classic cases (like the man with amnesia known as H.M.), I refer the reader to original sources for details. Other stories are based on what are called single-case studies, which involve individuals who manifest a rare or unusual syndrome.

A tension exists in neurology between those who believe that the most valuable lessons about the brain can be learned from statistical analyses involving large numbers of patients and those who believe that doing the right kind of experiments on the right patients—even a single patient—can yield much more useful information. This is really a silly debate since its resolution is obvious: It's a good idea to begin with experiments on single cases and then to confirm the findings through studies of additional patients. By way of analogy, imagine that I cart a pig into your living room and tell you that it can talk. You might say, "Oh, really? Show me." I then wave my wand and the pig starts talking. You might respond, "My God! That's amazing!" You are not likely to say, "Ah, but that's just one pig. Show me a few more and then I might believe you." Yet this is precisely the attitude of many people in my field.

I think it's fair to say that, in neurology, most of the major discoveries that have withstood the test of time were, in fact, based initially on single-case studies and demonstrations. More was learned about memory from a few days of studying a patient called H.M. than was gleaned from previous decades of research averaging data on many subjects. The same can be said about hemispheric specialization (the organization of the brain into a left brain and a right brain, which are specialized for different functions) and the experiments carried out on two patients with so-called split brains (in whom the left and right hemispheres were disconnected by cutting the fibers between them). More was learned from these two individuals than from the previous fifty years of studies on normal people.

In a science still in its infancy (like neuroscience and psychology) demonstration-style experiments play an especially important role. A classic example is Galileo's use of early telescopes. People often assume that Galileo invented the telescope, but he did not. Around 1607, a Dutch spectacle maker, Hans Lipperhey, placed two lenses in a cardboard tube and found that this arrangement made distant objects appear closer. The device was widely used as a child's toy and soon found its way into country fairs throughout Europe, including France. In 1609, when Galileo heard about this gadget, he immediately recognized its potential. Instead of spying on people and other terrestrial objects, he simply raised the tube to the sky—something that nobody else had done. First he aimed it at the moon and found that it was covered with craters, gullies and mountains—which told him that the so-called heavenly bodies are, contrary to conventional wisdom, not so perfect after all: They are full of flaws and imperfections, open to scrutiny by mortal eyes just like objects on earth. Next he directed the telescope at the Milky Way and noticed instantly that far from being a homogeneous cloud (as people believed), it was composed of millions of stars. But his most startling discovery occurred when he peered at Jupiter, which was known to be a planet or wandering star. Imagine his astonishment when he saw three tiny dots near Jupiter (which he initially assumed were new stars) and witnessed that after a few days one disappeared. He then waited for a few more days and gazed once again at Jupiter, only to find that not only had the missing dot reappeared, but there was now an extra dot—a total of four dots instead of three. He understood in a flash that the four dots were Jovian satellites—moons just like ours—that orbited the planet. The implications were immense. In one stroke, Galileo had proved that not all celestial bodies orbit the earth, for here were four that orbited another planet, Jupiter. He thereby dethroned the geocentric theory of the universe, replacing it with the Copernican view that the sun, not the earth, was at the center of the known universe. The clinching evidence came when he directed his telescope at Venus and found that it looked like a crescent moon going though all the phases, just like our moon, except that it took a year rather than a month to do so. Again, Galileo deduced from this that all the planets were orbiting the sun and that Venus was interposed between the earth and the sun. All this from a simple cardboard tube with two lenses. No equations, no graphs, no quantitative measurements: "just" a demonstration.

When I relate this example to medical students, the usual reaction is, Well, that was easy during Galileo's time, but surely now in the twentieth century all the major discoveries have already been made and we can't do any new research without expensive equipment and detailed quantitative methods. Rubbish! Even now amazing discoveries are staring at you all the time, right under your nose. The difficulty lies in realizing this. For example, in recent decades all medical students were taught that ulcers are caused by stress, which leads to excessive acid production that erodes the mucosal lining of the stomach and duodenum, producing the characteristic craters or wounds that we call ulcers. And for decades the treatment was either antacids, histamine receptor blockers, vagotomy (cutting the acid-secreting nerve that innervates the stomach) or even gastrectomy (removal of part of the stomach.) But then a young resident physician in Australia, Dr. Bill Marshall, looked at a stained section of a human ulcer under a microscope and noticed that it was teeming with *Helicobacter pylori*—a common bacterium that is found in a certain proportion of healthy individuals. Since he regularly saw these bacteria in ulcers, he started wondering whether perhaps they actually *caused* ulcers. When he mentioned this idea to his professors, he was told, "No way. That can't be true. We all know ulcers are caused by stress. What you are seeing is just a secondary infection of an ulcer that was already in place."

But Dr. Marshall was not dissuaded and proceeded to challenge the conventional wisdom. First he carried out an epidemiological study, which showed a strong correlation between the distribution of *Helicobacter* species in patients and the incidence of duodenal ulcers. But this finding did not convince his colleagues, so out of sheer desperation, Marshall swallowed a culture of the bacteria, did an endoscopy on himself a few weeks later and demonstrated that his gastrointestinal tract was studded with ulcers! He then conducted a formal clinical trial and showed that ulcer patients who were treated with a combination of antibiotics, bismuth and metronidazole (Flagyl, a bactericide) recovered at a much higher rate—and had fewer relapses—than did a control group given acid-blocking agents alone.

I mention this episode to emphasize that a single medical student or resident whose mind is open to new ideas and who works without sophisticated equipment can revolutionize the practice of medicine. It is in this spirit that we should all undertake our work, because one never knows what nature is hiding.

I'd also like to say a word about speculation, a term that has acquired a pejorative connotation among some scientists. Describing someone's idea as "mere speculation" is often considered insulting. This is unfortunate. As the English biologist Peter Medawar has noted, "An imaginative conception of what *might* be true is the starting point of all great discoveries in science." Ironically, this is sometimes true even when the speculation turns out to be wrong. Listen to Charles Darwin: "False facts are highly injurious to the progress of science for they often endure long; but false hypotheses do little harm, as everyone takes a salutary pleasure in proving their falseness; and when this is done, one path toward error is closed and the road to truth is often at the same time opened."

Every scientist knows that the best research emerges from a dialectic between speculation and healthy skepticism. Ideally the two should coexist in the same brain, but they don't have to. Since there are people who represent both extremes, all ideas eventually get tested ruthlessly. Many are rejected (like cold fusion) and others promise to turn our views topsy turvy (like the view that ulcers are caused by bacteria).

Several of the findings you are going to read about began as hunches and were later confirmed by other groups (the chapters on phantom limbs, neglect syndrome, blindsight and Capgras' syndrome). Other chapters describe work at an earlier stage, much of which is frankly speculative (the chapter on denial and temporal lobe epilepsy). Indeed, I will take you at times to the very limits of scientific inquiry.

I strongly believe, however, that it is always the writer's responsibility to spell out clearly when he is speculating and when his conclusions are clearly warranted by his observations. I've made every effort to preserve this distinction throughout the book, often adding qualifications, disclaimers and caveats in the text and especially in the notes. In striking this balance between fact and fancy, I hope to stimulate your intellectual curiosity and to widen your horizons, rather than to provide you with hard and fast answers to the questions raised.

The famous saying "May you live in interesting times" has a special meaning now for those of us who study the brain and human behavior. On the one hand, despite two hundred years of research, the most basic questions about the human mind—How do we recognize faces? Why do we cry? Why do we laugh? Why do we dream? and Why do we enjoy music and art?—remain unanswered, as does the really big question: What is consciousness? On the other hand, the advent of novel experimental approaches and imaging techniques is sure to transform our understanding of the human brain. What a unique privilege it will be for our generation—and our children's—to witness what I believe will be the greatest revolution in the history of the human race: understanding ourselves. The prospect of doing so is at once both exhilarating and disquieting.

There is something distinctly odd about a hairless neotenous primate that has evolved into a species that can look back over its own shoulder and ask questions about its origins. And odder still, the brain can not only discover how other brains work but also ask questions about its own existence: Who am I? What happens after death? Does my mind arise exclusively from neurons in my brain? And if so, what scope is there for free will? It is the peculiar recursive quality of these questions—as the brain struggles to understand itself—that makes neurology fascinating.

Contents

By the deficits, we may know the talents, by the exceptions, we may discern the rules, by studying pathology we may construct a model of health. And—most important—from this model may evolve the insights and tools we need to affect our own lives, mold our own destinies, change ourselves and our society in ways that, as yet, we can only imagine.

—LAURENCE MILLER

The world shall perish not for lack of wonders, but for lack of wonder.

—J.B.S. HALDANE

CHAPTER 1

The Phantom Within

For in and out, above, about, below,
'Tis nothing but a Magic Shadow-show
Play'd in a Box whose Candle is the Sun,
Round which we Phantom Figures come and go.

—The Rubáiyát of Omar Khayyám

I know, my dear Watson, that you share my love
of all that is bizarre and outside the conventions
and humdrum routines of everyday life.

—*Sherlock Holmes*

A man wearing an enormous bejeweled cross dangling on a gold chain sits in my office, telling me about his conversations with God, the "real meaning" of the cosmos and the deeper truth behind all surface appearances. The universe is suffused with spiritual messages, he says, if you just allow yourself to tune in. I glance at his medical chart, noting that he has suffered from temporal lobe epilepsy since early adolescence, and that is when "God began talking" to him. Do his religious experiences have anything to do with his temporal lobe seizures?

An amateur athlete lost his arm in a motorcycle accident but continues to feel a "phantom arm" with vivid sensations of movement. He can wave the missing arm in midair, "touch" things and even reach out and "grab" a coffee cup. If I pull the cup away from him suddenly, he yelps in pain. "Ouch! I can feel it being wrenched from my fingers," he says, wincing.

A nurse developed a large blind spot in her field of vision, which is troubling enough. But to her dismay, she often sees cartoon characters cavorting within the blind spot itself. When she looks at me seated across from her, she sees Bugs Bunny in my lap, or Elmer Fudd, or the Road Runner. Or sometimes she sees cartoon versions of real people she's always known.

A schoolteacher suffered a stroke that paralyzed the left side of her body, but she insists that her left arm is *not* paralyzed. Once, when I asked her whose arm was lying in the bed next to her, she explained that the limb belonged to her brother.

A librarian from Philadelphia who had a different kind of stroke began to laugh uncontrollably. This went on for a full day, until she literally died laughing.

And then there is Arthur, a young man who sustained a terrible head injury in an automobile crash and soon afterward claimed that his father and mother had been replaced by duplicates who looked exactly like his real parents. He recognized their faces but they seemed odd, unfamiliar. The only way Arthur could make any sense out of the situation was to assume that his parents were impostors.

None of these people is "crazy"; sending them to psychiatrists would be a waste of time. Rather, each of them suffers from damage to a specific part of the brain that leads to bizarre but highly characteristic changes in behavior. They hear voices, feel missing limbs, see things that no one else does, deny the obvious and make wild, extraordinary claims about other people and the world we all live in. Yet for the most part they are lucid, rational and no more insane than you or I.

Although enigmatic disorders like these have intrigued and perplexed physicians throughout history, they are usually chalked up as curiosities—case studies stuffed into a drawer labeled "file and forget." Most neurologists who treat such patients are not particularly interested in explaining these odd behaviors. Their goal is to alleviate symptoms and to make people well again, not necessarily to dig deeper or to learn how the brain works. Psychiatrists often invent ad hoc theories for curious syndromes, as if a bizarre condition requires an equally bizarre explanation. Odd symptoms are blamed on the patient's upbringing (bad thoughts from childhood) or even on the patient's mother (a bad nurturer). *Phantoms in the Brain* takes the opposite viewpoint. These patients, whose stories you will hear in detail, are our guides into the inner workings of the human brain—yours and mine. Far from being curiosities, these syndromes illustrate fundamental principles of how the normal human mind and brain work, shedding light on the nature of body image, language, laughter, dreams, depression and other hallmarks of human nature. Have you ever wondered why some jokes are funny and others are not, why you make an explosive sound when you laugh, why you are inclined to believe or disbelieve in God, and why you feel erotic sensations when someone sucks your toes? Surprisingly, we can now begin to provide scientific answers to at least some of these questions. Indeed, by studying these patients, we can even address lofty "philosophical" questions about the nature of the self: Why do you endure as one person through space and time, and what brings about the seamless unity of subjective experience? What does it mean to make a choice or to will an action? And more generally, how does the activity of tiny wisps of protoplasm in the brain lead to conscious experience?

Philosophers love to debate questions like these, but it's only now becoming clear that such issues can be tackled experimentally. By moving these patients out of the clinic and into the laboratory, we can conduct experiments that help reveal the deep architecture of our brains. Indeed, we can pick up where Freud left off, ushering in what might be called an era of experimental epistemology (the study of how the brain represents knowledge and belief) and cognitive neuropsychiatry (the interface between mental and physical disorders of the brain), and start experimenting on belief systems, consciousness, mind-body interactions and other hallmarks of human behavior.

I believe that being a medical scientist is not all that different from being a sleuth. In this book, I've attempted to share the sense of mystery that lies at the heart of all scientific pursuits and is especially characteristic of the forays we make in trying to understand our own minds. Each story begins with either an account of a patient displaying seemingly inexplicable symptoms or a broad question about human nature, such as why we laugh or why we are so prone to self-deception. We then go step by step through the same sequence of ideas that I followed in my own mind as I tried to tackle these cases. In some instances, as with phantom limbs, I can claim to have genuinely solved the mystery. In others—as in the chapter on God—the final answer remains elusive, even though we come tantalizingly close. But whether the case is solved or not, I hope to convey the spirit of intellectual adventure that accompanies this pursuit and makes neurology the most fascinating of all disciplines. As Sherlock Holmes told Watson, "The game is afoot!"

Consider the case of Arthur, who thought his parents were impostors. Most physicians would be tempted to conclude that he was just crazy, and, indeed, that is the most common explanation for this type of disorder, found in many textbooks. But, by simply showing him photographs of different people and measuring the extent to which he starts sweating (using a device similar to the lie detector test), I was able to figure out exactly what had gone wrong in his brain (see chapter 9). This is a recurring theme in this book: We begin with a set of symptoms that seem bizarre and incomprehensible and then end up—at least in some cases—with an intellectually satisfying account in terms of the neural circuitry in the patient's brain. And in doing so, we have often not only discovered something new about how the brain works but simultaneously opened the doors to a whole new direction of research.

•

But before we begin, I think it's important for you to understand my personal approach to science and why I am drawn to curious cases. When I give talks to lay audiences around the country, one question comes up again and again: "When are you brain scientists ever going to come up with a unified theory for how the mind works? There's Einstein's general theory of relativity and Newton's universal law of gravitation in physics. Why not one for the brain?"

My answer is that we are not yet at the stage where we can formulate grand unified theories of mind and brain. Every science has to go through an initial "experiment" or phenomena-driven stage—in which its practitioners are still discovering the basic laws—before it reaches a more sophisticated theory-driven stage. Consider the evolution of ideas about electricity and magnetism. Although people had vague notions about lodestones and magnets for centuries and used them both for making compasses, the Victorian physicist Michael Faraday was the first to study magnets systematically. He did two very simple experiments with astonishing results. In one experiment—which any schoolchild can repeat—he simply placed a bar magnet behind a sheet of paper, sprinkled powdered iron filings on the surface of the paper and found that they spontaneously aligned themselves along the magnetic lines of force (this was the very first time anyone had demonstrated the existence of fields in physics). In the second experiment, Faraday moved a bar magnet to and fro in the center of a coil of wire, and, lo and behold, this action produced an electrical current in the wire. These informal demonstrations—and this book is full of examples of this sort—had deep implications:[1] They linked magnetism and electricity for the first time. Faraday's own interpretation of these effects remained qualitative, but his experiments set the stage for James Clerk Maxwell's famous electromagnetic wave equations several decades later—the mathematical formalisms that form the basis of all modern physics.

My point is simply that neuroscience today is in the Faraday stage, not in the Maxwell stage, and there is no point in trying to jump ahead. I would love to be proved wrong, of course, and there is certainly no harm in trying to construct formal theories about the brain, even if one fails (and there is no shortage of people who are trying). But for me, the best research strategy might be characterized as "tinkering." Whenever I use this word, many people look rather shocked, as if one couldn't possibly do sophisticated science by just playing around with ideas and without an overarching theory to guide one's hunches. But that's exactly what I mean (although these hunches are far from random; they are always guided by intuition).

I've been interested in science as long as I can remember. When I was eight or nine years old, I started collecting fossils and seashells, becoming obsessed with taxonomy and evolution. A little later I set up a small chemistry lab under the stairway in our house and enjoyed watching iron filings "fizz" in hydrochloric acid and listening to the hydrogen "pop" when I set fire to it. (The iron displaced the hydrogen from the hydrochloric acid to form iron chloride and hydrogen.) The idea that you could learn so much from a simple experiment and that everything in the universe is based on such interactions was fascinating. I remember that when a teacher told me about Faraday's simple experiments, I was intrigued by the notion that you could accomplish so much with so little. These experiences left me with a permanent distaste for fancy equipment and the realization that you don't necessarily need complicated machines to generate scientific revolutions; all you need are some good hunches.[2]

Another perverse streak of mine is that I've always been drawn to the exception rather than to the rule in every science that I've studied. In high school I wondered why iodine is the only element that turns from a solid to a vapor directly when heated, without first melting and going through a liquid stage. Why does Saturn have rings and not the other planets? Why does water alone expand when it turns to ice, whereas every other liquid shrinks when it solidifies? Why do some animals not have sex? Why can tadpoles regenerate lost limbs though an adult frog cannot? Is it because the tadpole is younger, or is it because it's a tadpole? What would happen if you delayed metamorphosis by blocking the action of thyroid hormones (you could put a few drops of thiouracil into the aquarium) so that you ended up with a very old tadpole? Would the geriatric tadpole be able to regenerate a missing limb? (As a schoolboy I made some feeble attempts to answer this, but, to my knowledge, we don't know the answer even to this day.)[3]

Of course, looking at such odd cases is not the only way—or even the best way—of doing science; it's a lot of fun but it's not everyone's cup of tea. But it's an eccentricity that has remained with me since childhood, and fortunately I have been able to turn it into an advantage. Clinical neurology, in particular, is full of such examples that have been ignored by the "establishment" because they don't really fit received wisdom. I have discovered, to my delight, that many of them are diamonds in the rough.

For example, those who are suspcious of the claims of mind-body medicine should consider multiple personality disorders. Some clinicians say that patients can actually "change" their eye structure when assuming different personas—a nearsighted person becomes farsighted, a blue-eyed person becomes brown-eyed—or that the patient's blood chemistry changes along with personality (high blood glucose level with one and normal glucose level with another). There are also case descriptions of people's hair turning white, literally overnight, after a severe psychological shock and of pious nuns' developing stigmata on their palms in ecstatic union with Jesus. I find it surprising that despite three decades of research, we are not even sure whether these phenomena are real or bogus. Given all the hints that there is something interesting going on, why not examine these claims in greater detail? Are they like alien abduction and spoon bending, or are they genuine anomalies—like X rays or bacterial transformation[4]—that may someday drive paradigm shifts and scientific revolutions?

I was personally drawn into medicine, a discipline full of ambiguities, because its Sherlock Holmes style of inquiry greatly appealed to me. Diagnosing a patient's problem remains as much an art as a science, calling into play powers of observation, reason and all the human senses. I recall one professor, Dr. K.V. Thiruvengadam, instructing us how to identify disease by just smelling the patient—the unmistakable, sweetish nail polish breath of diabetic ketosis; the freshly baked bread odor of typhoid fever; the stale-beer stench of scrofula; the newly plucked chicken feathers aroma of rubella; the foul smell of a lung abscess; and the ammonialike Windex odor of a patient in liver failure. (And today a pediatrician might add the grape juice smell of *Pseudomonas* infection in children and the sweaty-feet smell of isovaleric acidemia.) Inspect the fingers carefully, Dr. Thiruvengadam told us, because a small change in the angle between the nail bed and the finger can herald the onset of a malignant lung cancer long before more ominous clinical signs emerge. Remarkably, this telltale sign—clubbing—disappears instantly on the operating table as the surgeon removes the cancer, but, even to this day, we have no idea why it occurs. Another teacher of mine, a professor of neurology, would insist on our diagnosing Parkinson's disease with our eyes closed—by simply listening to the patients' footsteps (patients with this disorder have a characteristic shuffling gait). This detectivelike aspect of clinical medicine is a dying art in this age of high-tech medicine, but it planted a seed in my mind. By carefully observing, listening, touching and, yes, even smelling the patient, one can arrive at a reasonable diagnosis and merely use laboratory tests to confirm what is already known.

Finally, when studying and treating a patient, it is the physician's duty always to ask himself, "What does it *feel like* to be in the patient's shoes?" "What if I were him?" In doing this, I have never ceased to be amazed at the courage and fortitude of many of my patients or by the fact that, ironically, tragedy itself can sometimes enrich a patient's life and give it new meaning. For this reason, even though many of the clinical tales you will hear are tinged with sadness, equally often they are stories of the triumph of the human spirit over adversity, and there is a strong undercurrent of optimism. For example, one patient I saw—a neurologist from New York—suddenly at the age of sixty started experiencing epileptic seizures arising from his right temporal lobe. The seizures were alarming, of course, but to his amazement and delight he found himself becoming fascinated by poetry, for the first time in his life. In fact, he began thinking in verse, producing a voluminous outflow of rhyme. He said that such a poetic view gave him a new lease on life, a fresh start just when he was starting to feel a bit jaded. Does it follow from this example that all of us are unfulfilled poets, as many new age gurus and mystics assert? Do we each have an untapped potential for beautiful verse and rhyme hidden in the recesses of our right hemisphere? If so, is there any way we can unleash this latent ability, short of having seizures?

•

Before we meet the patients, crack mysteries and speculate about brain organization, I'd like to take you on a short guided tour of the human brain. These anatomical signposts, which I promise to keep simple, will help you understand the many new explanations for why neurological patients act the way they do.

It's almost a cliché these days to say that the human brain is the most

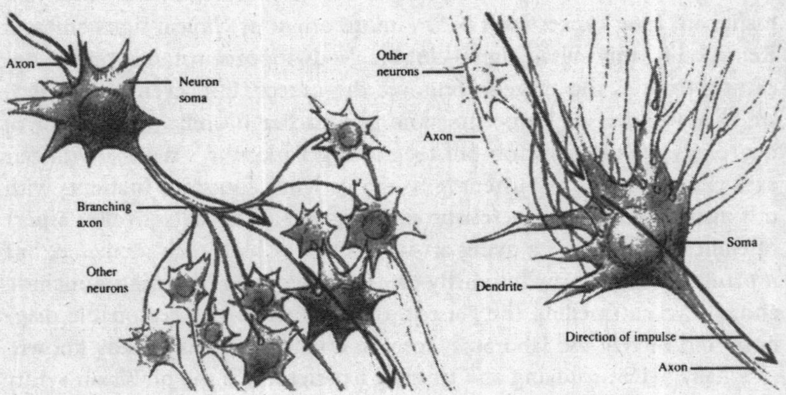

Figure 1.1

complexly organized form of matter in the universe, and there is actually some truth to this. If you snip away a section of brain, say, from the convoluted outer layer called the neocortex and peer at it under a microscope, you'll see that it is composed of neurons or nerve cells—the basic functional units of the nervous system, where information is exchanged. At birth, the typical brain probably contains over one hundred billion neurons, whose number slowly diminishes with age.

Each neuron has a cell body and tens of thousands of tiny branches called dendrites, which receive information from other neurons. Each neuron also has a primary axon (a projection that can travel long distances in the brain) for sending data out of the cell, and axon terminals for communication with other cells.

If you look at Figure 1.1, you'll notice that neurons make contacts with other neurons, at points called synapses. Each neuron makes anywhere from a thousand to ten thousand synapses with other neurons. These can be either on or off, excitatory or inhibitory. That is, some synapses turn on the juice to fire things up, whereas others release juices that calm everything down, in an ongoing dance of staggering complexity. A piece of your brain the size of a grain of sand would contain one hundred thousand neurons, two million axons and one billion synapses, all "talking to" each other. Given these figures, it's been calculated that the number of possible brain states—the number of permutations and combinations of activity that are theoretically possible—exceeds the number of elementary particles in the universe. Given this complexity,

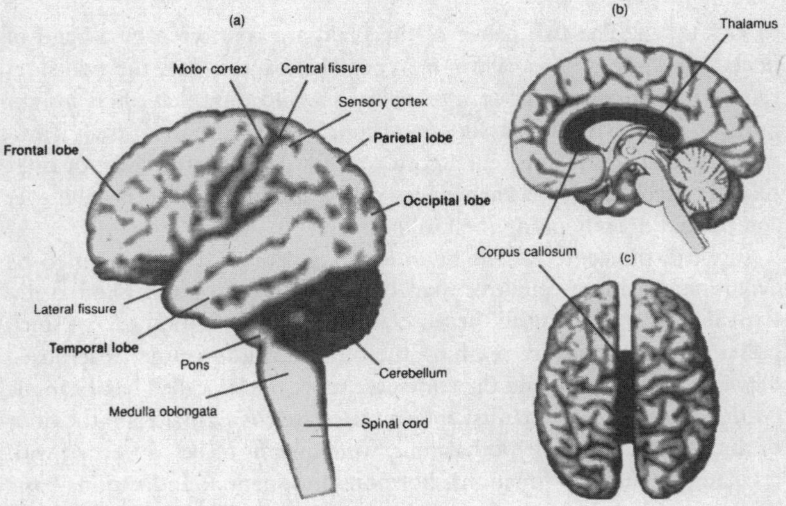

Figure 1.2 *Gross anatomy of the human brain. (a) Shows the left side of the left hemisphere. Notice the four lobes: frontal, parietal, temporal and occipital. The frontal is separated from the parietal by the central or rolandic sulcus (furrow or fissure), and the temporal from the parietal by the lateral or sylvian fissure. (b) Shows the inner surface of the left hemisphere. Notice the conspicuous corpus callosum (black) and the thalamus (white) in the middle. The corpus callosum bridges the two hemispheres. (c) Shows the two hemispheres of the brain viewed down the top.* (a) Ramachandran; (b) and (c) redrawn from Zeki, 1993.

how do we begin to understand the functions of the brain? Obviously, understanding the *structure* of the nervous system is vital to understanding its functions[5]—and so I will begin with a brief survey of the anatomy of the brain, which, for our purposes here, begins at the top of the spinal cord. This region, called the medulla oblongata, connects the spinal cord to the brain and contains clusters of cells or nuclei that control critical functions like blood pressure, heart rate and breathing. The medulla connects to the pons (a kind of bulge), which sends fibers into the cerebellum, a fist-sized structure at the back of the brain that helps you carry out coordinated movements. Atop these are the two enormous cerebral hemispheres—the famous walnut-shaped halves of the brain. Each half is divided into four lobes—frontal, temporal, parietal and occipital—that you will learn much more about in coming chapters (Figure 1.2).

Each hemisphere controls the movements of the muscles (for example, those in your arm and leg) on the opposite side of your body. Your right brain makes your left arm wave and your left brain allows your right leg to kick a ball. The two halves of the brain are connected by a band of fibers called the corpus callosum. When this band is cut, the two sides can no longer communicate; the result is a syndrome that offers insight into the role each side plays in cognition. The outer part of each hemisphere is composed of cerebral cortex: a thin, convoluted sheet of cells, six layers thick, that is scrunched into ridges and furrows like a cauliflower and packed densely inside the skull.

Right in the center of the brain is the thalamus. It is thought to be evolutionarily more primitive than the cerebral cortex and is often described as a "relay station" because all sensory information except smell passes through it before reaching the outer cortical mantle. Interposed between the thalamus and the cortex are more nuclei, called basal ganglia (with names like the putamen and caudate nucleus). Finally, on the floor of the thalamus is the hypothalamus, which seems to be concerned with regulating metabolic functions, hormone production, and various basic drives such as aggression, fear, and sexuality.

These anatomical facts have been known for a long time, but we still have no clear idea of how the brain works.[6] Many older theories fall into two warring camps—modularity and holism—and the pendulum has swung back and forth between these two extreme points of view for the last three hundred years. At one end of the spectrum are modularists, who believe that different parts of the brain are highly specialized for mental capacities. Thus there is a module for language, one for memory, one for math ability, one for face recognition and maybe even one for detecting people who cheat. Moreover, they argue, these modules or regions are largely autonomous. Each does its own job, set of computations, or whatever, and then—like a bucket brigade—passes its output to the next module in line, not "talking" much to other regions.

At the other end of the spectrum we have "holism," a theoretical approach that overlaps with what these days is called "connectionism." This school of thought argues that the brain functions as a whole and that any one part is as good as any other part. The holistic view is defended by the fact that many areas, especially cortical regions, can be recruited for multiple tasks. Everything is connected to everything else, say the holists, and so the search for distinct modules is a waste of time.

My own work with patients suggests that these two points of view are not mutually exclusive—that the brain is a dynamic structure that employs both "modes" in a marvelously complex interplay. The grandeur of the human potential is visible only when we take all the possibilities into account, resisting the temptation to fall into polarized camps or to ask whether a given function is localized or not localized.[7] As we shall see, it's much more useful to tackle each problem as it comes along and not get hung up taking sides.

Each view in its extreme form is in fact rather absurd. As an analogy, suppose you are watching the program *Baywatch* on television. Where is *Baywatch* localized? Is it in the phosphor glowing on the TV screen or in the dancing electrons inside the cathode-ray tube? Is it in the electromagnetic waves being transmitted through air? Or is it on the celluloid film or video tape in the studio from which the show is being transmitted? Or maybe it's in the camera that's looking at the actors in the scene?

Most people recognize right away that this is a meaningless question. You might be tempted to conclude therefore that *Baywatch* is not localized (there is no *Baywatch* "module") in any one place—that it permeates the whole universe—but that, too, is absurd. For we know it is *not* localized on the moon or in my pet cat or in the chair I'm sitting on (even though some of the electromagnetic waves may reach these locations). Clearly the phosphor, the cathode-ray tube, the electromagnetic waves and the celluloid or tape are all much more directly involved in this scenario we call *Baywatch* than is the moon, a chair or my cat.

This example illustrates that once you understand what a television program really is, the question "Is it localized or not localized?" recedes into the background, replaced with the question "How does it work?" But it's also clear that looking at the cathode-ray tube and electron gun may eventually give you hints about how the television set works and picks up the *Baywatch* program as it is aired, whereas examining the chair you are sitting on never will. So localization is not a bad place to start, so long as we avoid the pitfall of thinking that it holds all the answers.

So it is with many of the currently debated issues concerning brain function. Is language localized? Is color vision? Laughter? Once we understand these functions better, the question of "where" becomes less important than the question of "how." As it now stands, a wealth of empirical evidence supports the idea that there are indeed specialized parts or modules of the brain for various mental capacities. But the real secret to understanding the brain lies not only in unraveling the structure and function of each module but in discovering how they interact with each other to generate the whole spectrum of abilities that we call human nature.

Here is where the patients with bizarre neurological conditions come into the picture. Like the anomalous behavior of the dog that did not bark when the crime was being committed, providing Sherlock Holmes with a clue as to who might have entered the house on the night of the murder, the odd behavior of these patients can help us solve the mystery of how various parts of the brain create a useful representation of the external world and generate the illusion of a "self" that endures in space and time.

•

To help you get a feel for this way of doing science, consider these colorful cases—and the lessons drawn from them—taken from the older neurological literature.

More than fifty years ago a middle-aged woman walked into the clinic of Kurt Goldstein, a world-renowned neurologist with keen diagnostic skills. The woman appeared normal and conversed fluently; indeed, nothing was obviously wrong with her. But she had one extraordinary complaint—every now and then her left hand would fly up to her throat and try to strangle her. She often had to use her right hand to wrestle the left hand under control, pushing it down to her side—much like Peter Sellers portraying Dr. Strangelove. She sometimes even had to sit on the murderous hand, so intent was it on trying to end her life.

Not surprisingly, the woman's primary physician decided she was mentally disturbed or hysterical and sent her to several psychiatrists for treatment. When they couldn't help, she was dispatched to Dr. Goldstein, who had a reputation for diagnosing difficult cases. After Goldstein examined her, he established to his satisfaction that she was not psychotic, mentally disturbed or hysterical. She had no obvious neurological deficits such as paralysis or exaggerated reflexes. But he soon came up with an explanation for her behavior: Like you and me, the woman had two cerebral hemispheres, each of which is specialized for different mental capacities and controls movements on the opposite side of the body. The two hemispheres are connected by a band of fibers called the corpus callosum that allows the two sides to communicate and stay "in sync." But unlike most of ours, this woman's right hemisphere (which controlled her left hand) seemed to have some latent suicidal tendencies—a genuine urge to kill herself. Initially these urges may have been held in check by "brakes"—inhibitory messages sent across the corpus callosum from the more rational left hemisphere. But if she had suffered, as Goldstein surmised, damage to the corpus callosum as the result of a stroke, that inhibition would be removed. The right side of her brain and its murderous left hand were now free to attempt to strangle her.

This explanation is not as far-fetched as it seems, since it's been well known for some time that the right hemisphere tends to be more emotionally volatile than the left. Patients who have a stroke in the left brain are often anxious, depressed or worried about their prospects for recovery. The reason seems to be that with the left brain injured, their right brain takes over and frets about everything. In contrast, people who suffer damage to the right hemisphere tend to be blissfully indifferent to their own predicament. The left hemisphere just doesn't get all that upset. (More on this in Chapter 7.)

When Goldstein arrived at his diagnosis, it must have seemed like science fiction. But not long after that office visit, the woman died suddenly, probably from a second stroke (no, not from strangling herself). An autopsy confirmed Goldstein's suspicions: Prior to her Strangelovean behavior, she had suffered a massive stroke in her corpus callosum, so that the left side of her brain could not "talk to" nor exert its usual control over the right side. Goldstein had unmasked the dual nature of brain function, showing that the two hemispheres are indeed specialized for different tasks.

Consider next the simple act of smiling, something we all do every day in social situations. You see a good friend and you grin. But what happens when that friend aims a camera at your face and asks you to smile on command? Instead of a natural expression, you produce a hideous grimace. Paradoxically, an act that you perform effortlessly dozens of times each day becomes extraordinarily difficult to perform when someone simply asks you to do it. You might think it's because of embarrassment. But that can't be the answer because if you walk over to any mirror and try smiling, I assure you that the same grimace will appear.

The reason these two kinds of smiles differ is that different brain regions handle them, and only one of them contains a specialized "smile circuit." A spontaneous smile is produced by the basal ganglia, clusters of cells found between the brain's higher cortex (where thinking and planning take place) and the evolutionarily older thalamus. When you encounter a friendly face, the visual message from that face eventually reaches the brain's emotional center or limbic system and is subsequently relayed to the basal ganglia, which orchestrate the sequences of facial muscle activity needed for producing a natural smile. When this circuit is activated, your smile is genuine. The entire cascade of events, once set in motion, happens in a fraction of a second without the thinking parts of your cortex ever being involved.

But what happens when someone asks you to smile while taking your photograph? The verbal instruction from the photographer is received and understood by the higher thinking centers in the brain, including the auditory cortex and language centers. From there it is relayed to the motor cortex in the front of the brain, which specializes in producing voluntary skilled movements, like playing a piano or combing your hair. Despite its apparent simplicity, smiling involves the careful orchestration of dozens of tiny muscles in the appropriate sequence. As far as the motor cortex (which is not specialized for generating natural smiles) is concerned, this is as complex a feat as playing Rachmaninoff though it never had lessons, and therefore it fails utterly. Your smile is forced, tight, unnatural.

Evidence for two different "smile circuits" comes from brain-damaged patients. When a person suffers a stroke in the right motor cortex—the specialized brain region that helps orchestrate complex movements on the left side of the body—problems crop up on the left. Asked to smile, the patient produces that forced, unnatural grin, but now it's even more hideous; it's a half smile on the right side of the face alone. But when this same patient sees a beloved friend or relative walk through the door, her face erupts into a broad, natural smile using both sides of the mouth and face. The reason is that her basal ganglia have not been damaged by the stroke, so the special circuit for making symmetrical smiles is intact.[8]

Very rarely, one encounters a patient who has apparently had a small stroke, which neither he nor anyone else notices until he tries to smile. All of a sudden, his loved ones are astonished to see that only one half of his face is grinning. And yet when the neurologist instructs him to smile, he produces a symmetrical, albeit unnatural grin—the exact converse of the previous patient. This fellow, it turns out, had a tiny stroke that only affected his basal ganglia selectively on one side of the brain.

Yawning provides further proof for specialized circuitry. As noted, many stroke victims are paralyzed on the right or left side of their bodies, depending on where the brain injury occurs. Voluntary movements on the opposite side are permanently gone. And yet when such a patient yawns, he stretches out both arms spontaneously. Much to his amazement, his paralyzed arm suddenly springs to life! It does so because a different brain pathway controls the arm movement during the yawn—a pathway closely linked to the respiratory centers in the brain stem.

Sometimes a tiny brain lesion—damage to a mere speck of cells among billions—can produce far-reaching problems that seem grossly out of proportion to the size of the injury. For example, you may think that memory involves the entire brain. When I say the word "rose," it evokes all sorts of associations: perhaps images of a rose garden, the first time someone ever gave you a rose, the smell, the softness of petals, a person named Rose and so on. Even the simple concept of "rose" has many rich associations, suggesting that the whole brain must surely be involved in laying down every memory trace.

But the unfortunate story of a patient known as H.M. suggests otherwise.[9] Because H.M. suffered from a particularly intractable form of epilepsy, his doctors decided to remove "sick" tissue from both sides of his brain, including two tiny seahorse-shaped structures (one on each side) called the hippocampus, a structure that controls the laying down of new memories. We only know this because after the surgery, H.M. could no longer form new memories, yet he could recall everything that happened before the operation. Doctors now treat the hippocampus with greater respect and would never knowingly remove it from both sides of the brain (Figure 1.3).

Although I have never worked directly with H.M., I have often seen patients with similar forms of amnesia resulting from chronic alcoholism or hypoxia (oxygen starvation in the brain following surgery). Talking to them is an uncanny experience. For example, when I greet the patient, he seems intelligent and articulate, talks normally and may even discuss philosophy with me. If I ask him to add or subtract, he can do so without trouble. He's not emotionally or psychologically disturbed and can discuss his family and their various activities with ease.

Then I excuse myself to go to the restroom. When I come back, there is not a glimmer of recognition, no hint that he's ever seen me before in his life.

"Do you remember who I am?"

"No."

I show him a pen. "What is this?"

"A fountain pen."

"What color is it?"

"It's red."

I put the pen under a pillow on a nearby chair and ask him, "What did I just do?"

He answers promptly, "You put the pen under that pillow."

Then I chat some more, perhaps asking about his family. One minute goes by and I ask, "I just showed you something. Do you remember what it was?"

He looks puzzled. "No."

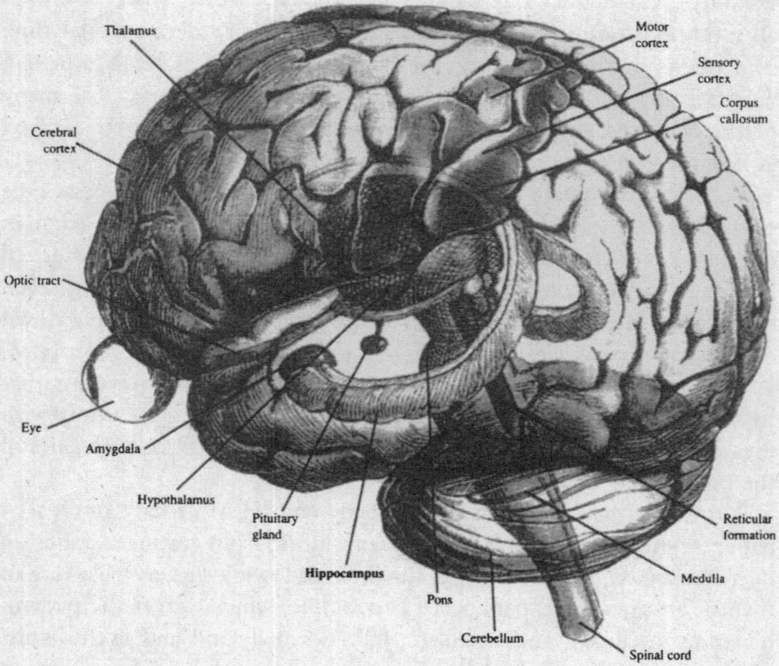

Figure 1.3 *Artist's rendering of a brain with the outer convoluted cortex rendered partially transparent to allow inner structures to be seen. The thalamus (dark) can be seen in the middle, and interposed between it and the cortex are clusters of cells called the basal ganglia (not shown). Embedded in the front part of the temporal lobe you can see the dark, almond-shaped amygdala, the "gateway" to the limbic system. In the temporal lobe you can also see the hippocampus (concerned with memory). In addition to the amygdala, other parts of the limbic system such as the hypothalamus (below the thalamus) can be seen. The limbic pathways mediate emotional arousal. The hemispheres are attached to the spinal cord by the brain stem (consisting of medulla, pons and midbrain), and below the occipital lobes is the cerebellum, concerned mainly with coordination of movements and timing.* From *Brain, Mind and Behavior* by Bloom and Laserson (1988) by Educational Broadcasting Corporation. Used with permission from W. H. Freeman and Company.

"Do you remember that I showed you an object? Do you remember where I put it?"

"No." He has absolutely no recollection of my hiding the pen sixty seconds earlier.

Such patients are, in effect, frozen in time in the sense they remember only events that took place before the accident that injured them neurologically. They may recall their first baseball game, first date and college graduation in elaborate detail, but nothing after the injury seems to be recorded. For example, if post accident they come upon last week's newspaper, they read it every day as if it were a brand-new paper each time. They can read a detective novel again and again, each time enjoying the plot and the surprise ending. I can tell them the same joke half a dozen times and each time I come to the punch line, they laugh heartily (actually, my graduate students do this too).

These patients are telling us something very important—that a tiny brain structure called the hippocampus is absolutely vital for laying down new memory traces in the brain (even though the actual memory traces are not stored in the hippocampus). They illustrate the power of the modular approach: In helping to narrow the scope of inquiry, if you want to understand memory, look at the hippocampus. And yet, as we shall see, studying the hippocampus alone will never explain all aspects of memory. To understand how memories are retrieved at a moment's notice, how they are edited, pigeonholed (sometimes even censored!), we need to look at how the hippocampus interacts with other brain structures such as the frontal lobes, the limbic system (concerned with emotions) and the structures in the brain stem (which allow you to attend selectively to specific memories).

The role of the hippocampus in forming memories is clearly established, but are there brain regions specialized in more esoteric abilities like the "number sense" that is unique to humans? Not long ago I met a gentleman, Bill Marshall, who had suffered a stroke a week earlier. Cheerful and on his way to recovery, he was only too happy to discuss his life and medical condition. When I asked him to tell me about his family, he named each of his children, listed their occupations and gave many details about his grandchildren. He was fluent, intelligent and articulate—and not everyone is so soon after a stroke.

"What was your occupation?" I asked Bill.

Bill replied, "I used to be an Air Force pilot."

"What kind of plane did you fly?"

He named the plane and said, "It was the fastest man-made thing on this planet at that time." Then he told me how fast it flew and said that it had been made before the introduction of jet engines.

At one point I said, "Okay, Bill, can you subtract seven from one hundred? What's one hundred minus seven?"

He said, "Oh. One hundred minus seven?"

"Yeah."

"Hmmm, one hundred minus seven."

"Yes, one hundred minus seven."

"So," said Bill. "One hundred. You want me to take away seven from one hundred. One hundred minus seven."

"Yes."

"Ninety six?"

"No."

"Oh," he said.

"Let's try something else. What's seventeen minus three?"

"Seventeen minus three? You know I'm not very good at this kind of thing," said Bill.

"Bill," I said, "is the answer going to be a smaller number or a bigger number?"

"Oh, a smaller number," he said, showing that he knew what subtraction is.

"Okay, so what's seventeen minus three?"

"Is it twelve?" he said at last.

I started wondering whether Bill had a problem understanding what a number is or the nature of numbers. Indeed, the question of numbers is old and deep, going back to Pythagoras.

I asked him, "What is infinity?"

"Oh, that's the largest number there is."

"Which number is bigger: one hundred and one or ninety-seven?

He answered immediately: "One hundred and one is larger."

"Why?"

"Because there are more digits."

This meant that Bill still understood, at least tacitly, sophisticated numerical concepts like place value. Also, even though he couldn't subtract three from seventeen, his answer wasn't completely absurd. He said "twelve," not seventy-five or two hundred, implying that he was still capable of making ballpark estimates.

Then I decided to tell him a little story: "The other day a man walked into the new dinosaur exhibit hall at the American Museum of Natural History in New York and saw a huge skeleton on display. He wanted to know how old it was, so he went up to an old curator sitting in the corner and said, 'I say, old chap, how old are these dinosaur bones?'

"The curator looked at the man and said, 'Oh they're sixty million and three years old, sir.'

" 'Sixty million and three years old? I didn't know you could get that precise with aging dinosaur bones. What do you mean, sixty million and three years old?'

" 'Oh, well,' he said, 'they gave me this job three years ago and at that time they told me the bones were sixty million years old.' "

Bill laughed out loud at the punch line. Obviously he understood far more about numbers than one might have guessed. It requires a sophisticated mind to understand that joke, given that it involves what philosophers call the "fallacy of misplaced concreteness."

I turned to Bill and asked, "Well, why do you think that's funny?"

"Well, you know," he said, "the level of accuracy is inappropriate."

Bill understands the joke and the idea of infinity, yet he can't subtract three from seventeen. Does this mean that each of us has a number center in the region of the left angular gyrus (where Bill's stroke injury was located) of our brain for adding, subtracting, multiplying and dividing? I think not. But clearly this region—the angular gyrus—is somehow necessary for numerical computational tasks but is not needed for other abilities such as short-term memory, language or humor. Nor, paradoxically, is it needed for understanding the numerical concepts underlying such computations. We do not yet know how this "arithmetic" circuit in the angular gyrus works, but at least we now know where to look.[10]

Many patients, like Bill, with dyscalculia also have an associated brain disorder called finger agnosia: They can no longer name which finger the neurologist is pointing to or touching. Is it a complete coincidence that both arithmetic operations and finger naming occupy adjacent brain regions, or does it have something to do with the fact that we all learn to count by using our fingers in early childhood? The observation that in some of these patients one function can be retained (naming fingers) while the other (adding and subtracting) is gone doesn't negate the argument that these two might be closely linked and occupy the same anatomical niche in the brain. It's possible, for instance, that the two functions are laid down in close proximity and were dependent on each other during the learning phase, but in the adult each function can survive without the other. In other words, a child may need to wiggle his or her fingers subconsciously while counting, whereas you and I may not need to do so.

These historical examples and case studies gleaned from my notes support the view that specialized circuits or modules do exist, and we shall encounter several additional examples in this book. But other equally interesting questions remain and we'll explore these as well. How do the modules actually work and how do they "talk to" each other to generate conscious experience? To what extent is all this intricate circuitry in the brain innately specified by your genes or to what extent is it acquired gradually as the result of your early experiences, as an infant interacts with the world? (This is the ancient "nature versus nurture" debate, which has been going on for hundreds of years, yet we have barely scratched the surface in formulating an answer.) Even if certain circuits are hard-wired from birth, does it follow that they cannot be altered? How much of the adult brain is modifiable? To find out, let's meet Tom, one of the first people who helped me explore these larger questions.

CHAPTER 2

"Knowing Where to Scratch"

My intention is to tell
of bodies changed
to different forms.

The heavens and all below them,
Earth and her creatures,
All change,
And we, part of creation,
Also must suffer change.

—OVID

Tom Sorenson vividly recalls the horrifying circumstances that led to the loss of his arm. He was driving home from soccer practice, tired and hungry from the exercise, when a car in the opposite lane swerved in front of him. Brakes squealed, Tom's car spun out of control and he was thrown from the driver's seat onto the ice plant bordering the freeway. As he was hurled through the air, Tom looked back and saw that his hand was still in the car, "gripping" the seat cushion—severed from his body like a prop in a Freddy Krueger horror film.

As a result of this gruesome mishap, Tom lost his left arm just above the elbow. He was seventeen years old, with just three months to go until high school graduation.

In the weeks afterward, even though he knew that his arm was gone, Tom could still feel its ghostly presence below the elbow. He could wiggle each "finger," "reach out" and "grab" objects that were within arm's reach. Indeed, his phantom arm seemed to be able to do anything that the real arm would have done automatically, such as warding off blows, breaking falls or patting his little brother on the back. Since Tom had been left-handed, his phantom would reach for the receiver whenever the telephone rang.

Tom was not crazy. His impression that his missing arm was still there is a classic example of a phantom limb—an arm or leg that lingers indefinitely in the minds of patients long after it has been lost in an accident or removed by a surgeon. Some wake up from anesthesia and are incredulous when told that their arm had to be sacrificed, because they still vividly *feel* its presence.[1] Only when they look under the sheets do they come to the shocking realization that the limb is really gone. Moreover, some of these patients experience excruciating pain in the phantom arm, hand or fingers, so much so that they contemplate suicide. The pain is not only unrelenting, it's also untreatable; no one has the foggiest idea of how it arises or how to deal with it.

As a physician I was aware that phantom limb pain poses a serious clinical problem. Chronic pain in a real body part such as the joint aches of arthritis or lower backache is difficult enough to treat, but how do you treat pain in a nonexistent limb? As a scientist, I was also curious about why the phenomenon occurs in the first place: Why would an arm persist in the patient's mind long after it had been removed? Why doesn't the mind simply accept the loss and "reshape" the body image? To be sure, this does happen in a few patients, but it usually takes years or decades. Why decades—why not just a week or a day? A study of this phenomenon, I realized, might not only help us understand the question of how the brain copes with a sudden and massive loss, but also help address the more fundamental debate over nature versus nurture—the extent to which our body image, as well as other aspects of our minds, are laid down by genes and the extent to which they are modified by experience.

The persistence of sensation in limbs long after amputation had been noticed as far back as the sixteenth century by the French surgeon Ambroise Paré, and, not surprisingly, there is an elaborate folklore surrounding this phenomenon. After Lord Nelson lost his right arm during an unsuccessful attack on Santa Cruz de Tenerife, he experienced compelling phantom limb pains, including the unmistakable sensation of fingers digging into his phantom palm. The emergence of these ghostly sensations in his missing limb led the sea lord to proclaim that his phantom was "direct evidence for the existence of the soul." For if an arm can exist after it is removed, why can't the whole person survive physical annihilation of the body? It is proof, Lord Nelson claimed, for the existence of the spirit long after it has cast off its attire.

•

The eminent Philadelphia physician Silas Weir Mitchell[2] first coined the phrase "phantom limb" after the Civil War. In those preantibiotic days, gangrene was a common result of injuries and surgeons sawed infected limbs off thousands of wounded soldiers. They returned home with the phantoms, setting off new rounds of speculation about what might be causing them. Weir Mitchell himself was so surprised by the phenomenon that he published the first article on the subject under a pseudonym in a popular magazine called *Lippincott's Journal* rather than risk facing the ridicule from his colleagues that might have ensued had he published in a professional medical journal. Phantoms, when you think about it, are a rather spooky phenomenon.

Since Weir Mitchell's time there have been all kinds of speculations about phantoms, ranging from the sublime to the ridiculous. As recently as fifteen years ago, a paper in the *Canadian Journal of Psychiatry* stated that phantom limbs are merely the result of wishful thinking. The authors argued that the patient desperately wants his arm back and therefore experiences a phantom—in much the same way that a person may have recurring dreams or may even see "ghosts" of a recently deceased parent. This argument, as we shall see, is utter nonsense.

A second, more popular explanation for phantoms is that the frayed and curled-up nerve endings in the stump (neuromas) that originally supplied the hand tend to become inflamed and irritated, thereby fooling higher brain centers into thinking that the missing limb is still there. Though there are far too many problems with this nerve irritation theory, because it's a simple and convenient explanation, most physicians still cling to it.

There are literally hundreds of fascinating case studies, which appear in the older medical journals. Some of the described phenomena have been confirmed repeatedly and still cry out for an explanation, whereas others seem like far-fetched products of the writer's own imagination. One of my favorites is about a patient who started experiencing a vivid phantom arm soon after amputation—nothing unusual so far—but after a few weeks developed a peculiar, gnawing sensation in his phantom. Naturally he was quite puzzled by the sudden emergence of these new sensations, but when he asked his physician why this was happening, the doctor didn't know and couldn't help. Finally, out of curiosity, the fellow asked, "Whatever happened to my arm after you removed it?" "Good question," replied the doctor, "you need to ask the surgeon." So the fellow called the surgeon, who said, "Oh, we usually send the limbs to the morgue." So the man called the morgue and asked, "What do you do with amputated arms?" They replied, "We send them either to the incinerator or to pathology. Usually we incinerate them."

"Well, what did you do with this particular arm? With *my* arm?" They looked at their records and said, "You know, it's funny. We didn't incinerate it. We sent it to pathology."

The man called the pathology lab. "Where is my arm?" he asked again. They said, "Well, we had too many arms, so we just buried it in the garden, out behind the hospital."

They took him to the garden and showed him where the arm was buried. When he exhumed it, he found it was crawling with maggots and exclaimed, "Well, maybe that's why I'm feeling these bizarre sensations in my arm." So he took the limb and incinerated it. And from that day on, his phantom pain disappeared.

Such stories are fun to tell, especially around a campfire at night, but they do very little to dispel the real mystery of phantom limbs. Although patients with this syndrome have been studied extensively since the turn of the century, there's been a tendency among physicians to regard them as enigmatic, clinical curiosities and almost no experimental work has been done on them. One reason for this is that clinical neurology historically has been a descriptive rather than an experimental science. Neurologists of the nineteenth and early twentieth centuries were astute clinical observers, and many valuable lessons can be learned from reading their case reports. Oddly enough, however, they did not take the next obvious step of doing experiments to discover what might be going on in the brains of these patients; their science was Aristotelian rather than Galilean.[3] Given how immensely successful the experimental method has been in almost every other science, isn't it high time we imported it into neurology?

Like most physicians, I was intrigued by phantoms the very first time I encountered them and have been puzzled by them ever since. In addition to phantom arms and legs—which are common among amputees—I had also encountered women with phantom breasts after radical mastectomy and even a patient with a phantom appendix: The characteristic spasmodic pain of appendicitis did not abate after surgical removal, so much so that the patient refused to believe that the surgeon had cut it out! As a medical student, I was just as baffled as the patients themselves, and the textbooks I consulted only deepened the mystery. I read about a patient who experienced phantom erections after his penis had been amputated, a woman with phantom menstrual cramps following hysterectomy, and a gentleman who had a phantom nose and face after the trigeminal nerve innervating his face had been severed in an accident.

All these clinical experiences lay tucked away in my brain, dormant, until about six years ago, when my interest was rekindled by a scientific paper published in 1991 by Dr. Tim Pons of the National Institutes of Health, a paper that propelled me into a whole new direction of research and eventually brought Tom into my laboratory. But before I continue with this part of the story, we need to look closely at the anatomy of the brain—particularly at how various body parts such as limbs are mapped onto the cerebral cortex, the great convoluted mantle on the surface of the brain. This will help you understand what Dr. Pons discovered and, in turn, how phantom limbs emerge.

Of the many strange images that have remained with me from my medical school days, perhaps none is more vivid than that of the deformed little man you see in Figure 2.1 draped across the surface of the cerebral cortex—the so-called Penfield homunculus. The homunculus is the artist's whimsical depiction of the manner in which different points on the body surface are mapped onto the surface of the brain—the grotesquely deformed features are an attempt to indicate that certain body parts such as the lips and tongue are grossly overrepresented.

The map was drawn from information gleaned from real human brains. During the 1940s and 1950s, the brilliant Canadian neurosurgeon Wilder Penfield performed extensive brain surgeries on patients under local anesthetic (there are no pain receptors in the brain, even though it is a mass of nerve tissue). Often, much of the brain was exposed during the operation and Penfield seized this opportunity to do experiments that had never been tried before. He stimulated specific regions of the patients' brains with an electrode and simply asked them what they felt. All kinds of sensations, images, and even memories were elicited by the electrode and the areas of the brain that were responsible could be mapped.

Among other things, Penfield found a narrow strip running from top to bottom down both sides of the brain where his electrode produced sensations localized in various parts of the body. Up at the top of the brain, in the crevice that separates the two hemispheres, electrical stimulation elicited sensations in the genitals. Nearby stimuli evoked sensa-

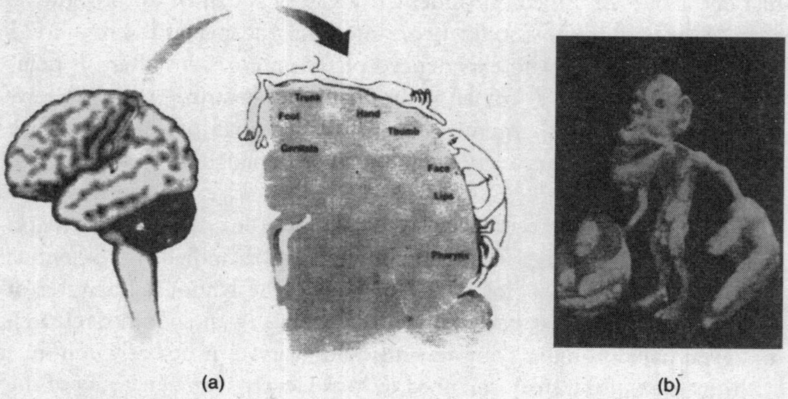

Figure 2.1 *(a) The representation of the body surface on the surface of the human brain (as discovered by Wilder Penfield) behind the central sulcus. There are many such maps, but for clarity only one is shown here. The homunculus ("little man") is upside down for the most part, and his feet are tucked onto the medial surface (inner surface) of the parietal lobe near the very top, whereas the face is down near the bottom of the outer surface. The face and hand occupy a disproportionately large share of the map. Notice, also that the face area is below the hand area instead of being where it should—near the neck—and that the genitals are represented below the foot. Could this provide an anatomical explanation of foot fetishes? (b) A whimsical three-dimensional model of the Penfield homunculus—the little man in the brain—depicting the representation of body parts. Notice the gross overrepresentation of mouth and hands.* Reprinted with permission from the British Museum, London.

tions in the feet. As Penfield followed this strip down from the top of the brain, he discovered areas that receive sensations from the legs and trunk, from the hand (a large region with a very prominent representation of the thumb), the face, the lips and finally the thorax and voicebox. This "sensory homunculus," as it is now called, forms a greatly distorted representation of the body on the surface of the brain, with the parts that are particularly important taking up disproportionately large areas. For example, the area involved with the lips or with the fingers takes up as much space as the area involved with the entire trunk of the body. This is presumably because your lips and fingers are highly sensitive to touch and are capable of very fine discrimination, whereas your trunk is considerably less sensitive, requiring less cortical space. For the most part, the map is orderly though upside down: The foot is represented at the top and the outstretched arms are at the bottom. However, upon close examination, you will see that the map is not entirely continuous. The face is not near the neck, where it should be, but is below the hand. The genitals, instead of being between the thighs, are located below the foot.[4]

These areas can be mapped out with even greater precision in other animals, particularly in monkeys. The researcher inserts a long thin needle made of steel or tungsten into the monkey's somatosensory cortex—the strip of brain tissue described earlier. If the needle tip comes to lie right next to the cell body of a neuron and if that neuron is active, it will generate tiny electrical currents that are picked up by the needle electrode and amplified. The signal can be displayed on an oscilloscope, making it possible to monitor the activity of that neuron.

For example, if you put an electrode into the monkey's somatosensory cortex and touch the monkey on a specific part of its body, the cell will fire. Each cell has its territory on the body surface—its own small patch of skin, so to speak—to which it responds. We call this the cell's receptive field. A map of the entire body surface exists in the brain, with each half of the body mapped onto the opposite side of the brain.

While animals are logical experimental subjects in which to examine the detailed structure and function of the brain's sensory regions, they have one obvious problem: Monkeys can't talk. Therefore, they cannot tell the experimenter, as Penfield's patients could, what they are feeling. Thus a large and important dimension is lost when animals are used in such experiments.

But despite this obvious limitation, a great deal can be learned by doing the right kinds of experiments. For instance, as we've noted, one important question concerns nature versus nurture: Are these body maps on the surface of the brain fixed, or can they change with experience as we grow from newborns to infancy, through adolescence and into old age? And even if the maps are already there at birth, to what extent can they be modified in the adult?[5]

It was these questions that prompted Tim Pons and his colleagues to embark on their research. Their strategy was to record signals from the brains of monkeys who had undergone dorsal rhizotomy—a procedure in which all the nerve fibers carrying sensory information from one arm into the spinal cord are completely severed.[6] Eleven years after the surgery, they anesthetized the animals, opened their skulls and recorded from the somatosensory map. Since the monkey's paralyzed arm was not sending messages to the brain, you would not expect to record any signals when you touch the monkey's useless hand and record from the "hand area" of the brain. There should be a big patch of silent cortex corresponding to the affected hand.

Indeed, when the researchers stroked the useless hand, there was no activity in this region. But to their amazement they found that when they touched the monkey's face, the cells in the brain corresponding to the "dead" hand started firing vigorously. (So did cells corresponding to the face, but those were expected to fire.) It appeared that sensory information from the monkey's face not only went to the face area of the cortex, as it would in a normal animal, but it had also invaded the territory of the paralyzed hand!

The implications of this finding are astonishing: It means that you *can* change the map; you can alter the brain circuitry of an adult animal, and connections can be modified over distances spanning a centimeter or more.

Upon reading Pons's paper, I thought, "My God! Might this be an explanation for phantom limbs?" What did the monkey actually "feel" when its face was being stroked? Since its "hand" cortex was also being excited, did it perceive sensations as arising from the useless hand as well as the face? Or would it use higher brain centers to reinterpret the sensations correctly as arising from the face alone? The monkey of course was silent on the subject.

It takes years to train a monkey to carry out even very simple tasks, let alone signal what part of its body is being touched. Then it occurred to me that you don't have to use a monkey. Why not answer the same question by touching the face of a human patient who has lost an arm? I telephoned my colleagues Dr. Mark Johnson and Dr. Rita Finkelstein in orthopedic surgery and asked, "Do you have any patients who have recently lost an arm?"

That is how I came to meet Tom. I called him up right away and asked whether he would like to participate in a study. Although initially shy and reticent in his mannerisms, Tom soon became eager to participate in our experiment. I was careful not to tell him what we hoped to find, so as not to bias his responses. Even though he was distressed by "itching" and painful sensations in his phantom fingers, he was cheerful, apparently pleased that he had survived the accident.

With Tom seated comfortably in my basement laboratory, I placed a blindfold over his eyes because I didn't want him to see where I was touching him. Then I took an ordinary Q-tip and started stroking various parts of his body surface, asking him to tell me where he felt the sensations. (My graduate student, who was watching, thought I was crazy.)

I swabbed his cheek. "What do you feel?"

"You are touching my cheek."

"Anything else?"

"Hey, you know it's funny," said Tom. "You're touching my missing thumb, my phantom thumb."

I moved the Q-tip to his upper lip. "How about here?"

"You're touching my index finger. And my upper lip."

"Really? Are you sure?"

"Yes. I can feel it both places."

"How about here?" I stroked his lower jaw with the swab.

"That's my missing pinkie."

I soon found a complete map of Tom's phantom hand—on his face! I realized that what I was seeing was perhaps a direct perceptual correlate of the remapping that Tim Pons had seen in his monkeys. For there is no other way of explaining why touching an area so far away from the stump—namely, the face—should generate sensations in the phantom hand; the secret lies in the peculiar mapping of body parts in the brain, with the face lying right beside the hand.[7]

I continued this procedure until I had explored Tom's entire body surface. When I touched his chest, right shoulder, right leg or lower back, he felt sensations only in those places and not in the phantom. But I also found a second, beautifully laid out "map" of his missing hand—tucked onto his left upper arm a few inches above the line of amputation (Figure 2.2). Stroking the skin surface on this second map also evoked precisely localized sensations on the individual fingers: Touch here and he says, "Oh, that's my thumb," and so on.

Why were there two maps instead of just one? If you look again at the Penfield map, you'll see that the hand area in the brain is flanked below by the face area and above by the upper arm and shoulder area. Input from Tom's hand area was lost after the amputation, and consequently, the sensory fibers originating from Tom's face—which normally activate only the face area in his cortex—now invaded the vacated territory of the hand and began to drive the cells there. Therefore, when I touched Tom's face, he also felt sensations in his phantom hand. But if the invasion of the hand cortex also results from sensory fibers that normally innervate the brain region above the hand cortex (that is, fibers that originate in the upper arm and shoulder), then touching points on

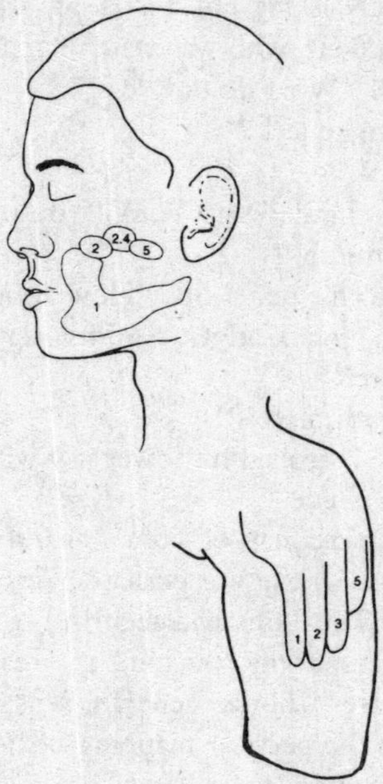

Figure 2.2 *Points on the body surface that yielded referred sensations in the phantom hand (this patient's left arm had been amputated ten years prior to our testing him). Notice that there is a complete map of all the fingers (labeled 1 to 5) on the face and a second map on the upper arm. The sensory input from these two patches of skin is now apparently activating the hand territory of the brain (either in the thalamus or in the cortex). So when these points are touched, the sensations are felt to arise from the missing hand as well.*

the upper arm should also evoke sensations in the phantom hand. And indeed I was able to map out these points on the arm above Tom's stump. So, this sort of arrangement is precisely what one would expect: One cluster of points on the face that evoke sensations in the phantom and a second cluster on the upper arm, corresponding to the two body parts that are represented on either side (above and below) of the hand representation in the brain.[8]

It's not often in science (especially neurology) that you can make a simple prediction like this and confirm it with a few minutes of exploration using a Q-tip. The existence of two clusters of points suggests strongly that remapping of the kind seen in Pons's monkeys also occurs in the human brain. But there was still a nagging doubt: How can we be sure that such changes are actually taking place—that the map is really changing in people like Tom? To obtain more direct proof, we took advantage of a modern neuroimaging technique called magnetoencephalography (MEG), which relies on the principle that if you touch different body parts, the localized electrical activity evoked in the Penfield map can be measured as changes in magnetic fields on the scalp. The major advantage of the technique is that it is noninvasive; one does not have to open the patient's scalp to peer inside the brain.

Using MEG, it is relatively easy in just a two-hour session to map out the entire body surface on the brain surface of any person willing to sit under the magnet. Not surprisingly, the map that results is quite similar to the original Penfield homunculus map, and there is very little variation from person to person in the gross layout of the map. When we conducted MEGs on four arm amputees, however, we found that the maps had changed over large distances, just as we had predicted. For example, a glance at Figure 2.3 reveals that the hand area (hatched) is missing in the right hemisphere and has been invaded by the sensory input from the face (in white) and upper arm (in gray). These observations, which I made in collaboration with a medical student, Tony Yang, and the neurologists Chris Gallen and Floyd Bloom, were in fact the first direct demonstration that such large-scale changes in the organization of the brain could occur in adult humans.

The implications are staggering. First and foremost, they suggest that brain maps can change, sometimes with astonishing rapidity. This finding flatly contradicts one of the most widely accepted dogmas in neurology—the fixed nature of connections in the adult human brain. It had always been assumed that once this circuitry, including the Penfield map, has been laid down in fetal life or in early infancy, there is very little one can do to modify it in adulthood. Indeed, this presumed absence of plasticity in the adult brain is often invoked to explain why there is so little recovery of function after brain injury and why neurological ailments are so notoriously difficult to treat. But the evidence from Tom shows—contrary to what is taught in textbooks—that new, highly precise and functionally effective pathways can emerge in the adult brain as early as four weeks after injury. It certainly doesn't follow that revolutionary new treatments for neurological syndromes will emerge from this discovery right away, but it does provide some grounds for optimism.

Second, the findings may help explain the very existence of phantom limbs. The most popular medical explanation, noted earlier, is that nerves that once supplied the hand begin to innervate the stump. Moreover,

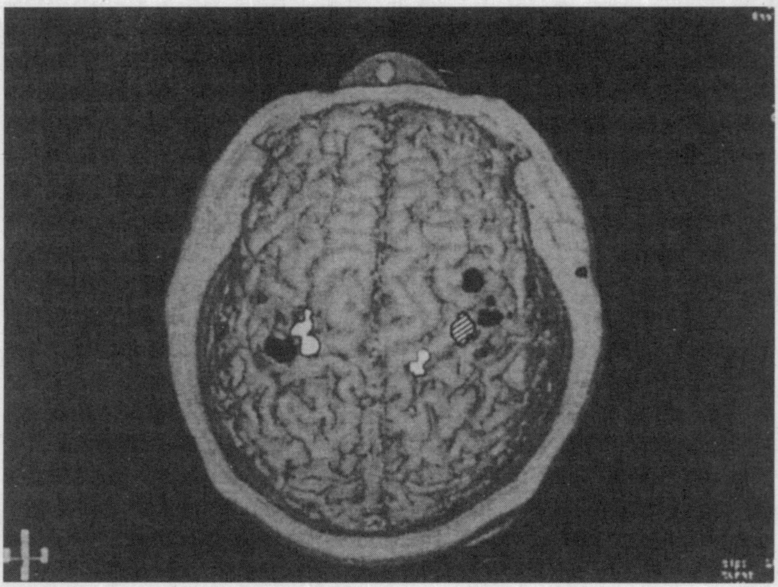

Figure 2.3 *Magnetoencephalography (MEG) image superimposed on a magnetic resonance (MR) image of the brain in a patient whose right arm was amputated below the elbow. The brain is viewed from the top. The right hemisphere shows normal activation of the hand (hatched), face (black) and upper arm (white) areas of the cortex corresponding to the Penfield map. In the left hemisphere there is no activation corresponding to the missing right hand, but the activity from the face and upper arm has now "spread" to this area.*

these frayed nerve endings form little clumps of scar tissue called neuromas, which can be very painful. When neuromas are irritated, the theory goes, they send impulses back to the original hand area in the brain so that the brain is "fooled" into thinking the hand is still there: hence the phantom limb and the notion that the accompanying pain arises because the neuromas are painful.

On the basis of this tenuous reasoning, surgeons have devised various treatments for phantom limb pain in which they cut and remove neuromas. Some patients experience temporary relief, but surprisingly, both the phantom and the associated pain usually return with a vengeance. To alleviate this problem, sometimes surgeons perform a second or even a third amputation (making the stump shorter and shorter), but when you think about this, it's logically absurd. Why would a second amputation help? You'd simply expect a second phantom, and indeed that's usually what happens; it's an endless regress problem.

Surgeons even perform dorsal rhizotomies to treat phantom limb pain, cutting the sensory nerves going into the spinal cord. Sometimes it works; sometimes it doesn't. Others try the even more drastic procedure of cutting the back of the spinal cord itself—a cordotomy—to prevent impulses from reaching the brain, but that, too, is often ineffective. Or they will go all the way into the thalamus, a brain relay station that processes signals before they are sent to the cortex, and again find that they have not helped the patient. They can chase the phantom farther and farther into the brain, but of course they'll never find it.

Why? One reason, surely, is that the phantom doesn't exist in any one of these areas; it exists in more central parts of the brain, where the remapping has occurred. To put it crudely, the phantom emerges not from the stump but from the face and jaw, because every time Tom smiles or moves his face and lips, the impulses activate the "hand" area of his cortex, creating the illusion that his hand is still there. Stimulated by all these spurious signals, Tom's brain literally hallucinates his arm, and perhaps this is the essence of a phantom limb. If so, the only way to get rid of the phantom would be to remove his jaw. (And if you think about it, that wouldn't help either. He'd probably end up with a phantom jaw. It's that endless regress problem again.)

But remapping can't be the whole story. For one thing, it doesn't explain why Tom or other patients experience the feeling of being able to move their phantoms voluntarily or why the phantom can change its posture. Where do these movement sensations originate? Second, remapping doesn't account for what both doctor and patient are most seriously concerned about—the genesis of phantom pain. We'll explore these two subjects in the next chapter.

When we think of sensations arising from skin we usually only think of touch. But, in fact, distinct neural pathways that mediate sensations of warmth, cold and pain also originate on the skin surface. These sensations have their own target areas or maps in the brain, but the paths used by them may be interlaced with each other in complicated ways. If so, could such remapping also occur in these evolutionarily older pathways quite independently of the remapping that occurs for touch? In other words, is the remapping seen in Tom and in Pons's monkeys peculiar to touch, or does it point to a very general principle—would it occur for sensations like warmth, cold, pain or vibration? And if such remapping were to occur would there be instances of accidental "cross-wiring" so that a touch sensation would evoke warmth or pain? Or would they remain segregated? The question of how millions of neural connections in the brain are hooked up so precisely during development—and the extent to which this precision is preserved when they are reorganized after injury—is of great interest to scientists who are trying to understand the development of pathways in the brain.

To investigate this, I placed a drop of warm water on Tom's face. He felt it there immediately but also said that his phantom hand felt distinctly warm. Once, when the water accidentally trickled down his face, he exclaimed with considerable surprise that he could actually feel the warm water trickling down the length of his phantom arm. He demonstrated this to me by using his normal hand to trace out the path of the water down his phantom. In all my years in neurology clinics, I had never seen anything quite so remarkable—a patient systematically mislocalizing a complex sensation such as a "trickle" from his face to his phantom hand.

These experiments imply that highly precise and organized new connections can be formed in the adult brain in a few days. But they don't tell us how these new pathways actually emerge, what the underlying mechanisms are at the cellular level.

I can think of two possibilities. First, the reorganization could involve sprouting—the actual growth of new branches from nerve fibers that normally innervate the face area toward cells in the hand area in the cortex. If this hypothesis were true, this would be quite remarkable since it is difficult to see how highly organized sprouting could take place over relatively long distances (in the brain several millimeters might as well be a mile) and in such a short period. Moreover, even if sprouting occurs, how would the new fibers "know" where to go? One can imagine a higgledy-piggledy jumble of connections, but not precisely organized pathways.

The second possibility is that there is in fact a tremendous redundancy of connections in the normal adult brain but that most of them are nonfunctional or have no obvious function. Like reserve troops, they may be called into action only when needed. Thus even in healthy normal adult brains there might be sensory inputs from the face to the brain's face map *and* to the hand map area as well. If so, we must assume that this occult or hidden input is ordinarily inhibited by the sensory fibers arriving from the real hand. But when the hand is removed, this silent input originating from the skin on the face is unmasked and allowed to express itself so that touching the face now activates the hand area and leads to sensations in the phantom hand. Thus every time Tom whistles, he might feel a tingling in his phantom arm.

We have no way at present of easily distinguishing between these two theories, although my hunch is that both mechanisms are at work. After all, we had seen the effect in Tom in less than four weeks and this seems too short a time for sprouting to take place. My colleague at the Massachusetts General Hospital Dr. David Borsook[9] has seen similar effects in a patient just twenty-four hours after amputation, and there is no question of sprouting's occurring in such a short period. The final answer to this will come from simultaneously tracking perceptual changes and brain changes (using imaging) in a patient over a period of several days. If Borsook and I are right, the completely static picture of these maps that you get from looking at textbook diagrams is highly misleading and we need to rethink the meaning of brain maps completely. Far from signaling a specific location on the skin, each neuron in the map is in a state of dynamic equilibrium with other adjacent neurons; its significance depends strongly on what other neurons in the vicinity are doing (or not doing).

These findings raise an obvious question: What if some body part is lost other than the hand? Will the same kind of remapping occur? When my studies on Tom were first published, I got many letters and phone calls from amputees wanting to know more. Some of them had been told that phantom sensations are imaginary and were relieved to learn that that isn't true. (Patients always find it comforting to know that there is a logical explanation for their otherwise inexplicable symptoms; nothing is more insulting to a patient than to be told that his pain is "all in the mind.")

One day I got a call from a young woman in Boston. "Dr. Ramachandran," she said, "I'm a graduate student at Beth Israel Hospital and for several years I've been studying Parkinson's disease. But recently I decided to switch to the study of phantom limbs."

"Wonderful," I said. "The subject has been ignored far too long. Tell me what you are studying."

"Last year I had a terrible accident on my uncle's farm. I lost my left leg below the knee and I've had a phantom limb ever since. But I'm calling to thank you because your article made me understand what is going on." She cleared her throat. "Something really strange happened to me after the amputation that didn't make sense. Every time I have sex I experience these strange sensations in my phantom foot. I didn't dare tell anybody because it's so weird. But when I saw your diagrams, that in the brain the foot is next to the genitals, it became instantly clear to me."

She had experienced and understood, as few of us ever will, the remapping phenomenon. Recall that in the Penfield map the foot is beside the genitals. Therefore, if a person loses a leg and is then stimulated in the genitals, she will experience sensations in the phantom leg. This is what you'd expect if input from the genital area were to invade the territory vacated by the foot.

The next day the phone rang again. This time it was an engineer from Arkansas.

"Is this Dr. Ramachandran?"

"Yes."

"You know, I read about your work in the newspaper, and it's really exciting. I lost my leg below the knee about two months ago but there's still something I don't understand. I'd like your advice."

"What's that?"

"Well, I feel a little embarrassed to tell you this."

I knew what he was going to say, but unlike the graduate student, he didn't know about the Penfield map.

"Doctor, every time I have sexual intercourse, I experience sensations in my phantom foot. How do you explain that? My doctor said it doesn't make sense."

"Look," I said. "One possibility is that the genitals are right next to the foot in the body's brain maps. Don't worry about it."

He laughed nervously. "All that's fine, doctor. But you still don't understand. You see, I actually experience my orgasm in my foot. And therefore it's much bigger than it used to be because it's no longer just confined to my genitals."

Patients don't make up such stories. Ninety-nine percent of the time they're telling the truth, and if it seems incomprehensible, it's usually because we are not smart enough to figure out what's going on in their brains. This gentleman was telling me that he sometimes enjoyed sex *more* after his amputation. The curious implication is that it's not just the tactile sensation that transferred to his phantom but the erotic sensations of sexual pleasure as well. (A colleague suggested I title this book "The Man Who Mistook His Foot for a Penis.")

This makes me wonder about the basis of foot fetishes in normal people, a subject that—although not exactly central to our mental life—everyone is curious about. (Madonna's book, *Sex,* has a whole chapter devoted to the foot.) The traditional explanation for foot fetishes comes, not surprisingly, from Freud. The penis resembles the foot, he argues, hence the fetish. But if that's the case, why not some other elongated body part? Why not a hand fetish or a nose fetish? I suggest that the reason is quite simply that in the brain the foot lies right next to the genitalia. Maybe even many of us so-called normal people have a bit of cross-wiring, which would explain why we like to have our toes sucked. The journeys of science are often tortuous with many unexpected twists and turns, but I never suspected that I would begin seeking an explanation for phantom limbs and end up explaining foot fetishes as well.

Given these assumptions, other predictions follow.[10] What happens when the penis is amputated? Carcinoma of the penis is sometimes treated with amputation, and many of these patients experience a phantom penis—sometimes even phantom erections! In such cases you would expect that stimulation of the feet would be felt in the phantom penis. Would such a patient find tap dancing especially enjoyable?

What about mastectomy? An Italian neurologist, Dr. Salvatore Aglioti, recently found that a certain proportion of women with radical mastectomies experience vivid phantom breasts. So, he asked himself, what body parts are mapped next to the breast? By stimulating adjacent regions on the chest he found that parts of the sternum and clavicle, when touched, produce sensations in the phantom nipple. Moreover, this remapping occurred just two days after surgery.

Aglioti also found to his surprise that one third of the women with radical mastectomies tested reported tingling, erotic sensations in their phantom nipples when their earlobes were stimulated. But this happened only in the phantom breast, not in the real one on the other side. He speculated that in one of the body maps (there are others besides the Penfield map) the nipple and ear are next to each other. This makes you wonder why many women report feeling erotic sensations when their ears are nibbled during sexual foreplay. Is it a coincidence, or does it have something to do with brain anatomy? (Even in the original Penfield map, the genital area of women is mapped right next to the nipples.)

A less titillating example of remapping also involving the ear came from Dr. A. T. Caccace, a neurologist who told me about an extraordinary phenomenon called gaze tinnitus.

People with this condition have a weird problem. When they look to the left (or right), they hear a ringing sound. When they look straight ahead, nothing happens. Physicians have known about this syndrome for a long time but were stymied by it. Why does it happen when the eyes deviate? Why does it happen at all?

After reading about Tom, Dr. Caccace was struck by the similarity between phantom limbs and gaze tinnitus, for he knew that his patients had suffered damage to the auditory nerve—the major conduit connecting the inner ear to the brain stem. Once in the brain stem the auditory nerve hooks up with the auditory nucleus, which is right next to another structure called the oculomotor nerve nucleus. This second, adjacent structure sends commands to the eyes, instructing them to move. Eureka! The mystery is solved.[11] Because of the patient's damage, the auditory nucleus no longer gets input from one ear. Axons from the eye movement center in the cortex invade the auditory nucleus so that every time the person's brain sends a command to move the eyes, that command is sent inadvertently to the auditory nerve nucleus and translated into a ringing sound.

The study of phantom limbs offers fascinating glimpses of the architecture of the brain, its astonishing capacity for growth and renewal[12] and may even explain why playing footsie is so enjoyable. But about half the people with phantom limbs also experience the most unpleasant manifestation of the phenomenon—phantom limb pain. Real pain, such as the pain of cancer, is hard enough to treat; imagine the challenge of treating pain in a limb that isn't there! There is very little that can be done, at the moment, to alleviate such pain, but perhaps the remapping that we observed with Tom may help explain why it happens. We know, for instance, that intractable phantom pain may develop weeks or months after the limb is amputated. Perhaps as the brain adjusts and cells slowly make new connections, there is a slight error in the remapping so that some of the sensory input from touch receptors is accidentally connected to the pain areas of the brain. If this were to happen, then every time the patient smiled or accidentally brushed his cheek, the touch sensations would be experienced as excruciating pain. This is almost certainly not the whole explanation for phantom pain (as we shall see in the next chapter), but it's a good place to start.

As Tom left my office one day, I couldn't resist asking him an obvious question. During the last four weeks, had he ever noticed any of these peculiar referred sensations in his phantom hand when his face had been touched—when he shaved every morning, for example?

"No, I haven't," he replied, "but you know, my phantom hand sometimes itches like crazy and I never know what to do about it. But now," he said, tapping his cheek and winking at me, "I know exactly where to scratch!"

CHAPTER 3

Chasing the Phantom

You never identify yourself with the shadow cast by your body, or with its reflection, or with the body you see in a dream or in your imagination. Therefore you should not identify yourself with this living body, either.

—*SHANKARA (A.D. 788–820),* Viveka Chudamani
(Vedic scriptures)

When a reporter asked the famous biologist J.B.S. Haldane what his biological studies had taught him about God, Haldane replied, "The creator, if he exists, must have an inordinate fondness for beetles," since there are more species of beetles than any other group of living creatures. By the same token, a neurologist might conclude that God is a cartographer. He must have an inordinate fondness for maps, for everywhere you look in the brain maps abound. For example, there are over thirty different maps concerned with vision alone. Likewise for tactile or somatic sensations—touch, joint and muscle sense—there are several maps, including, as we saw in the previous chapter, the famous Penfield homunculus, a map draped across a vertical strip of cortex on the sides of the brain. These maps are largely stable throughout life, thus helping ensure that perception is usually accurate and reliable. But, as we have seen, they are also being constantly updated and refined in response to vagaries of sensory input. Recall that when Tom's arm was amputated, the large patch of cortex corresponding to his missing hand was "taken over" by sensory input from his face. If I touch Tom's face, the sensory message now goes to two areas—the original face area (as it should) but also the original "hand area." Such brain map alterations may help explain the appearance of Tom's phantom limb soon after amputation. Every time he smiles or experiences some spontaneous activity of facial nerves, the activity stimulates his "hand area," thereby fooling him into thinking that his hand is still there.

But this cannot be the whole story. First, it doesn't explain why so many people with phantoms claim that they can move their "imaginary" limbs voluntarily. What is the source of this illusion of movement? Second, it doesn't explain the fact that these patients sometimes experience intense agony in the missing limb, the phenomenon called phantom pain. Third, what about a person who is born without an arm? Does remapping also occur in his brain, or does the hand area of the cortex simply never develop because he never had an arm? Would he experience a phantom? Can someone be *born* with phantom limbs?

The idea seems preposterous, but if there's one thing I've learned over the years it's that neurology is full of surprises. A few months after our first report on phantoms had been published, I met Mirabelle Kumar, a twenty-five-year-old Indian graduate student, referred to me by Dr. Sathyajit Sen, who knew about my interest in phantoms. Mirabelle was born without arms. All she had were two short stumps dangling from her shoulders. X rays revealed that these stumps contained the head of the humerus or upper arm bone, but that there were no signs of a radius or ulna. Even the tiny bones of her hands were missing, although she did have a hint of rudimentary fingernails in the stump.

Mirabelle walked into my office on a hot summer day, her face flushed from walking up three flights of stairs. An attractive, cheerful young lady, she was also extremely direct with a "don't pity me" attitude writ large on her face.

As soon as Mirabelle was seated, I began asking simple questions: where she was from, where she went to school, what she was interested in and so forth. She quickly lost patience and said, "Look, what do you really want to know? You want to know if I have phantom limbs, right? Let's cut the crap."

I said, "Well, yes, as a matter of fact, we do experiments on phantom limbs. We're interested in . . ."

She interrupted. "Yes. Absolutely. I've never had arms. All I've ever had are these." Deftly, using her chin to help her in a practiced move, she took off her prosthetic arms, clattered them onto my desk and held up her stumps. "And yet I've always experienced the most vivid phantom limbs, from as far back in my childhood as I can remember."

I was skeptical. Could it be that Mirabelle was just engaging in wishful thinking? Maybe she had a deep-seated desire to conform, to be normal. I was beginning to sound like Freud. How could I be sure she was not making it up?

I asked her, "How do you know that you have phantom limbs?"

"Well, because as I'm talking to you, they are gesticulating. They point to objects when I point to things, just like your arms and hands."

I leaned forward, captivated.

"Another interesting thing about them, doctor, is that they're not as long as they should be. They're about six to eight inches too short."

"How do you know that?"

"Because when I put on my artificial arms, my phantoms are much shorter than they should be," said Mirabelle, looking me squarely in the eye. "My phantom fingers should fit into the artificial fingers, like a glove, but my arm is about six inches too short. I find this incredibly frustrating because it doesn't feel natural. I usually end up asking the prosthetist to reduce the length of my artificial arms, but he says that would look short and funny. So we compromise. He gives me limbs that are shorter than most but not so absurdly short that they look strange." She pointed to one of her prosthetic arms lying on the desk, so I could see. "They're a little bit shorter than normal arms, but most people don't notice it."

To me this was proof that Mirabelle's phantoms were not wishful thinking. If she wanted to be like other people, why would she want shorter-than-normal arms? There must be something going on inside her brain that was giving rise to the vivid phantom experience.

Mirabelle had another point. "When I walk, doctor, my phantom arms don't swing like normal arms, like your arms. They stay frozen on the side, like this." She stood up, letting her stumps drop straight down on both sides. "But when I talk," she said, "my phantoms gesticulate. In fact, they're moving now as I speak."

This is not as mysterious as it sounds. The brain region responsible for smooth, coordinated swinging of the arms when we walk is quite different from the one that controls gesturing. Perhaps the neural circuitry for arm swinging cannot survive very long without continuous nurturing feedback from the limbs. It simply drops out or fails to develop when the arms are missing. But the neural circuitry for gesticulation—activated during spoken language—might be specified by genes during development. (The relevant circuitry probably antedates spoken language.) Remarkably, the neural circuitry that generates these commands in Mirabelle's brain seems to have survived intact, despite the fact that she has received no visual or kinesthetic feedback from those "arms" at any point in her life. Her body keeps telling her, "There are no arms, there are no arms," yet she continues to experience gesticulation.

This suggests that the neural circuitry for Mirabelle's body image must have been laid down at least partly by genes and is not strictly dependent on motor and tactile experience. Some early medical reports claim that patients with limbs missing from birth do not experience phantoms. What I saw in Mirabelle, however, implies that each of us has an internally hard-wired image of the body and limbs at birth—an image that can survive indefinitely, even in the face of contradictory information from the senses.[1]

In addition to these spontaneous gesticulations, Mirabelle can also generate voluntary movements in her phantom arms, and this is also true of patients who lose arms in adulthood. Like Mirabelle, most of these patients can "reach out" and "grab" objects, point, wave good-bye, shake hands, or perform elaborate skilled maneuvers with the phantom. They know it sounds crazy since they realize that the arm is gone, but to them these sensory experiences are very real.

I didn't realize how compelling these felt movements could be until I met John McGrath, an arm amputee who telephoned me after he had seen a television news story on phantom limbs. An accomplished amateur athlete, John had lost his left arm just below the elbow three years earlier. "When I play tennis," he said, "my phantom will do what it's supposed to do. It'll want to throw the ball up when I serve or it will try to give me balance in a hard shot. It's always trying to grab the phone. It even waves for the check in restaurants," he said with a laugh.

John had what is known as a telescoped phantom hand. It felt as if it were attached directly to his stump with no arm in between. However, if an object such as a teacup were placed a foot or two away from the stump, he could try to reach for it. When he did this, his phantom no longer remained attached to the stump but felt as if it were zooming out to grab the cup.

On a whim I started thinking, What if I ask John to reach out and grab this cup but pull it away from him before he "touches" it with his phantom? Will the phantom stretch out, like a cartoon character's rubbery arm, or will it stop at a natural arm's length? How far can I move the cup away before John will say he can't reach it? Could he grab the moon? Or will the physical limitations that apply to a real arm also apply to the phantom?

I placed a coffee cup in front of John and asked him to grab it. Just as he said he was reaching out, I yanked away the cup.

"Ow!" he yelled. "Don't do that!"

"What's the matter? "

"Don't do that," he repeated. "I had just got my fingers around the cup handle when you pulled it. That really hurts!"

Hold on a minute. I wrench a real cup from phantom fingers and the person yells, ouch! The fingers were illusory, of course, but the pain was real—indeed, so intense that I dared not repeat the experiment.

My experience with John started me wondering about the role of vision in sustaining the phantom limb experience. Why would merely "seeing" the cup be pulled away result in pain? But before we answer this question, we need to consider why anyone would experience movements in a phantom limb. If you close your eyes and move your arm, you can of course feel its position and movement quite vividly partly because of joint and muscle receptors. But neither John nor Mirabelle has such receptors. Indeed, they have no arm. So where do these sensations originate?

Ironically, I got the first clue to this mystery when I realized that many phantom limb patients—perhaps one third of them—are *not* able to move their phantoms. When asked, they say, "My arm is cast in cement, doctor" or "It's immobilized in a block of ice." "I try to move my phantom, but I can't," said Irene, one of our patients. "It won't obey my mind. It won't obey my command." Using her intact arm, Irene mimicked the position of her phantom arm, showing me how it was frozen in an odd, twisted position. It had been that way for a whole year. She always worried that she would "bump" it when entering doorways, and that it would hurt even more.

How can a phantom—a nonexistent limb—be paralyzed? It sounds like an oxymoron.

I looked up the case sheets and found that many of these patients had had preexisting pathology in the nerves entering the arm from the spinal cord. Their arms really had been paralyzed, held in a sling or cast for a few months and later been amputated simply because they were constantly getting in the way. Some patients were advised to get rid of it, perhaps in a misguided attempt to eliminate the pain in the arm or to correct postural abnormalities caused by the paralyzed arm or leg. Not surprisingly, after the operations these patients often experience a vivid phantom limb, but to their dismay the phantom remains locked in the same position as before the amputation, as though a memory of the paralysis is carried over into the phantom limb.

So here we have a paradox. Mirabelle never had arms in her entire life, yet she can move her phantoms. Irene had just lost her arm a year earlier and yet she cannot generate a flicker of movement. What's going on here?

To answer this question we need to take a closer look at the anatomy and physiology of the motor and sensory systems in the human brain. Consider what happens when you or I close our eyes and gesticulate. We have a vivid sense of our body and of the position of our limbs and their movements. Two eminent English neurologists, Lord Russell Brain and Henry Head (yes, these are their real names), coined the phrase "body image" for this vibrant, internally constructed ensemble of experiences—the internal image and memory of one's body in space and time. To create and maintain this body image at any given instant, your parietal lobes combine information from many sources: the muscles, joints, eyes and motor command centers.

When you decide to move your hand, the chain of events leading to its movements originates in the frontal lobes—especially in the vertical strip of cortical tissue called the motor cortex. This strip lies just in front of the furrow that separates the frontal lobe from the parietal lobe. Like the sensory homunculus that occupies the region just behind this furrow, the motor cortex contains an upside-down "map" of the whole body—except that it is concerned with sending signals to the muscles rather than receiving signals from the skin.

Experiments show that the primary motor cortex is concerned mainly with simple movements like wiggling your finger or smacking your lips. An area immediately in front of it, called the supplementary motor area, appears to be in charge of more complex skills such as waving good-bye and grabbing a banister. This supplementary motor area acts like a kind of master of ceremonies, passing specific instructions about the proper sequence of required movements to the motor cortex. Nerve impulses that will then direct these movements travel from the motor cortex down the spinal cord to the muscles on the opposite side of the body, allowing you to wave good-bye or put on lipstick.

Every time a "command" is sent from the supplementary motor area to the motor cortex, it goes to the muscles and they move.[2] At the same time, identical copies of the command signal are sent to two other major "processing" areas—the cerebellum and the parietal lobes—informing them of the intended action.

Once these command signals are sent to the muscles, a feedback loop is set in motion. Having received a command to move, the muscles execute the movement. In turn, signals from the muscle spindles and joints are sent back up to the brain, via the spinal cord, informing the cerebellum and parietal lobes that "yes, the command is being performed correctly." These two structures help you compare your intention with your actual performance, behaving like a thermostat in a servo-loop, and modifying the motor commands as needed (applying brakes if they are too fast and increasing the motor outflow if it's too slow). Thus intentions are transformed into smoothly coordinated movements.

Now let's return to our patients to see how all this relates to the phantom experience. When John decides to move his phantom arm, the front part of his brain still sends out a command message, since this particular part of John's brain doesn't "know" that his arm is missing—even though John "the person" is unquestionably aware of the fact. The commands continue to be monitored by the parietal lobe and are felt as movements. But they are phantom movements carried out by a phantom arm.

Thus the phantom limb experience seems to depend on signals from at least two sources. The first is remapping; recall that sensory input from the face and upper arm activates brain areas that correspond to the "hand." Second, each time the motor command center sends signals to the missing arm, information about the commands is also sent to the parietal lobe containing our body image. The convergence of information from these two sources results in a dynamic, vibrant image of the phantom arm at any given instant—an image that is continuously updated as the arm "moves."

In the case of an actual arm there is a third source of information, namely, the impulses from the joints, ligaments and muscle spindles of that arm. The phantom arm of course lacks these tissues and their signals, but oddly enough this fact does not seem to prevent the brain from being fooled into thinking that the limb is moving—at least for the first few months or years after amputation.

This takes us back to an earlier question. How can a phantom limb be paralyzed? Why does it remain "frozen" after amputation? One possibility is that when the actual limb is paralyzed, lying in a sling or brace, the brain sends its usual commands—move that arm, shake that leg.

The command is monitored by the parietal lobe, but this time it does not receive the proper visual feedback. The visual system says, "nope, this arm is not moving." The command is sent out again—arm, move. The visual feedback returns, informing the brain repeatedly that the arm isn't moving. Eventually the brain learns that the arm does not move and a kind of "learned paralysis" is stamped onto the brain's circuitry. Exactly where this occurs is not known, but it may lie partly in motor centers and partly in parietal regions concerned with body image. Whatever the physiological explanation turns out to be, when the arm is later amputated, the person is stuck with that revised body image: a paralyzed phantom.

If you can learn paralysis, is it possible that you can unlearn it? What if Irene were to send a "move now" message to her phantom arm, and every time she did so she got back a visual signal that it was moving; that, yes, it was obeying her command? But how can she get visual feedback when she doesn't have an arm? Can we trick her eyes into actually seeing a phantom?

I thought about virtual reality. Maybe we could create the visual illusion that the arm was restored and was obeying her commands. But that technology, costing over half a million dollars, would exhaust my entire research budget with one purchase. Fortunately, I thought of a way to do the experiment with an ordinary mirror purchased from a five-and-dime store.

To enable patients like Irene to perceive real movement in their nonexistent arms, we constructed a virtual reality box. The box is made by placing a vertical mirror inside a cardboard box with its lid removed. The front of the box has two holes in it, through which the patient inserts her "good hand" (say, the right one) and her phantom hand (the left one). Since the mirror is in the middle of the box, the right hand is now on the right side of the mirror and the phantom is on the left side. The patient is then asked to view the reflection of her normal hand in the mirror and to move it around slightly until the reflection appears to be superimposed on the felt position of her phantom hand. She has thus created the illusion of observing two hands, when in fact she is only seeing the mirror reflection of her intact hand. If she now sends motor commands to both arms to make mirror symmetric movements, as if she were conducting an orchestra or clapping, she of course "sees" her phantom moving as well. Her brain receives confirming visual feedback that the phantom hand is moving correctly in response to her command. Will this help restore voluntary control over her paralyzed phantom?

The first person to explore this new world was Philip Martinez. In 1984 Philip was hurled off his motorcycle, going at forty-five miles an hour down the San Diego freeway. He skidded across the median, landed at the foot of a concrete bridge and, getting up in a daze, he had the presence of mind to check himself for injuries. A helmet and leather jacket prevented the worst, but Philip's left arm had been severely torn near his shoulder. Like Dr. Pons's monkeys, he had a brachial avulsion—the nerves supplying his arm had been yanked off the spinal column. His left arm was completely paralyzed and lay lifeless in a sling for one year. Finally, doctors advised amputation. The arm was just getting in the way and would never regain function.

Ten years later, Philip walked into my office. Now in his midthirties, he collects a disability benefit and has made a rather impressive reputation for himself as a pool player, known among his friends as the "one-armed bandit."

Philip had heard about my experiments with phantom limbs in local press reports. He was desperate. "Dr. Ramachandran," he said, "I'm hoping you can help me." He glanced down at his missing arm. "I lost it ten years ago. But ever since I've had a terrible pain in my phantom elbow, wrist and fingers." Interviewing him further, I discovered that during the decade, Philip had never been able to move his phantom arm. It was always fixed in an awkward position. Was Philip suffering from learned paralysis? If so, could we use our virtual reality box to resurrect the phantom visually and restore movements?

I asked Philip to place his right hand on the right side of the mirror in the box and imagine that his left hand (the phantom) was on the left side. "I want you to move your right and left arms simultaneously," I instructed.

"Oh, I can't do that," said Philip. "I can move my right arm but my left arm is frozen. Every morning when I get up, I try to move my phantom because it's in this funny position and I feel that moving it might help relieve the pain. But," he said, looking down at his invisible arm, "I have never been able to generate a flicker of movement in it."

"Okay, Philip, but try anyway."

Philip rotated his body, shifting his shoulder, to "insert" his lifeless phantom into the box. Then he put his right hand on the other side of the mirror and attempted to make synchronous movements. As he gazed into the mirror, he gasped and then cried out, "Oh, my God! Oh, my God, doctor! This is unbelievable. It's mind-boggling!" He was jumping up and down like a kid. "My left arm is plugged in again. It's as if I'm in the past. All these memories from so many years ago are flooding back into my mind. I can move my arm again. I can feel my elbow moving, my wrist moving. It's all moving again."

After he calmed down a little I said, "Okay, Philip, now close your eyes."

"Oh, my," he said, clearly disappointed. "It's frozen again. I feel my right hand moving, but there's no movement in the phantom."

"Open your eyes."

"Oh, yes. Now it's moving again."

It was as though Philip had some temporary inhibition or block of the neural circuits that would ordinarily move the phantom and the visual feedback had overcome this block. More amazing still, these bodily sensations of the arm's movements were revived instantly,[3] even though they had never been felt in the preceding ten years!

Though Philip's response was exciting and provided some support for my hypothesis about learned paralysis, I went home that night and asked myself, "So what? So we have this guy moving his phantom limb again. But it's a perfectly useless ability if you think about it—precisely the sort of arcane thing that many of us medical researchers are sometimes accused of working on." I wouldn't win a prize, I realized, for getting someone to move a phantom limb.

But maybe learned paralysis is a more widespread phenomenon.[4] It might happen to people with real limbs that are paralyzed, say, from a stroke. Why do people lose the use of an arm after a stroke? When a blood vessel supplying the brain gets clogged, the fibers that extend from the front part of the brain down to the spinal cord are deprived of oxygen and sustain damage, leaving the arm paralyzed. But in the early stages of a stroke, the brain swells, temporarily causing some nerves to die off but leaving others simply stunned and "off-line," so to speak. During this time, when the arm is nonfunctional, the brain receives visual feedback: "Nope, the arm is not moving." After the swelling subsides, it's possible that the patient's brain is stuck with a form of learned paralysis. Could the mirror contraption be used to overcome at least that component of the paralysis that is due to learning? (Obviously there is nothing one can do with mirrors to restore paralysis caused by actual destruction of fibers.)

But before we could implement this kind of novel therapy for stroke patients, we needed to ensure that the effect is more than a mere temporary illusion of movement in the phantom. (Recall that when Philip closed his eyes, the sense of movement in his phantom disappeared.)

What if the patient were to practice with the box in order to receive continuous visual feedback for several days? Is it conceivable that the brain would "unlearn" its perception of damage and that movements would be permanently restored?

I went back the next day and asked Philip, "Are you willing to take this device home and practice with it?"

"Sure," said Philip. "I'd love to take it home. I find it very exciting that I can move my arm again, even if only momentarily."

So Philip took the mirror home. A week later I telephoned him. "What's happening?"

"Oh, it's fun, doctor. I use it for ten minutes every day. I put my hand inside, wave it around and see how it feels. My girlfriend and I play with it. It's very enjoyable. But when I close my eyes, it still doesn't work. And if I don't use the mirror, it doesn't work. I know you want my phantom to start moving again, but without the mirror it doesn't."

Three more weeks passed until one day Philip called me, very excited and agitated. "Doctor," he exclaimed, "it's gone!"

"What's gone?" (I thought maybe he had lost the mirror box.)

"My phantom is gone."

"What are you talking about?"

"You know, my phantom arm, which I had for ten years. It doesn't exist anymore. All I have is my phantom fingers and palm dangling from my shoulder!"

My immediate reaction was, Oh, no! I have apparently permanently altered a person's body image using a mirror. How would this affect his mental state and well-being? "Philip—does it bother you?"

"No no no no no no," he said. "On the contrary. You know the excruciating pain I always had in my elbow? The pain that tortured me several times a week? Well, now I don't have an elbow and I don't have that pain anymore. But I still have my fingers dangling from my shoulder and they still hurt." He paused, apparently to let this sink in. "Unfortunately," he added, "your mirror box doesn't work anymore because my fingers are up too high. Can you change the design to eliminate my fingers?" Philip seemed to think I was some kind of magician.

I wasn't sure I could help Philip with his request, but I realized that this was probably the first example in medical history of a successful "amputation" of a phantom limb! The experiment suggests that when Philip's right parietal lobe was presented with conflicting signals—visual feedback telling him that his arm is moving again while his muscles are telling him the arm is not there—his mind resorted to a form of denial. The only way his beleaguered brain could deal with this bizarre sensory conflict was to say, "To hell with it, there is no arm!" And as a huge bonus, Philip lost the associated pain in his phantom elbow as well, for it may be impossible to experience a disembodied pain in a nonexistent phantom. It's not clear why his fingers didn't disappear, but one reason might be that they are overrepresented—like the huge lips on the Penfield map—in the somatosensory cortex and may be more difficult to deny.

•

Movements and paralysis of phantom limbs are hard enough to explain, but even more puzzling is the agonizing pain that many patients experience in the phantom soon after amputation, and Philip had brought me face to face with this problem. What confluence of biological circumstances could cause pain to erupt in a nonexistent limb? There are several possibilities.

The pain could be caused by scar tissue or neuromas—little curled-up clusters or clumps of nerve tissue in the stump. Irritation of these clumps and frayed nerve endings could be interpreted by the brain as pain in the missing limb. When neuromas are removed surgically, phantom pain sometimes vanishes, at least temporarily, but then insidiously it often returns.

The pain could also result in part from remapping. Keep in mind that remapping is ordinarily modality-specific: That simply means that the sense of touch follows touch pathways, and the feeling of warmth follows warmth pathways, and so on. (As we noted, when I lightly stroke Tom's face with a Q-tip, he feels me touching his phantom. When I dribble ice water on his cheek, he feels cold on his phantom hand and when I warm up the water he feels heat in the phantom as well as on his face.) This probably means that remapping doesn't happen randomly. The fibers concerned with each sense must "know" where to go to find their appropriate targets. Thus in most people, including you, me and amputees, one does not get cross-wiring.

But imagine what might happen if a slight error were to occur during the remapping process—a tiny glitch in the blueprint—so that some of the touch input is hooked up accidentally to pain centers. The patient might experience severe pain every time regions around his face or upper arm (rather than neuromas) were brushed, even lightly. Such trivial touches could generate excruciating pain, all because a few fibers are in the wrong place, doing the wrong thing.

Abnormal remapping could also cause pain two other ways. When we experience pain, special pathways are activated simultaneously both to carry the sensation and to amplify it or dampen it down as needed. Such "volume control" (sometimes called gate control) is what allows us to modulate our responses to pain effectively in response to changing demands (which might explain why acupuncture works or why women in some cultures don't experience pain during labor). Among amputees, it's entirely possible that these volume control mechanisms have gone awry as a result of remapping—resulting in an echolike "wha wha" reverberation and amplification of pain. Second, remapping is inherently a pathological or abnormal process, at least when it occurs on a large scale, as after the loss of a limb. It's possible that the touch synapses are not quite correctly rewired and their activity could be chaotic. Higher brain centers would then interpret the abnormal pattern of input as junk, which is perceived as pain. In truth, we really don't know how the brain translates patterns of nerve activity into conscious experience, be it pain, pleasure or color.

Finally, some patients say that the pain they felt in their limbs immediately prior to amputation persists as a kind of pain memory. For example, soldiers who have grenades blow up in their hands often report that their phantom hand is in a fixed position, clenching the grenade, ready to toss it. The pain in the hand is excruciating—the same they felt the instant the grenade exploded, seared permanently in their brains. In London I once met a woman who told me she had experienced chilblains—a frostbitelike pain due to cold weather—in her thumb for several months in her childhood. The thumb later became gangrenous and was amputated. She now has a vivid phantom thumb and experiences chilblains in it every time the weather turns cold. Another woman described arthritic pain in her phantom joints. She'd had the problem before her arm was amputated but it has continued in the absence of real joints, with the pain being worse when it gets damp and cold just as it had in the real joints before amputation.

One of my medical school professors told me a story that he swore was true, the tale of another physician, an eminent cardiologist, who developed a pulsating cramp in his leg caused by Buerger's disease—a malady that produces constriction of arteries and intense, pulsing pain in the calf muscles.

Despite many attempts at treatment, nothing eased the pain. Out of sheer despair, the physician decided to have his leg amputated. He simply couldn't live with the pain any longer. He consulted a surgeon colleague and scheduled the operation, but to the surgeon's astonishment, he said he had a special request: "After you amputate my leg, could you please pickle it in a jar of formaldehyde and give it to me?" This was eccentric, to say the least, but the surgeon agreed, amputated the leg, put it in a jar of preservative and gave it to the physician, who then put it in his office and said, "Hah, at last, I can look at this leg and laugh at it and say, 'I finally got rid of you!' "

But the leg had the last laugh. The pulsatile pains returned with a vengeance in the phantom leg. The good doctor stared at his floating limb in disbelief while it stared back at him, as if to mock all his efforts to rid himself of it.

There are many such stories in circulation, illustrating the astonishing specificity of pain memories and their tendency to surface when a limb is amputated. If this is the case, one can imagine being able to reduce the incidence of pain after amputation simply by injecting the limb with a local anesthetic before surgery. (This has been tried with some success.)

•

Pain is one of the most poorly understood of all sensory experiences. It is a source of great frustration to patient and physician alike and can emerge in many different guises. One especially enigmatic complaint frequently heard from patients is that every now and then the phantom hand becomes curled into a tight, white-knuckled fist, fingers digging into palm with all the fury of a prizefighter ready to deliver a knockout blow.

Robert Townsend is an intelligent, fifty-five-year-old engineer whose cancer caused him to lose his left arm six inches above the elbow. When I saw him seven months after the amputation, he was experiencing a vivid phantom limb that would often go into an involuntary clenching spasm. "It's like my nails are digging into my phantom hand," said Robert. "The pain is unbearable." Even if he concentrated all his attention on it, he could not open his invisible hand to relieve the spasm.

We wondered whether using the mirror box could help Robert eliminate his spasms. Like Philip, Robert looked into the box, positioned his good hand to superimpose its reflection over his phantom hand and, after making a fist with the normal hand, tried to unclench both hands simultaneously. The first time he did this, Robert exclaimed that he could feel the phantom fist open along with his good fist, simply as a result of the visual feedback. Better yet, the pain disappeared. The phantom then remained unclenched for several hours until a new spasm occurred spontaneously. Without the mirror, his phantom would throb in pain for forty minutes or more. Robert took the box home and tried the same trick each time that the clenching spasm recurred. If he did not use the box, he could not unclench his fist despite trying with all his might. If he used the mirror, the hand opened instantly.

We have tried this treatment in over a dozen patients and it works for half of them. They take the mirrored box home and whenever a spasm occurs, they put their good hand into the box and open it and the spasm is eliminated. But is it a cure? It's difficult to know. Pain is notoriously susceptible to the placebo effect (the power of suggestion). Perhaps the elaborate laboratory setting or the mere presence of a charismatic expert on phantom limbs is all you need in order to eliminate the pain and it has nothing to do with mirrors. We tested this possibility on one patient by giving him a harmless battery pack that generates an electric current. Whenever the spasms and abnormal postures occurred, he was asked to rotate the dial on the unit of his "transcutaneous electrical simulator" until he began to feel a tingling in his left arm (which was his good arm). We told him that this would immediately restore voluntary movements in the phantom and provide relief from the spasms. We also told him that the procedure had worked on other patients in his predicament.

He said, "Really? Wow, I can't wait to try it."

Two days later he was back, obviously annoyed. "It's useless," he exclaimed. "I tried it five times and it just doesn't work. I turned it up to full strength even though you told me not to."

When I gave him the mirror to try that same afternoon, he was able to open his phantom hand instantly. The spasms were eliminated and so too was the "digging sensation" of nails biting into his palm. This is a mind-boggling observation if you think about it. Here is a man with no hand and no fingernails. How does one get nonexistent nails digging into a nonexistent palm, resulting in severe pain? Why would a mirror eliminate the phantom spasm?

Consider what happens in your brain when motor commands are sent from the premotor and motor cortex to make a fist. Once your hand is clenched, feedback signals from muscles and joints of your hand are sent back through the spinal cord to your brain saying, Slow down, enough. Any more pressure and it could hurt. This proprioceptive feedback applies brakes, automatically, with astonishing speed and precision.

If the limb is missing, however, this damping feedback is not possible. The brain therefore keeps sending the message, Clench more, clench more. Motor output is amplified even further (to a level that far exceeds anything you or I would ever experience) and the overflow or "sense of effort" may itself be experienced as pain. The mirror may work by providing visual feedback to unclench the hand, so that the clenching spasm is abolished.

But why the sensation of digging fingernails? Just think of the numerous occasions when you actually clenched your fist and felt your nails biting in your palm. These occasions must have created a memory link in your brain (psychologists call it a Hebbian link) between the motor command to clench and the unmistakable sensation of "nails digging," so you can readily summon up this image in your mind. Yet even though you can imagine the image quite vividly, you don't actually feel the sensation and say, "Ouch, that hurts." Why not? The reason, I believe, is that you have a real palm and the skin on the palm says there is no pain. You can imagine it but you don't feel it because you have a normal hand sending real feedback and in the clash between reality and illusion, reality usually wins.

But the amputee doesn't have a palm. There are no countermanding signals from the palm to forbid the emergence of these stored pain memories. When Robert imagines that his nails are digging into his hand, he doesn't get contradictory signals from his skin surface saying, "Robert, you fool, there's no pain down here." Indeed, if the motor commands themselves are linked to the sense of nail digging, it's conceivable that the amplification of these commands leads to a corresponding amplification of the associated pain signals. This might explain why the pain is so brutal.

The implications are radical. Even fleeting sensory associations such as the one between clenching our hands and digging our fingernails into our palms are laid down as permanent traces in the brain and are only unmasked under certain circumstances—experienced in this case as phantom limb pain. Moreover, these ideas imply that pain is an *opinion* on the organism's state of health rather than a mere reflexive response to an injury. There is no direct hotline from pain receptors to "pain centers" in the brain. On the contrary, there is so much interaction between different brain centers, like those concerned with vision and touch, that even the mere visual appearance of an opening fist can actually feed all the way back into the patient's motor and touch pathways, allowing him to feel the fist opening, thereby killing an illusory pain in a nonexistent hand.

If pain is an illusion, how much influence do senses like vision have over our subjective experiences? To find out, I tried a somewhat diabolical experiment on two of my patients. When Mary came into the lab, I asked her to place her phantom right hand, palm down, into the mirror box. I then asked her to put a gray glove on her good left hand and place it in the other side of the box, in a mirror image position. After making sure she was comfortable I instructed one of my graduate students to hide under the curtained table and put his gloved left hand into the same side of the box where Mary's good hand rested, above hers on a false platform. When Mary looked into the box she could see not only the student's gloved left hand (which looked exactly like her own left hand) but also its reflection in the mirror, as if she were looking at her own phantom right hand wearing a glove. When the student now made a fist or used his index finger pad to touch the ball of his thumb, Mary felt her phantom moving vividly. As in our previous two patients, vision was enough to trick her brain into experiencing movements in her phantom limb.

What would happen if we fooled Mary into thinking that her fingers were occupying anatomically impossible positions? The box permitted this illusion. Again, Mary put her phantom right hand, palm down, in the box. But the student now did something different. Instead of placing his left hand into the other side of the box, in an exact mirror image of the phantom, he inserted his right hand, palm up. Since the hand was gloved, it looked exactly like her "palm-down" phantom right hand. Then the student flexed his index finger to touch his palm. To Mary, peering into the box, it appeared as if her phantom index finger were bending backward to touch the back of her wrist—in the wrong direction![5] What would her reaction be?

When Mary saw her finger twisted backward, she said, "One would have thought it should feel peculiar, doctor, but it doesn't. It feels exactly like the finger is bending backward, like it isn't supposed to. But it doesn't feel peculiar or painful or anything like that."

Another subject, Karen, winced and said that the twisted phantom finger hurt. "It felt like somebody was grabbing and pulling my finger. I felt a twinge of pain," she said.

These experiments are important because they flatly contradict the theory that the brain consists of a number of autonomous modules acting as a bucket brigade. Popularized by artificial intelligence researchers, the idea that the brain behaves like a computer, with each module performing a highly specialized job and sending its output to the next module, is widely believed. In this view, sensory processing involves a one-way cascade of information sensory receptors on the skin and other sense organs to higher brain centers.

But my experiments with these patients have taught me that this is not how the brain works. Its connections are extraordinarily labile and dynamic. Perceptions emerge as a result of reverberations of signals between different levels of the sensory hierarchy, indeed even across different senses. The fact that visual input can eliminate the spasm of a nonexistent arm and then erase the associated memory of pain vividly illustrates how extensive and profound these interactions can be.

•

Studying patients with phantom limbs has given me insights into the inner working of the brain that go far beyond the simple questions I started with four years ago when Tom first walked into my office. We've actually witnessed (directly and indirectly) how new connections emerge in the adult brain, how information from different senses interacts, how the activity of sensory maps is related to sensory experience and more generally how the brain is continuously updating its model of reality in response to novel sensory inputs.

This last observation sheds new light on the so-called nature versus nurture debate by allowing us to ask the question, Do phantom limbs arise mainly from nongenetic factors such as remapping or stump neuromas, or do they represent the ghostly persistence of an inborn, genetically specified "body image"? The answer seems to be that the phantom emerges from a complex interaction between the two. I'll give you five examples to illustrate this.

In the case of below-the-elbow amputees, surgeons will sometimes cleave the stump into a lobster claw–like appendage, as an alternative to a standard metal hook. After the surgery, people learn to use their pincers at the stump to grasp objects, turn them around and otherwise manipulate the material world. Intriguingly, their phantom hand (some inches away from real flesh) also feels split in two—with one or more phantom fingers occupying each pincer, vividly mimicking the movements of the appendage. I know of one instance in which a patient underwent amputation of his pincers only to be left with a permanently cleaved phantom—striking evidence that a surgeon's scalpel can dissect a phantom.

After the original surgery in which the stump was split, this patient's brain must have reshaped his body image to include the two pincers—for why else would he experience phantom pincers?

The other two stories both entertain and inform. A girl who was born without forearms and who experienced phantom hands six inches below her stumps frequently used her *phantom* fingers to calculate and solve arithmetic problems. A sixteen-year-old girl who was born with her right leg two inches shorter than her left leg and who received a below-knee amputation at age six had the odd sensation of possessing four feet! In addition to one good foot and the expected phantom foot, she developed two supernumerary phantom feet, one at the exact level of amputation and a second one, complete with calf, extending all the way down to the floor, where it should be had the limb not been congenitally shorter.[6] Although researchers have used this example to illustrate the role of genetic factors in determining body image, one could equally use it to emphasize nongenetic influences, for why would your genes specify three separate images of one leg?

A fourth example that illustrates the complex interplay between genes and environment harks back to our observation that many amputees experience vivid phantom movements, both voluntary and involuntary, but in most the movements disappear eventually. Such movements are experienced at first because the brain continues sending motor commands to the missing limb (and monitors them) after amputation. But sooner or later, the lack of visual confirmation (Gee, there is no arm) causes the patient's brain to reject these signals and the movements are no longer experienced. But if this explanation is correct, how can we understand the continued presence of vivid limb movements in people like Mirabelle, who was born without arms? I can only guess that a normal adult has had a lifetime of visual and kinesthetic feedback, a process that leads the brain to expect such feedback even after amputation. The brain is "disappointed" if the expectation is not fulfilled—leading eventually to a loss of voluntary movements or even a complete loss of the phantom itself. The sensory areas of Mirabelle's brain, however, have never received such feedback. Consequently, there is no learned dependence on sensory feedback, and that lack might explain why the sensation of movements had persisted, unchanged, for twenty-five years.

The final example comes from my own country, India, which I visit every year. The dreaded disease leprosy is still quite common there and often leads to progressive mutilation and loss of limbs. At the leprosarium at Vellore, I was told that these patients who lose their arms do not experience phantoms, and I personally saw several cases and verified these claims. The standard explanation is that the patient gradually "learns" to assimilate the stump into his body image by using visual feedback, but if this is true, how does it account for the continued presence of phantoms in amputees? Perhaps the *gradual* loss of the limb or the simultaneous presence of progressive nerve damage caused by the leprosy bacterium is somehow critical. This might allow their brains more time to readjust their body image to match reality. Odder still, when such a patient develops gangrene in his stump and the diseased tissue is amputated, he *does* develop a phantom. But it's not a phantom of the old stump; it's a phantom of the entire hand! It's as though the brain has a dual representation, one of the original body image laid down genetically and one ongoing, up-to-date image that can incorporate subsequent changes. For some weird reason, the amputation disturbs the equilibrium and resurrects the original body image, which has always been competing for attention.[7]

I mention these bizarre examples because they imply that phantom limbs emerge from a complex interplay of both genetic and experiential variables whose relative contributions can be disentangled only by systematic empirical investigations. As with most nature/nurture debates, asking which is the more important variable is meaningless—despite extravagant claims to the contrary in the IQ literature. (Indeed, the question is no more meaningful than asking whether the wetness of water results mainly from the hydrogen molecules or from the oxygen molecules that constitute H_2O!) But the good news is that by doing the right kinds of experiments, you can begin to tease them apart, investigate how they interact and eventually help develop new treatments for phantom pain. It seems extraordinary even to contemplate the possibility that you could use a visual illusion to eliminate pain, but bear in mind that pain itself is an illusion—constructed entirely in your brain like any other sensory experience. Using one illusion to erase another doesn't seem very surprising after all.

•

The experiments I've discussed so far have helped us understand what is going on in the brains of patients with phantoms and given us hints as to how we might help alleviate their pain. But there is a deeper message here: *Your own body* is a phantom, one that your brain has temporarily constructed purely for convenience. I know this sounds astonishing so I will demonstrate to you the malleability of your own body image and how you can alter it profoundly in just a few seconds. Two of these experiments you can do on yourself right now, but the third requires a visit to a Halloween supply shop.

To experience the first illusion, you'll need two helpers. (I will call them Julie and Mina.) Sit in a chair, blindfolded, and ask Julie to sit on another chair in front of you, facing the same direction as you are. Have Mina stand on your right side and give her the following instructions: "Take my right hand and guide my index finger to Julia's nose. Move my hand in a rhythmic manner so that my index finger repeatedly strokes and taps her nose in a random sequence like a Morse code. At the same time, use your left hand to stroke my nose with the same rhythm and timing. The stroking and tapping of my nose and Julia's nose should be in perfect synchrony."

After thirty or forty seconds, if you're lucky, you will develop the uncanny illusion that you are touching your nose out there or that your nose has been dislocated and stretched out about three feet in front of your face. The more random and unpredictable the stroking sequence, the more striking the illusion will be. This is an extraordinary illusion; why does it happen? I suggest that your brain "notices" that the tapping and stroking sensations from your right index finger are perfectly synchronized with the strokes and taps felt on your nose. It then says, "The tapping on my nose is identical to the sensations on my right index finger; why are the two sequences identical? The likelihood that this is a coincidence is zero, and therefore the most probable explanation is that my finger must be tapping my nose. But I also know that my hand is two feet away from my face. So it follows that my nose must also be out there, two feet away."[8]

I have tried this experiment on twenty people and it works on about half of them (I hope it will work on you). But to me, the astonishing thing is that it works at all—that your certain knowledge that you have a normal nose, your image of your body and face constructed over a lifetime should be negated by just a few seconds of the right kind of sensory stimulation. This simple experiment not only shows how malleable your body image is but also illustrates the single most important principle underlying all of perception—that the mechanisms of perception are mainly involved in extracting statistical correlations from the world to create a model that is temporarily useful.

The second illusion requires one helper and is even spookier.[9] You'll need to go to a novelty or Halloween store to buy a dummy rubber hand. Then construct a two-foot by two-foot cardboard "wall" and place it on a table in front of you. Put your right hand behind the cardboard so that you cannot see it and put the dummy hand in front of the cardboard so you can see it clearly. Next have your friend stroke identical locations on both your hand and the dummy hand synchronously while you look at the dummy. Within seconds you will experience the stroking sensation as arising from the dummy hand. The experience is uncanny, for you know perfectly well that you're looking at a disembodied rubber hand, but this doesn't prevent your brain from assigning sensation to it. The illusion illustrates, once again, how ephemeral your body image is and how easily it can be manipulated.

Projecting your sensations on to a dummy hand is surprising enough, but, more remarkably, my student Rick Stoddard and I discovered that you can even experience touch sensations as arising from tables and chairs that bear no physical resemblance to human body parts. This experiment is especially easy to do since all you need is a single friend to assist you. Sit at your writing desk and hide your left hand under the table. Ask your friend to tap and stroke the surface of the table with his right hand (as you watch) and then use his hand simultaneously to stroke and tap your left hand, which is hidden from view. It is absolutely critical that you not see the movements of his left hand as this will ruin the effect (use a cardboard partition or a curtain if necessary). After a minute or so, you will start experiencing taps and strokes as emerging from the table surface even though your conscious mind knows perfectly well that this is logically absurd. Again, the sheer statistical improbability of the two sequences of taps and strokes—one seen on the table surface and one felt on your hand—lead the brain to conclude that the table is now part of your body. The illusion is so compelling that on the few occasions when I accidentally made a much longer stroke on the table surface than on the subject's hidden hand, the person exclaimed that his hand felt "lengthened" or "stretched" to absurd proportions.

Both these illusions are much more than amusing party tricks to try on your friends. The idea that you can actually *project* your sensations to external objects is radical and reminds me of phenomena such as out-of-body experiences or even voodoo (prick the doll and "feel" the pain). But how can we be sure the student volunteer isn't just being metaphorical when she says "I feel my nose out there" or "The table feels like my own hand." After all, I often have the experience of "feeling" that my car is part of my extended body image, so much so that I become infuriated if someone makes a small dent on it. But would I want to argue from this that the car had become part of my body?

These are not easy questions to tackle, but to find out whether the students really identified with the table surface, we devised a simple experiment that takes advantage of what is called the galvanic skin response or GSR. If I hit you with a hammer or hold a heavy rock over your foot and threaten to drop it, your brain's visual areas will dispatch messages to your limbic system (the emotional center) to prepare your body to take emergency measures (basically telling you to run from danger). Your heart starts pumping more blood and you begin sweating to dissipate heat. This alarm response can be monitored by measuring the changes in skin resistance—the so-called GSR—caused by the sweat. If you look at a pig, a newspaper or a pen there is no GSR, but if you look at something evocative—a Mapplethorpe photo, a *Playboy* centerfold or a heavy rock teetering above your foot—you will register a huge GSR.

So I hooked up the student volunteers to a GSR device while they stared at the table. I then stroked the hidden hand and the table surface simultaneously for several seconds until the student started experiencing the table as his own hand. Next I bashed the table surface with a hammer as the student watched. Instantly, there was a huge change in GSR as if I had smashed the student's own fingers. (When I tried the control experiment of stroking the table and hand out of sync, the subject did not experience the illusion and there was no GSR response.) It was as though the table had now become coupled to the student's own limbic system and been assimilated into his body image, so much so that pain and threat to the dummy are felt as threats to his own body, as shown by the GSR. If this argument is correct, then perhaps it's not all that silly to ask whether you identify with your car. Just punch it to see whether your GSR changes. Indeed the technique may give us a handle on elusive psychological phenomena such as the empathy and love that you feel for a child or spouse. If you are deeply in love with someone, is it possible that you have actually become part of that person? Perhaps your souls—and not merely your bodies—have become intertwined.

Now just think about what all this means. For your entire life, you've been walking around assuming that your "self" is anchored to a single body that remains stable and permanent at least until death. Indeed, the "loyalty" of your self to your own body is so axiomatic that you never even pause to think about it, let alone question it. Yet these experiments suggest the exact opposite—that your body image, despite all its appearance of durability, is an entirely transitory internal construct that can be profoundly modified with just a few simple tricks. It is merely a shell that you've temporarily created for successfully passing on your genes to your offspring.

CHAPTER 4

The Zombie in the Brain

He refused to associate himself with any investigation which did not tend towards the unusual, and even the fantastic.

—DR. JAMES WATSON

David Milner, a neuropsychologist at the University of St. Andrews in Fife, Scotland, was so eager to get to the hospital to test his newly arrived patient that he almost forgot to take along the case notes describing her condition. He had to rush back to his house through a cold winter rain to fetch the folder describing Diane Fletcher. The facts were simple but tragic: Diane had recently moved to northern Italy to work as a free-lance commercial translator. She and her husband had found one of those lovely old apartments near the medieval town center, with fresh paint, new kitchen appliances and a refurbished bathroom—a place nearly as luxurious as their permanent home back in Canada. But their adventure was short-lived. When Diane stepped into the shower one morning, she had no warning that the hot water heater was improperly vented. When the propane gas ignited to heat a steady flow of water flowing past red-hot burners, carbon monoxide built up in the small bathroom. Diane was washing her hair when the odorless fumes gradually overwhelmed her, causing her to lose consciousness and fall to the tile floor, her face a bright pink from the irreversible binding of carbon monoxide to hemoglobin in her blood. She had lain there for perhaps twenty minutes with water cascading over her limp body, when her husband returned to retrieve something he had forgotten. Had he not gone home, she would have died within the hour. But even though Diane survived and made an amazing recovery, her loved ones soon realized that parts of her had forever vanished, lost in patches of permanently atrophied brain tissue.

When Diane woke from the coma, she was completely blind. Within a couple of days she could recognize colors and textures, but not shapes of objects or faces—not even her husband's face or her own reflection in a handheld mirror. At the same time, she had no difficulty identifying people from their voices and could tell what objects were if they were placed in her hands.

Dr. Milner was consulted because of his long-standing interest in visual problems following strokes and other brain injuries. He was told that Diane had come to Scotland, where her parents live, to see whether something could be done to help her. When Dr. Milner began his routine visual tests, it was obvious that Diane was blind in every traditional sense of the word. She could not read the largest letters on an eye chart and when he showed her two or three fingers, she couldn't identify how many fingers he held up.

At one point, Dr. Milner held up a pencil. "What's this?" he asked.

As usual, Diane looked puzzled. Then she did something unexpected. "Here, let me see it," she said, reaching out and deftly taking the pencil from his hand. Dr. Milner was stunned, not by her ability to identify the object by feeling it but by her dexterity in taking it from his hand. As Diane reached for the pencil, her fingers moved swiftly and accurately toward it, grasped it and carried it back to her lap in one fluid motion. You'd never have guessed that she was blind. It was as if some other person—an unconscious zombie inside her—had guided her actions. (When I say zombie I mean a completely nonconscious being, but it's clear that the zombie is not asleep. It's perfectly alert and capable of making complex, skilled movements, like creatures in the cult movie *Night of the Living Dead*.)

Intrigued, Dr. Milner decided to do some experiments on Diane's covert ability. He showed her a straight line and asked, "Diane, is this line vertical, horizontal or slanted?"

"I don't know," she replied.

Then he showed her a vertical slit (actually a mail slot) and asked her to describe its orientation. Again she said, "I don't know."

When he handed her a letter and asked her to mail it through the slot, she protested, "Oh, I can't do that."

"Oh, come on, give it a try," he said. "Pretend that you're posting a letter."

Diane was reluctant. "Try it," he urged.

Diane took the letter from the doctor and moved it toward the slot, rotating her hand in such a way that the letter was perfectly aligned with the orientation of the slot. In yet another skilled maneuver, Diane popped the letter into the opening even though she could not tell you whether it was vertical, horizontal or slanted. She carried out this instruction without any conscious awareness, as if that very same zombie had taken charge of the task and effortlessly steered her hand toward the goal.[1]

Diane's actions are amazing because we usually think of vision as a single process. When someone who is obviously blind can reach out and grab a letter, rotate the letter into the correct position and mail it through an opening she cannot "see," the ability seems almost paranormal.

To understand what Diane is experiencing, we need to abandon all our commonsense notions about what seeing really is. In the next few pages, you will discover that there is a great deal more to perception than meets the eye.

Like most people, you probably take vision for granted. You wake up in the morning, open your eyes and, *voilà,* it's all out there in front of you. Seeing seems so effortless, so automatic, that we simply fail to recognize that vision is an incredibly complex—and still deeply mysterious—process. But consider, for a moment, what happens each time you glance at even the simplest scene. As my colleague Richard Gregory has pointed out, all you're given are two tiny upside-down two-dimensional images inside your eyeballs, but what you perceive is a single panoramic, right-side-up, three-dimensional world. How does this miraculous transformation come about?[2]

Many people cling to the misconception that seeing simply involves scanning an internal mental picture of some kind. For example, not long ago I was at a cocktail party and a young fellow asked me what I did for a living. When I told him that I was interested in how people see things—and how the brain is involved in perception—he looked perplexed. "What's there to study?" he asked.

"Well," I said, "what do you think happens in the brain when you look at an object?"

He glanced down at the glass of champagne in his hand. "Well, there is an upside-down image of this glass falling in my eyeball. The play of light and dark images activates photoreceptors on my retina, and the patterns are transmitted pixel by pixel through a cable—my optic nerve—and displayed on a screen in my brain. Isn't that how I see this glass of champagne? Of course, my brain would need to make the image upright again."

Though his knowledge of photoreceptors and and optics was impressive, his explanation—that there's a screen somewhere inside the brain where images are displayed—embodies a serious logical fallacy. For if you were to display an image of a champagne glass on an internal neural screen, you'd need another little person inside the brain to see that image. And that won't solve the problem either because you'd then need yet another, even tinier person inside his head to view that image, and so on and so forth, ad infinitum. You'd end up with an endless regress of eyes, images and little people without really solving the problem of perception.

So the first step in understanding perception is to get rid of the idea of images in the brain and to begin thinking about symbolic descriptions of objects and events in the external world. A good example of a symbolic description is a written paragraph like the ones on this page. If you had to convey to a friend in China what your apartment looks like, you wouldn't have to teletransport it to China. All you'd have to do would be to write a letter describing your apartment. Yet the actual squiggles of ink—the words and paragraphs in the letter—bear no physical resemblance to your bedroom. The letter is a symbolic description of your bedroom.

What is meant by a symbolic description in the brain? Not squiggles of ink, of course, but the language of nerve impulses. The human brain contains multiple areas for processing images, each of which is composed of an intricate network of neurons that is specialized for extracting certain types of information from the image. Any object evokes a pattern of activity—unique for each object—among a subset of these areas. For example, when you look at a pencil, a book or a face, a different pattern of nerve activity is elicited in each case, "informing" higher brain centers about what you are looking at. The patterns of activity symbolize or represent visual objects in much the same way that the squiggles of ink on the paper symbolize or represent your bedroom. As scientists trying

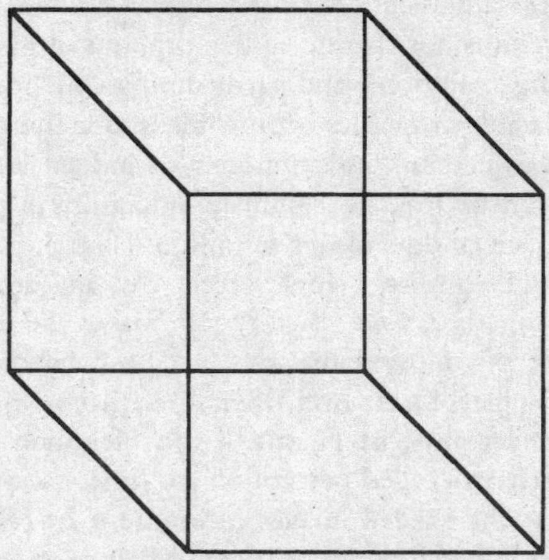

Figure 4.1 *A Necker cube. Notice that this skeleton drawing of a cube can be seen in one of two different ways—either pointing upward and to the left or downward and to the right. The perception can change even when the image on your retina is constant.*

to understand visual processes, our goal is to decipher the code used by the brain to create these symbolic descriptions, much as a cryptographer tries to crack an alien script.

Thus perception involves much more than replicating an image in your brain. If vision were simply a faithful copy of reality in the same way that a photograph captures a scene, then your perception should always remain constant if the retinal image is held constant. But this is not the case. Your perceptions can change radically even when the image on your retina stays the same. A striking example was discovered in 1832 by the Swiss crystallographer L. A. Necker. One day he was looking through a microscope at a cuboid crystal and suddenly the thing flipped on him. Each time he looked, it seemed to change the way it was facing—a physical impossibility. Necker was puzzled and wondered whether something inside his own head was flipping rather than the crystal itself. To test this strange notion, he made a simple line drawing of the crystal, and lo and behold, it, too, flipped (Figure 4.1). You can see it pointing up or down, depending on how your brain interprets the image, even though the image remains constant on your retina, not changing at all. Thus every act of perception, even something as simple as viewing a drawing of a cube, involves an act of judgment by the brain.

In making these judgments, the brain takes advantage of the fact that the world we live in is not chaotic and amorphous; it has stable physical properties. During evolution—and partly during childhood as a result of learning—these stable properties became incorporated into the visual areas of the brain as certain "assumptions" or hidden knowledge about the world that can be used to eliminate ambiguity in perception. For example, when a set of dots moves in unison—like the spots on a leopard—they usually belong to a single object. So, any time you see a set of dots moving together, your visual system makes the reasonable inference that they're not moving like this just by coincidence—that they probably are a single object. And, therefore, that's what you see. No wonder the German physicist Hermann von Helmholtz (the founding father of visual science) called perception an "unconscious inference."[3]

Take a look at the shaded images in Figure 4.2. These are just flat shaded disks, but you will notice that about half of them look like eggs bulging out at you, and the other half, randomly interspersed, look like hollow cavities. If you inspect them carefully, you'll notice that the ones that are light on top appear to bulge out at you, whereas the ones that are dark on top look like cavities. If you turn the page upside down, you'll see that they all reverse. The bulges become cavities and vice versa. The reason is that, in interpreting the shapes of shaded images, your visual system has a built-in assumption that the sun is shining from above, and that, in the real world, a convex object bulging toward you would be illuminated on the top whereas a cavity would receive light at the bottom. Given that we evolved on a planet with a single sun that usually shines from on high, this is a reasonable assumption.[4] Sure, it's sometimes on the horizon, but statistically speaking the sunlight usually comes from above and certainly never from below.

Not long ago, I was pleasantly surprised to find that Charles Darwin had been aware of this principle. The tail feathers of the argus pheasant have striking gray disk-shaped markings that look very much like those you see in Figure 4.3; they are, however, shaded left to right instead of up and down. Darwin realized that the bird might be using this as a sexual "come hither" in its courtship ritual, the striking metallic-looking disks on the feathers being the avian equivalent of jewelry. But if so, why was the shading left to right instead of up and down? Darwin conjectured correctly that perhaps during courtship the feathers stick up, and indeed this is precisely what happens, illustrating a striking harmony in the birds' visual system between its courtship ritual and the direction of sunlight.

Even more compelling evidence of the existence of all these extraor-

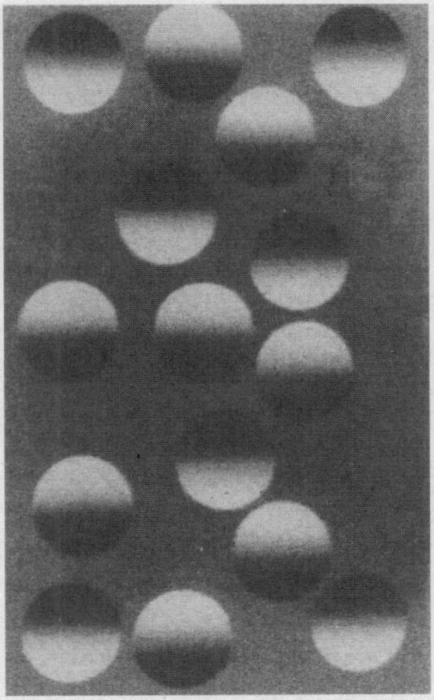

Figure 4.2 *A mixture of eggs and cavities. The shaded disks are all identical except that half of them are light on top and the rest are dark on top. The ones that are light on top are always seen as eggs bulging out from the paper, whereas the ones that are dark on top are seen as cavities. This is because the visual areas in your brain have a built-in sense that the sun is shining from above. If that were true, then only bulges (eggs) would be light on top and concavities would be light below.*

If you turn the page upside down the eggs will transform themselves into cavities and cavities into eggs. Adapted from Ramachandran, 1988a.

dinarily sophisticated processes in vision comes from neurology—from patients like Diane and others like her who have suffered highly selective visual deficits. If vision simply involves displaying an image on a neural screen, then in the case of neural damage, you would expect bits and pieces of the scene—or the whole scene—to be missing, depending on the extent of damage. But the defects are usually far more subtle than that. To understand what is really going on in the brains of these patients and why they suffer such peculiar problems, we need to look more closely at the anatomical pathways concerned with vision.

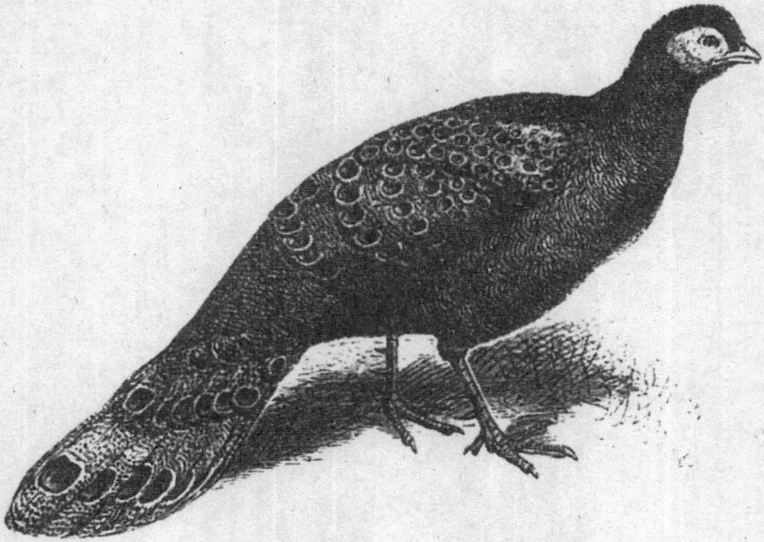

Figure 4.3 *The tail feathers of the argus pheasant have prominent disklike markings ordinarily shaded left to right instead of top to bottom. Charles Darwin pointed out that when the bird goes through its courtship ritual, the tail points up. The disks then are light on top—making them bulge out prominently like the eggs in Figure 4.2. This may be the closest thing to the avian equivalent of jewelry.* From *The Descent of Man* by Charles Darwin (1871), John Murray, London.

When I was a student, I was taught that messages from my eyeballs go through the optic nerve to the visual cortex at the back of my brain (to an area called the primary visual cortex) and that this is where seeing takes place. There is a point-to-point map of the retina in this part of the brain—each point in space seen by the eye has a corresponding point in this map. This mapping process was originally deduced from the fact that when people sustain damage to the primary visual cortex—say, a bullet passes through one small area—they get a corresponding hole or blind spot in their visual field. Moreover, because of some quirk in our evolutionary history, each side of your brain sees the opposite half of the world (Figure 4.4). If you look straight ahead, the entire world on your left is mapped onto your right visual cortex and the world to the right of your center of gaze is mapped onto your left visual cortex.[5]

But the mere existence of this map does not explain seeing, for as I noted earlier, there is no little man inside watching what is displayed on

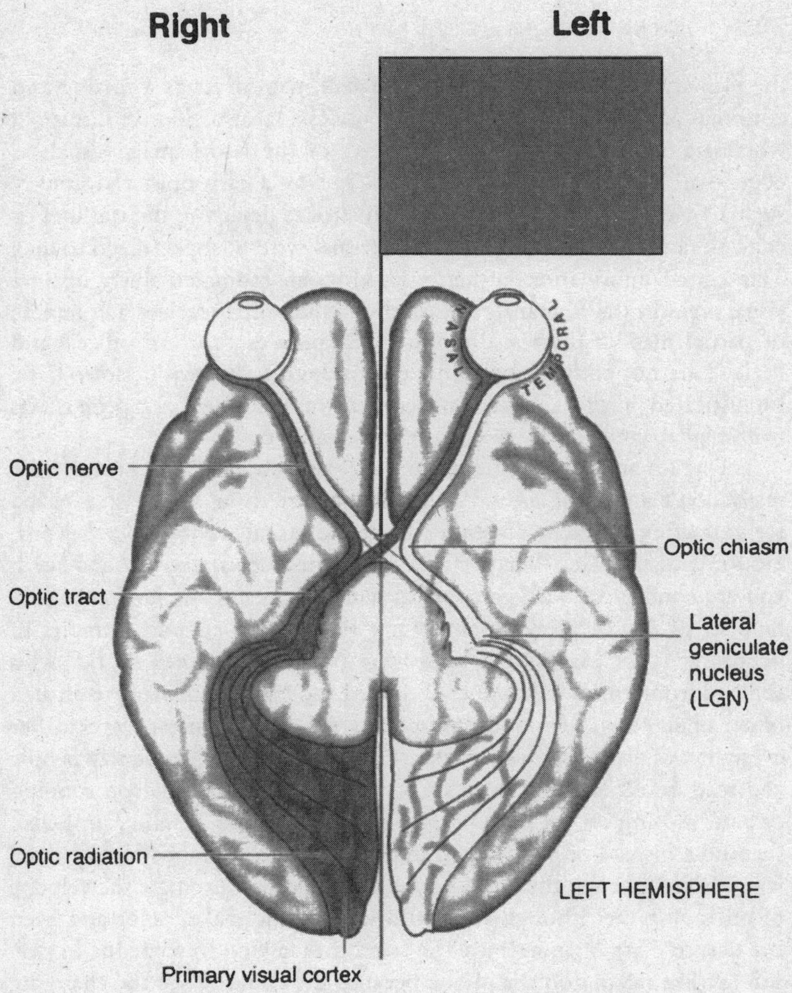

Figure 4.4 *Bottom of the human brain viewed from below. Notice the curious arrangement of fibers going from the retina to the visual cortex. A visual image in the left visual field (dark gray) falls on the right side of the right eye's retina as well as the right side of the left eye's retina. The outer (temporal) fibers from the right eye (dark gray) go then to the same right (visual) cortex without crossing at the optic chiasm. The inner (nasal) fibers of the left eye (dark gray) cross at the chiasm and go to the right visual cortex as well. So the right visual cortex "sees" the left side of the world.*

Because there is a systematic map of the retina in the visual cortex, a "hole" in the visual cortex will cause a corresponding blind spot (or scotoma) in the visual field. If the right visual cortex is completely removed, the patient will be completely blind in the left side of the world. Redrawn from S. Zeki, *A Vision of the Brain*, 1993. Reproduced with permission from Blackwell (Oxford).

the primary visual cortex. Instead, this first map serves as a sorting and editorial office where redundant or useless information is discarded wholesale and certain defining attributes of the visual image—such as edges—are strongly emphasized. (This is why a cartoonist can convey such a vivid picture with just a few pen strokes depicting the outlines or edge alone; he's mimicking what your visual system is specialized to do.) This edited information is then relayed to an estimated thirty distinct visual areas in the human brain, each of which thus receives a complete or partial map of the visual world. (The phrases "sorting office" and "relay" are not entirely appropriate since these early areas perform fairly sophisticated image analyses and contain massive feedback projections from higher visual areas. We'll take these up later.)

This raises an interesting question. Why do we need thirty areas?[6] We really don't know the answer, but they appear to be highly specialized for extracting different attributes from the visual scene—color, depth, motion and the like. When one or more areas are selectively damaged, you are confronted with paradoxical mental states of the kind seen in a number of neurological patients. One of the most famous examples in neurology is the case of a Swiss woman (whom I shall call Ingrid) who suffered from "motion blindness." Ingrid had bilateral damage to an area of her brain called the middle temporal (MT) area. In most respects, her eyesight was normal; she could name shapes of objects, recognize people and read books with no trouble. But if she looked at a person running or a car moving on the highway, she saw a succession of static, strobelike snapshots instead of the smooth impression of continuous motion. She was terrified to cross the street because she couldn't estimate the velocity of oncoming cars, though she could identify the make, color and even the license plate of any vehicle. She said that talking to someone in person felt like talking on the phone because she couldn't see the changing facial expressions associated with normal conversation. Even pouring a cup of coffee was an ordeal because the liquid would inevitably overflow and spill onto the floor. She never knew when to slow down, changing the angle of the coffeepot, because she couldn't estimate how fast the liquid was rising in the cup. All of these abilities ordinarily seem so effortless to you and me that we take them for granted. It's only when something goes wrong, as when this motion area is damaged, that we begin to realize how sophisticated vision really is.

Another example involves color vision. When patients suffer bilateral damage to an area called V4, they become completely color-blind (this is different from the more common from of congenital color blindness that arises because color-sensitive pigments in the eye are deficient). In his book *An Anthropologist on Mars*, Oliver Sacks describes an artist who went home one evening after suffering a stroke so small he didn't notice it at the time. But when he walked into his house, all his color paintings suddenly looked as if they had been done in black and white. In fact, the whole world was black and white and soon he realized that the paintings had not changed, but rather something had happened to him. When he looked at his wife, her face was a muddy gray color—he claimed she looked like a rat.

So that covers two of the thirty areas—MT and V4—but what about all the rest? Undoubtedly they're doing something equally important, but we have no clear ideas yet of what their functions might be. Yet despite the bewildering complexity of all these areas, the visual system appears to have a relatively simple overall organization. Messages from the eyeballs go through the optic nerve and immediately bifurcate along two pathways—one phylogenetically old and a second, newer pathway that is most highly developed in primates, including humans. Moreover, there appears to be a clear division of labor between these two systems.

The "older" pathway goes from the eye straight down to a structure called the superior colliculus in the brain stem, and from there it eventually gets to higher cortical areas especially in the parietal lobes. The "newer" pathway, on the other hand, travels from the eyes to a cluster of cells called the lateral geniculate nucleus, which is a relay station en route to the primary visual cortex (Figure 4.5). From there, visual information is transmitted to the thirty or so other visual areas for further processing.

Why do we have an old pathway and a new pathway?

One possibility is that the older pathway has been preserved as a sort of early warning system and is concerned with what is sometimes called "orienting behavior." For example, if a large looming object comes at me from the left, this older pathway tells me where the object is, enabling me to swivel my eyeballs and turn my head and body to look at it. This is a primitive reflex that brings potentially important events into my fovea, the high-acuity central region of my eyes.

At this stage I begin to deploy the phylogenetically newer system to determine what the object is, for only then can I decide how to respond to it. Should I grab it, dodge it, flee from it, eat it, fight it or make love to it? Damage to this second pathway—particularly in the primary visual cortex—leads to blindness in the conventional sense. It is most commonly brought on by a stroke—a leakage or blood clot in one of the

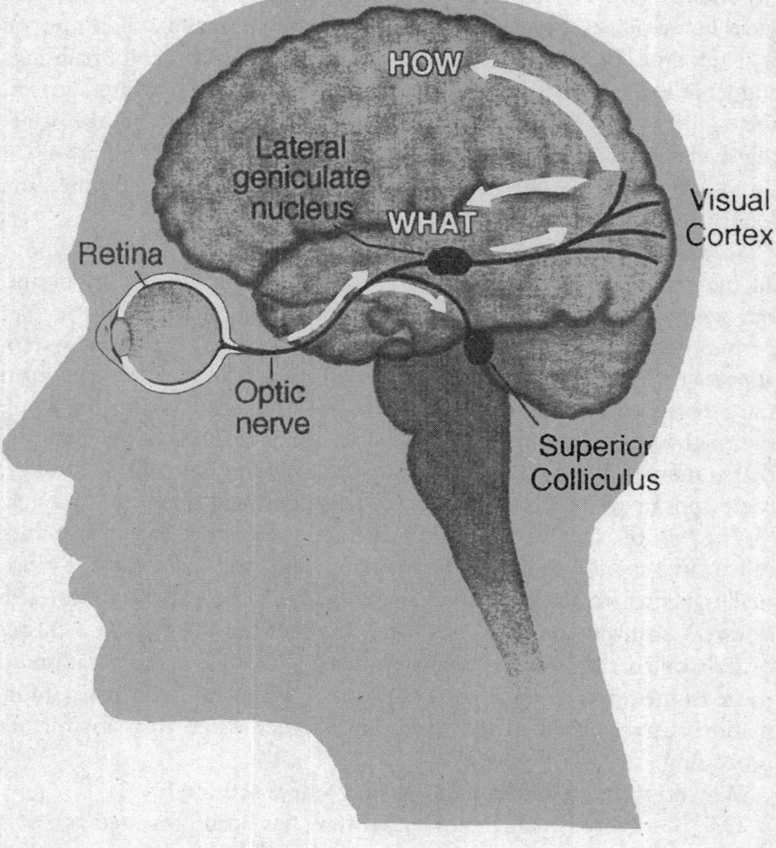

Figure 4.5 *The anatomical organization of the visual pathways. Schematic diagram of the left hemisphere viewed from the left side.*

The fibers from the eyeball diverge in two parallel "streams": a new pathway that goes to the lateral geniculate nucleus (shown here on the surface for clarity, though it is actually inside the thalamus, not the temporal lobe) and an old pathway that goes to the superior colliculus in the brain stem.

The "new" pathway then goes to the visual cortex and diverges again (after a couple of relays) into two pathways (white arrows)—a "how" pathway in the parietal lobes that is concerned with grasping, navigation and other spatial functions, and the second, "what" pathway in the temporal lobes concerned with recognizing objects. These two pathways were discovered by Leslie Ungerleider and Mortimer Mischkin of the National Institutes of Health. The two pathways are shown by white arrows.

main blood vessels supplying the brain. If the vessel happens to be a cerebral artery in the back of the brain, damage can occur in either the left or the right side of the primary visual cortex. When the right primary cortex is damaged, the person is blind in the left visual field, and if the left primary cortex is damaged, the right visual field is obliterated. This kind of blindness, called hemianopia, has been known about for a long time.

But it, too, holds surprises. Dr. Larry Weiskrantz, a scientist working at Oxford University in England, did a very simple experiment that stunned experts on vision.[7] His patient (known as D.B., whom I will call Drew) had an abnormal clump of blood vessels surgically removed from his brain along with some normal brain tissue in the same vicinity. Since the malformed clump was located in the right primary visual cortex, the procedure rendered Drew completely blind to the left half of the world. It did not matter whether he used his left eye or right eye—if he looked straight ahead, he could not see anything on the left side of the world. In other words, although he could see out of both eyes, neither eye could see its own left visual field.

After the surgery Drew's ophthalmologist, Dr. Mike Sanders, asked him to gaze straight ahead at a small fixation spot mounted in the center of a device that looks like an enormous translucent Ping-Pong ball. Drew's entire visual field was filled with a homogeneous background. Next, Dr. Sanders flashed spots of light onto different parts of the curved screen mounted on the inside of a ball and asked Drew whether he could see them. Each time a spot fell into his good visual field, he'd say, "Yes, yes, yes," but when the spot fell into his blind region he would say nothing. He didn't see it.

So far so good. Dr. Sanders and Dr. Weiskrantz then noticed something very odd. Drew was obviously blind in the left visual field, but if the experimenter put his hand in that region Drew reached out for it accurately! The two researchers asked Drew to stare straight ahead and put movable markers on the wall to the left of where he was looking, and again he was able to point to the markers, although he insisted that he did not actually "see" them. They held up a stick, in either a vertical or a horizontal position, in his blind field and asked him to guess which way the stick was oriented. Drew had no problem with this task, although he said again that he could not see the stick. After one such long series of "guesses," when he made virtually no errors, he was asked, "Do you know how well you have done?"

"No," he replied, "I didn't—because I couldn't see anything; I couldn't see a darn thing."

"Can you say how you guessed—what it was that allowed you to say whether it was vertical or horizontal?"

"No, I could not because I did not see anything; I just don't know."

Finally, he was asked, "So you really did not know you were getting them right?"

"No," Drew replied, with an air of incredulity.

Dr. Weiskrantz and his colleagues gave this phenomenon an oxymoronic name—"blindsight"—and went on to document it in other patients. The discovery is so surprising, however, that many people still don't accept that the phenomenon is possible.

Dr. Weiskrantz questioned Drew repeatedly about his "vision" in his blind left field, and most of the time Drew said that he saw nothing at all. If pressed, he might occasionally say that he had a "feeling" that a stimulus was approaching or receding or was "smooth" or "jagged." But Drew always stressed that he saw nothing in the sense of "seeing"; that he was typically guessing and that he was at a loss for words to describe any conscious perception. The researchers were convinced that Drew was a reliable and honest reporter, and when test objects fell near the cusp of his good visual field, he always said so promptly.

Without invoking extrasensory perception, how do you account for blindsight—a person's pointing to or correctly guessing the presence of an object that he cannot consciously perceive? Dr. Weiskrantz suggested that the paradox is resolved when you consider the division of labor between the two visual pathways that we considered earlier. In particular, even though Drew had lost his primary visual cortex—rendering him blind—his phylogenetically primitive "orienting" pathway was still intact, and perhaps it mediates blindsight. In other words, the spot of light in the blind region—even though it fails to activate the newer pathway, which is damaged—gets transmitted through the superior colliculus to higher brain centers such as the parietal lobes, guiding Drew's arm toward the "invisible" spot. This daring interpretation carries with it an extraordinary implication—that only the new pathway is capable of conscious awareness ("I see this"), whereas the old pathway can use visual input for all kinds of behavior, even though the person is completely unaware of what is going on. Does it follow, then, that consciousness is a special property of the evolutionarily more recent visual cortex pathway? If so, why does this pathway have privileged access to the mind? These are questions we'll consider in the last chapter.

•

What we have considered so far is the simple version of the perception story, but in fact the picture is a bit more complicated. It turns out that information in the "new" pathway—the one containing the primary visual cortex that purportedly leads to conscious experience (and is completely damaged in Drew)—once again diverges into two distinct streams. One is the "where" pathway, which terminates in the parietal lobe (on the sides of your brain above the ears); the other, sometimes called the "what" pathway, goes to the temporal lobe (underlying the temples). And it looks as though each of these two systems is also specialized for a distinct subset of visual functions.

Actually the term "where" pathway is a little misleading because this system specializes in not just "where"—in assigning spatial location to objects—but in all aspects of spatial vision: the ability of organisms to walk around the world, negotiate uneven terrain and avoid bumping into objects or falling into black pits. It probably enables an animal to determine the direction of a moving target, to judge the distance of approaching or receding objects and to dodge a missile. If you are a primate, it helps you reach out and grab an object with your fingers and thumb. Indeed, the Canadian psychologist Mel Goodale has suggested that this system should really be called the "vision for action pathway" or the "how pathway" since it seems to be mainly concerned with visually guided movements. (From here on I will call it the "how" pathway.)

Now you may scratch your head and say, My God, what's left? What remains is your ability to identify the object; hence the second pathway is called the "what" pathway. The fact that the majority of your thirty visual areas are in fact located in this system gives you some idea of its importance. Is this thing you are looking at a fox, a pear or a rose? Is this face an enemy, friend or mate? Is it Drew or Diane? What are the semantic and emotional attributes of this thing? Do I care about it? Am I afraid of it? Three researchers, Ed Rolls, Charlie Gross and David Perrett, have found that if you put an electrode into a monkey's brain to monitor the activity of cells in this system, there is a particular region where you find so-called face cells—each neuron fires only in response to the photograph of a particular face. Thus one cell may respond to the dominant male in the monkey troop, another to the monkey's mate, another to the surrogate alpha male—that is, to the human experimenter. This does not mean that a single cell is somehow responsible for the complete process of recognizing faces; the recognition probably relies on a network involving thousands of synapses. Nevertheless, face cells exist as a critical part of the network of cells involved in the recognition of faces and other objects. Once these cells are activated, their message is somehow relayed to higher areas in the temporal lobes concerned with "semantics"—all your memories and knowledge of that person. Where did we meet before? What is his name? When is the last time I saw this person? What was he doing? Added to this, finally, are all the emotions that the person's face evokes.

To illustrate further what these two streams—the what and how pathways—are doing in the brain, I'd like you to consider a thought experiment. In real life, people have strokes, head injuries or other brain accidents and may lose various chunks of the how and what streams. But nature is messy and rarely are losses confined exclusively to one stream and not the other. So let's assume that one day you wake up and your what pathway has been selectively obliterated (perhaps a malicious doctor entered in the night, knocked you out and removed both your temporal lobes). I'd venture to predict that when you woke up the entire world would look like a gallery of abstract sculpture, a Martian art gallery perhaps. No object you looked at would be recognizable or evoke emotions or associations with anything else. You'd "see" these objects, their boundaries and shapes, and you could reach out and grab them, trace them with your finger and catch one if I threw it at you. In other words, your how pathway would be functional. But you'd have no inkling as to what these objects were. It's a moot point as to whether you'd be "conscious" of any of them, for one could argue that the term consciousness doesn't mean anything unless you recognize the emotional significance and semantic associations of what you are looking at.

Two scientists, Heinrich Klüver and Paul Bucy at the University of Chicago, have actually carried out an experiment like this on monkeys by surgically removing their temporal lobes containing the what pathway. The animals can walk around and avoid bumping into cage walls—because their how pathway is intact—but if they are presented with a lit cigarette or razor blade, they will likely stuff it into their mouths and start chewing. Male monkeys will mount any other animal including chickens, cats or even human experimenters. They are not hypersexual, just indiscriminate. They have great difficulty in knowing what prey is, what a mate is, what food is and in general what the significance of any object might be.

Are there any human patients who have similar deficits? On rare occasions a person will sustain widespread damage to both temporal lobes and develop a cluster of symptoms similar to what we now call the Klüver-Bucy syndrome. Like the monkeys, they may put anything and everything into their mouths (much as babies do) and display indiscriminate sexual behavior, such as making lewd overtures to physicians or to patients in adjacent wheelchairs.

Such extremes of behavior have been known for a long time and lend credibility to the idea that there is a clear division of labor between these two systems—and that brings us back to Diane. Though her deficit is not quite so extreme, Diane also had dissociation between her what and how vision systems. She couldn't tell the difference between a horizontal and a vertical pencil or a slit because her what pathway had been selectively obliterated. But since her how pathway was still intact (as indeed was her evolutionarily older "orienting behavior" pathway), she was able to reach out and grab a pencil accurately or rotate a letter by the correct angle to post it into a slot that she could not see.

To make this distinction even more clear, Dr. Milner performed another ingenious experiment. After all, posting letters is a relatively easy, habitual act and he wanted to see how sophisticated the zombie's manipulative abilities really were. Placing two blocks of wood in front of Diane, a large and a small one, Dr. Milner asked her which was bigger. He found, not surprisingly, that she performed at chance level. But when he asked her to reach out and grab the object, once again her arm went unerringly toward it with thumb and index finger moving apart by the exact distance appropriate for that object. All this was verified by videotaping the approaching arm and conducting a frame-by-frame analysis of the tape. Again, it was as though there were an unconscious "zombie" inside Diane carrying out complicated computations that allowed her to move her hand and fingers correctly, whether she was posting a letter or simply grabbing objects of different sizes. The "zombie" corresponded to the how pathway, which was still largely intact, and the "person" corresponded to the what pathway, which was badly damaged. Diane can interact with the world spatially, but she is not consciously aware of the shapes, locations and sizes of most objects around her. She now lives in a country home, where she keeps a large herb garden, entertains friends and carries on an active, though protected, life.

But there's another twist to the tale, for even Diane's what pathway was not completely damaged. Although she couldn't recognize the shapes of objects—a line drawing of a banana would not look different from a drawing of a pumpkin—as I noted at the beginning of this chapter, she had no problem distinguishing colors or visual textures. She was good at "stuff" rather than "things" and knew a banana from a yellow zucchini by their visual textures. The reason for this might be that even within the areas constituting the what pathway, there are finer subdivisions concerned with color, texture and form, and the "color" and "texture" cells might be more resistant to carbon monoxide poisoning than the "form" cells. The evidence for the existence of such cells in the primate brain is still fiercely debated by physiologists, but the highly selective deficits and preserved abilities of Diane give us additional clues that exquisitely specialized regions of this sort do indeed exist in the human brain. If you're looking for evidence of modularity in the brain (and ammunition against the holist view), the visual areas are the best place to look.

Now let's go back to the thought experiment I mentioned earlier and turn it around. What might happen if the evil doctor removed your how pathway (the one that guides your actions) and left your what system intact? You'd expect to see a person who couldn't get her bearings, who would have great difficulty looking toward objects of interest, reaching out and grabbing things or pointing to interesting targets in her visual field. Something like this does happen in a curious disorder called Balint's syndrome, in which there is bilateral damage to the parietal lobes. In a kind of tunnel vision, the patient's eyes stay focused on any small object that happens to be in her foveal vision (the high-acuity region of the eye), but she completely ignores all other objects in the vicinity. If you ask her to point to a small target in her visual field, she'll very likely miss the mark by a wide margin—sometimes by a foot or more. But once she captures the target with her two foveas, she can recognize it effortlessly because her intact what pathway is engaged in full gear.

•

The discovery of multiple visual areas and the division of labor between the two pathways is a landmark achievement in neuroscience, but it barely begins to scratch the surface of the problem of understanding vision. If I toss a red ball at you, several far-flung visual areas in your brain are activated simultaneously, but what you see is a single unified picture of the ball. Does this unification come about because there is some later place in the brain where all this information is put together—what the philosopher Dan Dennett pejoratively calls a "Cartesian theatre"?[8] Or are there connections between these areas so that their simultaneous activation leads directly to a sort of synchronized firing pattern that in turn creates perceptual unity? This question, the so-called binding problem, is one of the many unsolved riddles in neuroscience. Indeed, the problem is so mysterious that there are philosophers who argue it is not even a legitimate scientific question. The problem arises, they argue, from peculiarities in our use of language or from logically flawed assumptions about the visual process.

Despite this reservation, the discovery of the how and what pathways and of multiple visual areas has generated a great deal of excitement, especially among young researchers entering the field.[9] It's now possible not only to record the activity of individual cells but also to watch many of these areas light up in the living human brain as a person views a scene—whether it's something simple like a white square on a black background or something more complex like a smiling face. Furthermore, the existence of regions that are highly specialized for a specific task gives us an experimental lever for approaching the question posed at the beginning of this chapter: How does the activity of neurons give rise to perceptual experience? For instance, we now know that cones in the retina first send their outputs to clusters of color-sensitive cells in the primary visual cortex fancifully called blobs and thin stripes (in the adjacent area 18) and from there to V4 (recall the man who mistook his wife for a hat) and that the processing of color becomes increasingly sophisticated as you go along this sequence. Taking advantage of the sequence and of all this detailed anatomical knowledge, we can ask, How does this specific chain of events result in our experience of color? Or, recalling Ingrid, who was motion blind, we can ask, How does the circuitry in the middle temporal area enable us to see motion?

As the British immunologist Peter Medawar has noted, science is the "art of the soluble," and one could argue that the discovery of multiple specialized areas in vision makes the problem of vision soluble, at least in the foreseeable future. To his famous dictum, I would add that in science one is often forced to choose between providing precise answers to piffling questions (how many cones are there in a human eye) or vague answers to big questions (what is the self), but every now and then you come up with a precise answer to a big question (such as the link between deoxyribonucleic acid [DNA] and heredity) and you hit the jackpot. It appears that vision is one of the areas in neuroscience where sooner or later we will have precise answers to big questions, but only time will tell.

In the meantime, we've learned a great deal about the structure and function of the visual pathways from patients like Diane, Drew and Ingrid. For example, even though Diane's symptoms initially seemed out-

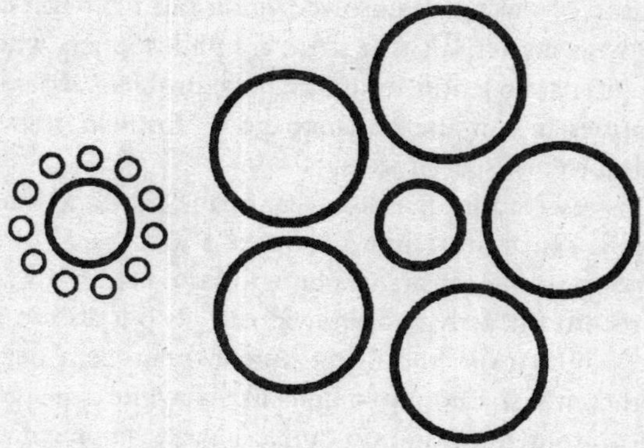

Figure 4.6 *The size-contrast illusion. The two central medium-sized disks are physically identical in size. Yet the one surrounded by the large disks looks smaller than the one surrounded by the little ones. When a normal person reaches out to grab the central disk, his/her fingers move exactly the same distance apart for either of them—even though they look different in size. The zombie—or the "how" pathway in the parietal lobes—is apparently not fooled by the illusion.*

landish, we can now begin to explain them in terms of what we learned about the two visual pathways—the what pathway and the how pathway. It's important to keep reminding ourselves, though, that the zombie exists not only in Diane but in all of us. Indeed, the purpose of our whole enterprise is not simply to explain Diane's deficits but to understand how your brain and my brain work. Since these two pathways normally work in unison, in a smooth coordinated fashion, it's hard to discern their separate contributions. But it's possible to devise experiments to show that they do exist and work to some extent independently even in you and me. To illustrate this, I'll describe one last experiment.

The experiment was carried out by Dr. Salvatore Aglioti,[10] who took advantage of a well-known visual illusion (Figure 4.6) involving two circular disks side by side, identical in size. One of them is surrounded by six tiny disks and the other by six giant disks. To most eyes, the two central disks do not look the same size. The one surrounded by big disks looks about 30 percent smaller than the one with small disks—an illusion called size contrast. It is one of many illusions used by Gestalt psychologists to show that perception is always relative—never absolute—always dependent on the surrounding context.

Instead of using a line drawing to get this effect, Dr. Aglioti set two medium-sized dominoes on a table. One was surrounded with larger dominoes and the second with smaller dominoes—just like the disks. As with the disks, when a student looked at the two central dominoes, one looked obviously smaller than the other. But the astonishing thing is that when he was asked to reach out and pick up one of the two central dominoes, his fingers moved the right distance apart as his hand approached the domino. A frame-by-frame analysis of his hand revealed that the fingers moved apart exactly the same amount for each of the two central dominoes, even though to his eyes (and to yours) one looks 30 percent bigger. Obviously, his hands knew something that his eyes did not, and this implies that the illusion is only "seen" by the object stream in his brain. The how stream—the zombie—is not fooled for a second, and so "it" (or he) was able to reach out and correctly grasp the domino.

This little experiment may have interesting implications for day-to-day activities and athletics. Marksmen say that if you focus too much on a rifle target, you will not hit the bull's-eye; you need to "let go" before you shoot. Most sports rely heavily on spatial orientation. A quarterback throws the ball toward an empty spot on the field, calculating where the receiver will be if he is not tackled. An outfielder starts running the moment he hears the crack of a baseball coming into contact with a bat, as his how pathway in the parietal lobe calculates the expected destination of the ball given this auditory input. Basketball players can even close their eyes and toss a ball into the basket if they stand on the same spot on the court each time. Indeed, in sports as in many aspects of life, it may pay to "release your zombie" and let it do its thing. There's no direct evidence that all of this mainly involves your zombie—the how pathway—but the idea can be tested with brain imaging techniques.

My eight-year-old son, Mani, once asked me whether maybe the zombie is smarter than we think, a fact that is celebrated in both ancient martial arts and modern movies like *Star Wars*. When young Luke Skywalker is struggling with his conscious awareness, Yoda advises, "Use the force. Feel it. Yes," and "No. Try not! Do or do not. There is no try." Was he referring to a zombie?

I answered, "No," but later began to have second thoughts. For in truth, we know so little about the brain that even a child's questions should be seriously entertained.

The most obvious fact about existence is your sense of being a single, unified self "in charge" of your destiny; so obvious, in fact, that you rarely pause to think about it. And yet Dr. Aglioti's experiment and observations on patients like Diane suggest that there is in fact another being inside you that goes about his or her business without your knowledge or awareness. And, as it turns out, there is not just one such zombie but a multitude of them inhabiting your brain. If so, your concept of a single "I" or "self" inhabiting your brain may be simply an illusion[11]—albeit one that allows you to organize your life more efficiently, gives you a sense of purpose and helps you interact with others. This idea will be a recurring theme in the rest of this book.

CHAPTER 5

The Secret Life of James Thurber

Is this a dagger which I see before me,
The handle toward my hand?
Come, let me clutch
  thee:
I have thee not, and yet I see thee still.
Art thou not fatal vision, sensible
To feeling as to sight? or art thou but
A dagger of the mind, a false creation,
Proceeding from the heat oppressed brain?

—William Shakespeare

When James Thurber was six years old, a toy arrow shot accidentally at him by his brother impaled his right eye and he never saw out of that eye again. Though the loss was tragic, it was not devastating; like most one-eyed people he was able to navigate the world successfully. But much to his distress, in the years after the accident his left eye also started progressively deteriorating so that by the time he was thirty-five he had become completely blind. Yet ironically, far from being an impediment, Thurber's blindness somehow stimulated his imagination so that his visual field, instead of being dark and dreary, was filled with hallucinations, creating for him a fantastic world of surrealistic images. Thurber fans adore "The Secret Life of Walter Mitty," wherein Mitty, a milquetoast of a man, bounces back and forth between flights of fantasy and reality as if to mimic Thurber's own curious predicament. Even the whimsical

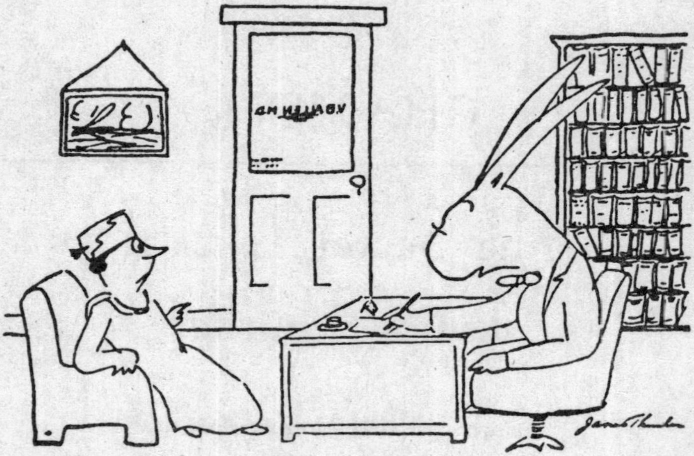

"You said a moment ago that everybody you look at seems to be a rabbit. Now just what do you mean by that, Mrs. Sprague?"

Figure 5.1 *One of James Thurber's well-known cartoons that appeared in* The New Yorker. *Could his visual hallucinations have been a source of inspiration for some of these cartoons?* By James Thurber, 1937, from *The New Yorker Collection.* All rights reserved.

cartoons for which he was so famous were probably provoked by his visual handicap (Figure 5.1).[1]

Thus James Thurber was not blind in the sense that you or I might think of blindness—a falling darkness like the blackest night sky, entirely devoid of moonlight and stars, or even a complete absence of vision—an unbearable void. For Thurber, blindness was brilliant, star-studded and sprinkled with pixie dust. He once wrote to his ophthalmologist:

> Years ago you told me about a nun of the middle centuries who confused her retinal disturbances with holy visitation, although she saw only about one tenth of the holy symbols I see. Mine have included a blue Hoover, golden sparks, melting purple blobs, a skein of spit, a dancing brown spot, snowflakes, saffron and light blue waves, and two eight balls, to say nothing of the corona, which used to halo street lamps and is now brilliantly discernible when a shaft of light breaks against a crystal bowl or a bright metal edge. This corona, usually triple, is like a chrysanthemum composed of thousands of radiating petals, each ten

> times as slender and each containing in order the colors of the prism. Man has devised no spectacle of light in any way similar to this sublime arrangement of colors or holy visitation.

Once, after Thurber's glasses shattered, he said, "I saw a Cuban flag flying over a national bank, I saw a gay old lady with a gray parasol walk right through the side of a truck, I saw a cat roll across a street in a small striped barrel. I saw bridges rise lazily into the air, like balloons."

Thurber knew how to use his visions creatively. "The daydreamer," he said, "must visualize the dream so vividly and insistently that it becomes, in effect, an actuality."

Upon seeing his whimsical cartoons and reading his prose, I realized that Thurber probably suffered from an extraordinary neurological condition called Charles Bonnet syndrome. Patients with this curious disorder usually have damage somewhere in their visual pathway—in the eye or in the brain—causing them to be either completely or partially blind. Yet paradoxically, like Thurber, they start experiencing the most vivid visual hallucinations as if to "replace" the reality that is missing from their lives. Unlike many other disorders you will encounter in this book, Charles Bonnet syndrome is extremely common worldwide and affects millions of people whose vision has become compromised by glaucoma, cataracts, macular degeneration or diabetic retinopathy. Many such patients develop Thurberesque hallucinations—yet oddly enough most physicians have never heard about the disorder.[2] One reason may be simply that people who have these symptoms are reluctant to mention them to anyone for fear of being labeled crazy. Who would believe that a blind person was seeing clowns and circus animals cavorting in her bedroom? When Grandma, sitting in her wheelchair in the nursing home, says, "What are all those water lilies doing on the floor?" her family is likely to think she's lost her mind.

If my diagnosis of Thurber's condition is correct, we must conclude that he wasn't just being metaphorical when he spoke of enhancing his creativity with his dreams and hallucinations; he really *did* experience all those haunting visions—a cat in a striped barrel did indeed cross his visual field, snowflakes danced and a lady walked through the side of the truck.

But the images that Thurber and other Charles Bonnet patients experience are very different from those that you or I could conjure up in our minds. If I asked you to describe the American flag or to tell me how many sides a cube has, you'd maybe shut your eyes to avoid distraction and conjure up a faint internal mental picture, which you'd then proceed to scan and describe. (People vary greatly in this ability; many undergraduates say that they can only visualize four sides on a cube.) But the Charles Bonnet hallucinations are much more vivid and the patient has no conscious control over them—they emerge completely unbidden, although like real objects they may disappear when the eyes are closed.

I was intrigued by these hallucinations because of the internal contradiction they represent. They seem so extraordinarily real to the patient—indeed some tell me that the images are more "real than reality" or that the colors are "supervivid"—and yet we know they are mere figments of the imagination. The study of this syndrome may thus allow us to explore that mysterious no-man's-land between seeing and knowing and to discover how the lamp of our imagination illuminates the prosaic images of the world. Or it may even help us investigate the more basic question of how and where in the brain we actually "see" things—how the complex cascade of events in the thirty-odd visual areas in my cortex enables me to perceive and comprehend the world.

•

What is visual imagination? Are the same parts of your brain active when you imagine an object—say, a cat—as when you look at it actually sitting in front of you? A decade ago, these might have been considered philosophical questions, but recently cognitive scientists have begun to probe these processes at the level of the brain itself and have come up with some surprising answers. It turns out that the human visual system has an astonishing ability to make educated guesses based on the fragmentary and evanescent images dancing in the eyeballs. Indeed, in the last chapter, I showed you many examples to illustrate that vision involves a great deal more than simply transmitting an image to a screen in the brain and that it is an active, constructive process. A specific manifestation of this is the brain's remarkable capacity for dealing with inexplicable gaps in the visual image—a process that is sometimes loosely referred to as "filling in." A rabbit viewed behind a picket fence, for instance, is not seen as a series of rabbit slices but as a single rabbit standing behind the vertical bars of the fence; your mind apparently fills in the missing rabbit segments. Even a glimpse of your cat's tail sticking out from underneath the sofa evokes the image of the whole cat; you certainly don't see a disembodied tail, gasp and panic or, like Lewis Carroll's Alice, wonder where the rest of the cat is. Actually, "filling in" occurs at several different stages of the visual process, and it's somewhat misleading to lump all of them together in one phrase. Even so, it's clear that the mind, like nature, abhors a vacuum and will apparently supply whatever information is required to complete the scene.

Migraine sufferers are well aware of this extraordinary phenomenon. When a blood vessel goes into a spasm, they temporarily lose a patch of visual cortex and this causes a corresponding blind region—a scotoma—in the visual field. (Recall there is a point-to-point map of the visual world in the visual field.) If a person having a migraine attack glances around the room and his scotoma happens to "fall" on a large clock or painting on the wall, the object will disappear completely. But instead of seeing an enormous void in its place, he sees a normal-looking wall with paint or wallpaper. The region corresponding to the missing object is simply covered with the same color of paint or wallpaper.

What does it actually feel like to have a scotoma? With most brain disorders you have to remain content with a clinical description, but you can get a clear sense of what is going on in migraine sufferers by simply examining your own blind spot. The existence of this natural blind spot of the eye was actually predicted by the seventeenth-century French scientist Edme Mariotte. While dissecting a human eye, Mariotte noticed the optic disk—the area of the retina where the optic nerve exits the eyeball. He realized that unlike other parts of the retina, the optic disk is not sensitive to light. Applying his knowledge of optics and eye anatomy, he deduced that every eye should be blind in a small portion of its visual field.

You can easily confirm Mariotte's conclusion by examining the illustration of a hatched disk on a light gray background (Figure 5.2). Close your right eye and hold this book about a foot away from your face and fixate your gaze on the little black dot on the page. Concentrate on the dot as you slowly move the page toward your left eye. At some critical distance, the hatched disk should fall within your natural blind spot and disappear completely![3] However, notice that when the disk disappears, you do not experience a big black hole or void in its place. You simply see this region as being "colored" by the same light gray background as the rest of the page—another striking example of filling in.[4]

You may be wondering why you've never noticed your blind spot before now. One reason is related to binocular vision, which you can test for yourself. After the hatched disk has disappeared, try opening the other eye and you will see that the disk pops back instantly into view. This happens because when both eyes are open the two blind spots don't

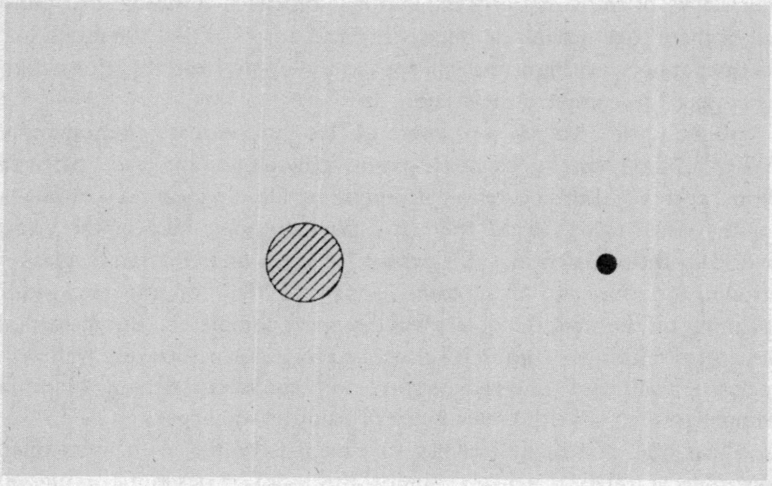

Figure 5.2 *Blind spot demonstration. Shut your right eye and look at the black dot on the right with your left eye. From about one and a half feet away, move the book slowly toward you. At a critical distance the circular hatched disk on the left will fall entirely on your blind spot and disappear completely. If you move the book closer still, the disk will reappear. You may need to "hunt" for the blind spot by moving the book to and fro several times until the disk disappears.*

Notice that when the disk disappears you don't see a dark void or hole in its place. The region is seen as being covered with the same light gray color as the background. This phenomenon is loosely referred to as "filling in."

overlap; the normal vision of your left eye compensates for the right eye's blind spot and vice versa. But the surprising thing is that even if you close one eye and glance around the room, you are still not aware of the blind spot unless you carefully look for it. Again, you don't notice the gap because your visual system obligingly fills in the missing information.[5]

But how sophisticated is this filling-in process? Are there clear limits as to what can be filled in and what cannot? And would answering this question give us hints about what type of neural brain machinery may be involved in allowing it to happen?

Bear in mind that the filling in is not just some odd quirk of the visual system that has evolved for the sole purpose of dealing with the blind spot. Rather, it appears to be a manifestation of a very general ability to construct surfaces and bridge gaps that might be otherwise distracting in an image—the same ability, in fact, that allows you to see a rabbit behind a picket fence as a complete rabbit, not a sliced-up one. In our natural blind spot we have an especially obvious example of filling in—one that provides us with a valuable experimental opportunity to examine the "laws" that govern the process. Indeed, you can actually discover these laws and explore the limits of filling in by playing with your own blind spot. (To me, this is one reason the study of vision is so exciting. It allows anyone armed with a sheet of paper, a pencil and some curiosity to peer into the inner workings of his own brain.)

First, you can decapitate your friends and enemies, using your natural blind spot. Standing about ten feet away from the person, close your right eye and look at his head with your left eye. Now, slowly start moving your left eye horizontally toward the right, away from the person's head, until your blind spot falls directly on his head. At this critical distance, his head should disappear. When King Charles II, the "science king" who founded the Royal Society, heard about the blind spot, he took great delight in walking around in his court decapitating his ladies in waiting or beheading criminals with his blind spot before they were actually guillotined. I must confess I sometimes sit in faculty meetings and enjoy decapitating our departmental chairman.

Next we can ask what will happen if you run a vertical black line through your blind spot. Again, close your right eye and stare at the black spot to the right of the picture (Figure 5.3) with your left eye. Then move the page gradually to and fro until the small hatched square on the center of the vertical line falls exactly inside your left eye's blind spot. (The hatched square should now disappear.) Since no information about this central portion of the line—falling on the blind spot—is available to the eye or the brain, do you perceive two short vertical lines with a gap in the middle, or do you "fill in" and see one continuous line? The answer is clear. You will always see a continuous vertical line. Perhaps neurons in your visual system are making a statistical estimate; they "realize" that it is extremely unlikely that two different lines are precisely lined up on either side of the blind spot in this manner simply by chance. So they "signal" to higher brain centers that this is probably a single continuous line. Everything that the visual system does is based on such educated guesswork.

But what if you try to confound the visual system by presenting internally contradictory evidence—for instance, by making the two line segments differ in some way? What if one line is black and the other is white (shown on a gray background)? Does your visual system still regard these two dissimilar segments as being parts of a single line and proceed to complete it? Surprisingly, the answer is again yes. You will see a con-

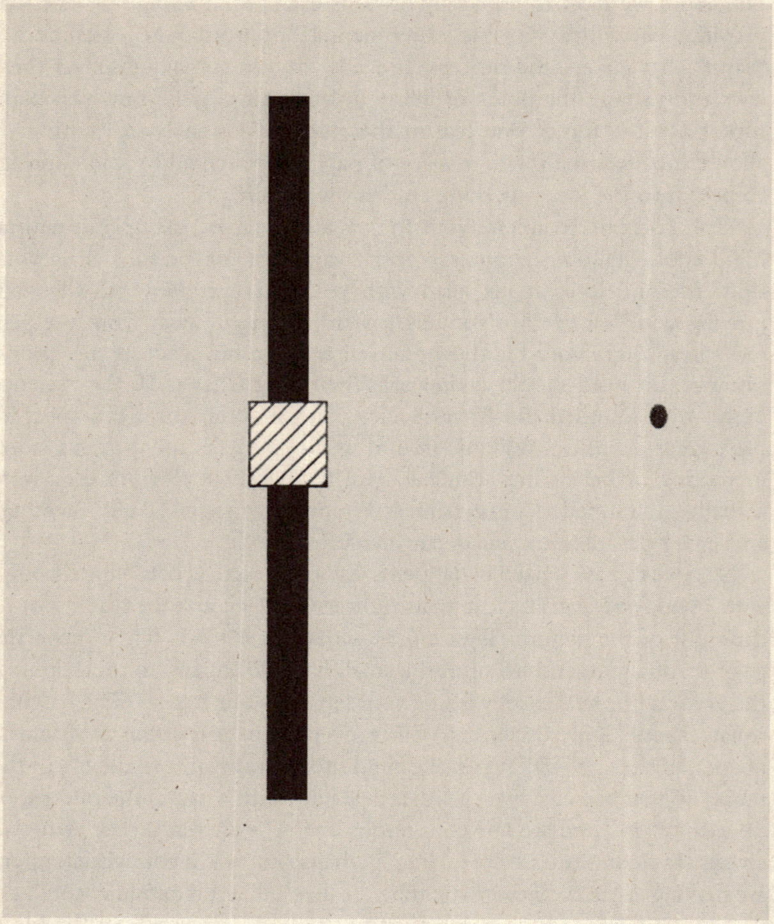

Figure 5.3 *A vertical black line running through the blind spot. Repeat the procedure described for Figure 5.2. Shut your right eye, look at the small black dot on the right with your left eye and move the page to and fro until the hatched square on the left falls on your blind spot and disappears. Does the vertical line look continuous, or does it have a gap in the middle? There is a lot of variation from person to person, but most people "complete" the line. If the illusion doesn't work for you, try aiming your blind spot at a single black-white edge (such as the edge of a black book on a white background) and you will see it complete.*

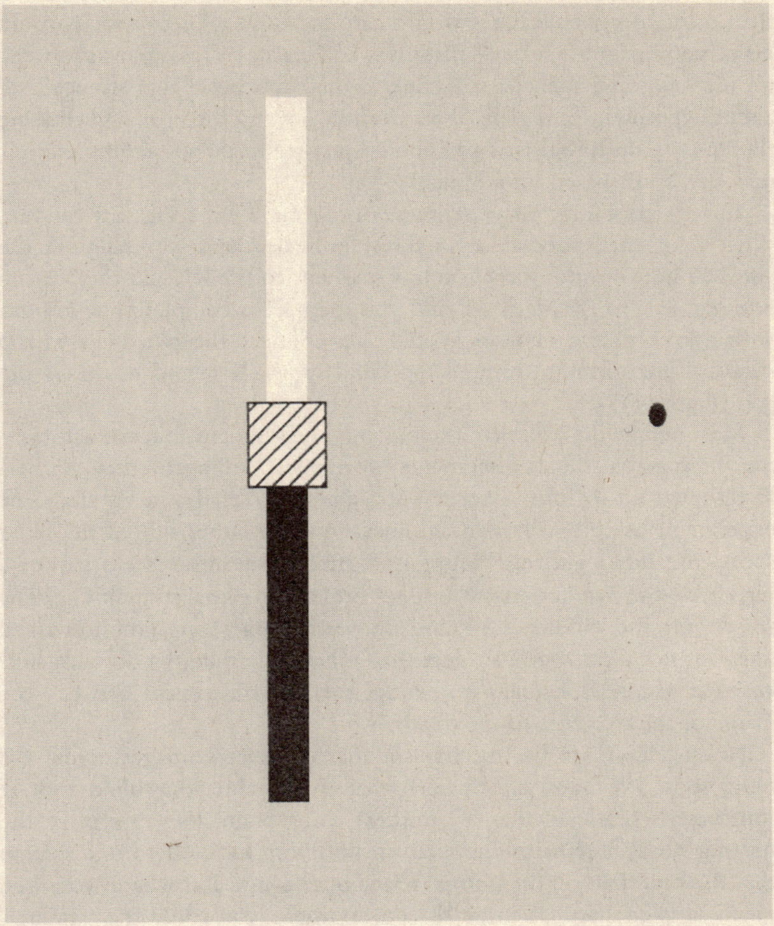

Figure 5.4 *The upper half of the line is white and the lower half black. Does your brain complete the vertical line in spite of this internally contradictory evidence?*

tinuous single straight line, black on top and white below, but smeared in the middle into a lustrous metallic gray (Figure 5.4). This is the compromise solution that the visual system seems to prefer.

People often assume that science is serious business, that it is always "theory driven," that you generate lofty conjectures based on what you already know and then proceed to design experiments specifically to test these conjectures. Actually real science is more like a fishing expedition than most of my colleagues would care to admit. (Of course, I would never say this in a National Institutes of Health [NIH] grant proposal, for most funding agencies still cling to the naive belief that science is all about hypothesis testing and then carefully dotting the "i's" and crossing the "t's." God forbid that you should just try to do something entirely new that's just based on a hunch!)

So let's continue our experiments on your blind spot, just for fun. What if you challenged your visual system by deliberately misaligning the two half lines—shifting the top line segment to the left and the bottom line segment to the right? Would you then see a complete line anyway with a kink in the middle? Would you connect the two lines with a diagonal line running through the blind spot? Or would you see a big gap (Figure 5.5)?[6]

Most people do complete the missing line segment, but the astonishing thing is that the two segments now appear collinear—they get perfectly lined up to form a vertical straight line! Yet if you try the same experiment using two horizontal lines—one on either side of the blind spot—you don't get this "lining-up" effect. You either see a gap or a big kink—the two lines don't fuse to form a horizontal straight line. The reason for the difference—lining up vertical lines but not horizontal lines—is not clear, but I suspect that it has something to do with stereoscopic vision: our ability to extract the tiny differences between the image of the two eyes to see depth.[7]

How "clever" is the mechanism that completes images across the blind spot? We have already seen that if you aim your blind spot at somebody's head (so that it vanishes), your brain doesn't replace the missing head; it remains chopped off until you look off to one side so that the head falls on the normal retina once again. But what if you used much simpler shapes than heads? For example, you could try "aiming" your blind spot at the corner of a square (Figure 5.6). Noticing the other three corners, does your visual system fill in the missing corner? If you try this experiment, you will notice that in fact the corner disappears or looks "bitten off" or smudged. Clearly the neural machinery that allows completion across the blind spot cannot deal with corners; there's a limit to what can and what cannot be filled in.[8]

Completing a corner is obviously too big a challenge for the visual system; perhaps it can cope only with very simple patterns such as homogeneous colors and straight lines. But you're in for a surprise. Try aiming your blind spot at the center of a bicycle wheel with radiating

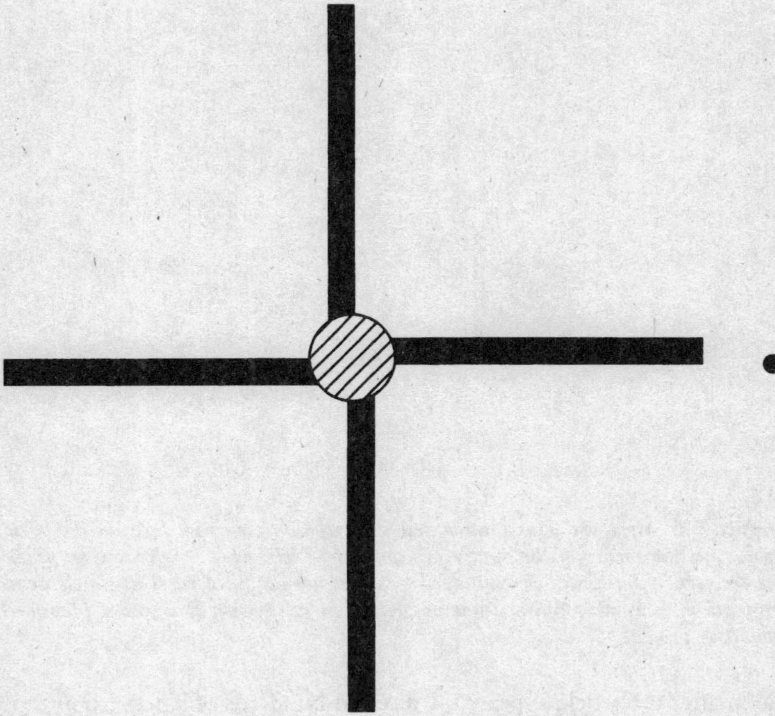

Figure 5.5 *Repeat the experiment, "aiming" your blind spot at a pattern that resembles a swastika—an ancient Indo-European peace symbol. The lines are deliberately misaligned, one on either side of the blind spot.*

Many people find that when the central hatched disk disappears, the two vertical lines get "lined up" and become collinear, whereas the two horizontal lines are not lined up—there is a slight bend or kink in the middle.

spokes (Figure 5.7). Notice that when you do this, unlike what you observed with the corner of the square, you do not see a gap or smudge. You do indeed "complete" the gap—you actually see the spokes converging into a vortex at the center of your blind spot.

So it appears that there are some things you can complete across the blind spot and other things you cannot, and it's relatively easy to discover these principles by simply experimenting with your own blind spot or a friend's.

Some years ago, Jonathan Piel, the former editor of *Scientific American*, invited me to write an article on the blind spot for that journal.

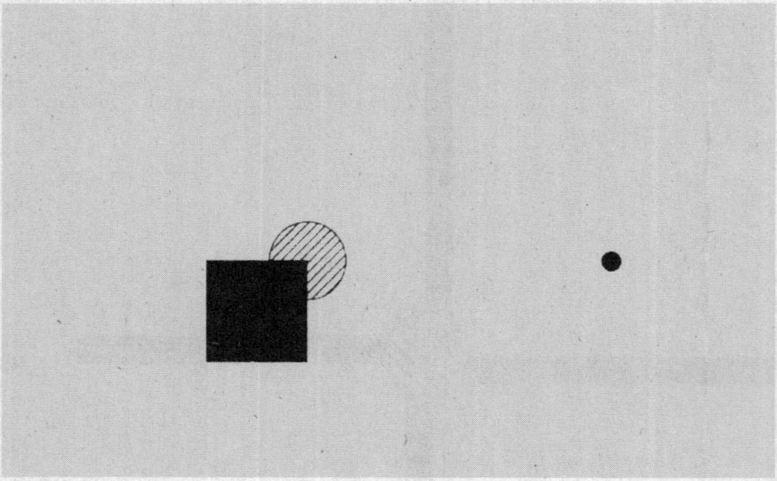

Figure 5.6 *Move the page toward you until the hatched disk falls on the blind spot. Does the corner of the square get completed? The answer is that most people see the corner "missing" or "smudged"; it does not get filled in. This simple demonstration shows that filling in is not based on guesswork; it is not a high-level cognitive process.*

Soon after the article appeared, I received hundreds of letters from readers who tried the various experiments I had described or had devised new ones of their own. These letters made me realize how intensely curious people are about the inner workings of their visual pathways. One chap even embarked on a whole new style of art and had a show of his own paintings at an art gallery. He had created various complex geometric designs, which you have to view with one eye, aiming your blind spot at a specific section of the painting. Like James Thurber, he had used his blind spot creatively to inspire his art.

•

I hope these examples have given you a feel for what it is like to "fill in" missing portions of the visual field. You have to bear in mind, though, that you have had a blind spot all your life and you might be especially skilled at this process. But what if you lost a patch of visual cortex as a result of disease or accident? What if a much larger hole in your visual field—a scotoma—suddenly appeared? Such patients do exist

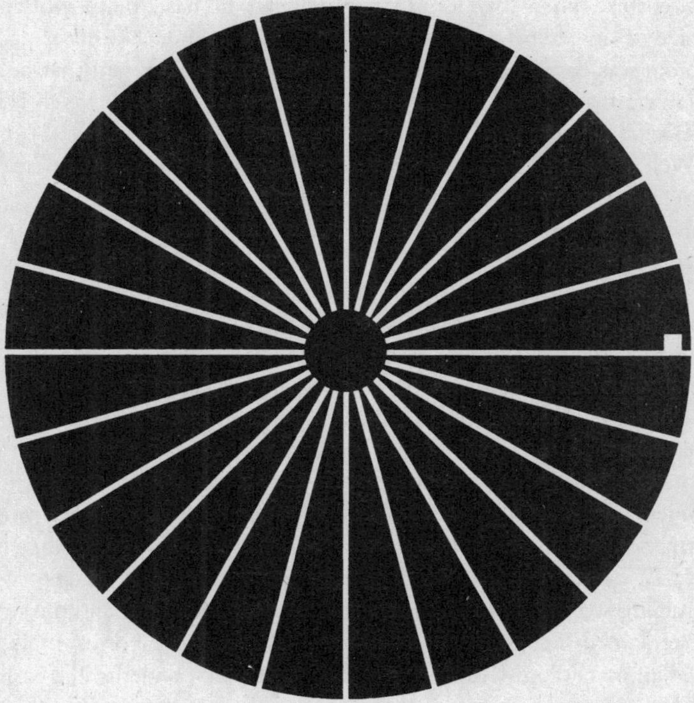

Figure 5.7 *Amazingly, when the blind spot is aimed at the center of a bicycle wheel, no gap is seen. People usually report that the spokes converge toward a vortex.*

and they present a valuable opportunity to study how far the brain can go in supplying the "missing information" when needed. Migraine patients have transient scotomas, but I decided it would be best to study someone who had a large permanent blind spot in his visual field, and that is how I met Josh.[9]

Josh was a large man with Brezhnev-like eyebrows, a barrel chest and meaty hands. Yet he exuded a natural twinkle and sense of humor that infused what would otherwise be a rather menacing body type with the burly sweetness of a teddy bear. Whenever Josh laughed, everyone in the room chuckled with him. Now in his early thirties, some years earlier he had suffered an industrial accident in which a steel rod penetrated the back of his skull, punching a hole in his right occipital pole in the primary visual cortex. When Josh looks straight ahead, he has a blind spot about the size of my palm to the left of where he's looking. No other part of his brain was damaged. When Josh came to see me, he said that he was well aware that he had a large blind spot.

"How do you know?" I asked.

"Well, one problem is that I often walk into the women's room."

"Why is that?"

"Because when I look at the sign WOMEN straight on, I don't see the 'w' and the 'o' to the left. I just see 'MEN.' " Josh insisted, however, that other than these occasional hints that something was wrong, his vision seemed surprisingly normal. In fact, given his deficit, he was surprised by the unitary nature of his visual world. "When I look at you," he said, "I don't see anything missing. No pieces are left out." He paused, knitted his eyebrows, studied my face and then broke into a huge smile. "If I pay careful attention, Dr. Ramachandran, I notice that one of your eyes and an ear are missing! Are you feeling okay?"

Unless he scrutinized his visual field, Josh seemed to fill in the missing information with no trouble. Although researchers have known for a long time that patients like Josh exist (and live quite normally except when frightening women in ladies' rooms), many psychologists and physicians have remained skeptical of the filling-in phenomenon. For example, the Canadian psychologist Justine Sergent claimed that patients like Josh are confabulating or engaging in a kind of unconscious guesswork when they say they can see normally. (He guesses that there is wallpaper in his scotoma because there is wallpaper everywhere else.) This type of guesswork, she said, would be very different from the types of true perceptual completion that you experienced when you had a line passing through your blind spot.[10] But I realized that Josh gave us the opportunity to find out what is really going on inside a scotoma. Why try to second-guess the mechanisms of vision from scratch when we could ask Josh?

Josh swept into the laboratory one drizzly, cold afternoon, propped an umbrella in one corner and lit up the room with his cheerfulness. He was dressed in a plaid shirt, loose jeans and beat-up running shoes, damp with mud from the walk into our building. We were going to have some fun today. Our strategy was simply to repeat on Josh all the experiments you just did on your own blind spot. First, we decided to see what would happen if we ran a line through his scotoma, where a big piece of the visual field was missing. Would he see the line as having a gap, or would he fill it in?

But before we did the experiment, we realized we had a minor technical problem. If we gave Josh an actual line, asked him to look straight ahead and tell us whether he saw a complete line or piece missing, he might "cheat" inadvertently. He might accidentally move his eyes a tiny amount, and the slight motion would bring the line into his normal visual field and would tell him that the line is complete. We wanted to avoid that so we simply presented Josh with two half lines on either side of his scotoma and asked him what he saw. Would he see a continuous line or two half lines? Recall that when you tried this little experiment using your own blind spot, you saw the lines as complete.

He considered for a moment and said, "Well, I see two lines, one above, one below and there's a big gap in the middle."

"Okay," I said. This was not going anywhere.

"Wait!" said Josh, squinting. "Wait a minute. You know what? They're growing toward each other."

"What?"

He held up his right index finger vertically, pointing upward, to mimic the bottom line and his left index finger pointing downward to mimic the top line. At first the two fingertips were two inches apart, and then Josh started moving them toward each other. "Okay," he said excitedly. "They're growing, growing, growing, growing together, and now there's one complete line." As he said this, his index fingers touched.

Not only is Josh filling in, but the filling in is happening in real time. He could watch it and describe it, contrary to claims that the phenomenon doesn't exist in people with scotomas.

Clearly some nerve circuits in Josh's brain were taking two half lines, lying on either side of the scotoma, as sufficient evidence that there is a complete line there, and these circuits are sending this message to higher centers in Josh's brain. So his brain could complete information across the huge, gaping hole right near his center of gaze in much the same way that you did across your natural blind spot.

Next we wondered what would happen when we deliberately misaligned the two lines. Would he complete it with a diagonal line? Or would his visual system simply give up? Presented with this display, Josh said, "No dice. They're not completed. I see a gap. Sorry."

"I know that; just tell me what happens."

A couple of seconds later Josh exclaimed, "Oh, my God, look what's happening!"

"What?"

"Hey, they started like this and now they're moving toward each other like this." He again held up his fingers to show the two lines moving sideways. "Now they're completely lined up, and now they're filling in like that. Okay, now it's complete." The whole process lasted five seconds, an eternity as far as the visual system is concerned. We repeated the experiment several times with identical results.

So it seemed fairly clear we are dealing with genuine perceptual completion here, for why else would it take so many seconds? If Josh were guessing, he should guess immediately. But how far could we push this? How sophisticated is the visual system's capacity to "insert" the missing information? What if we used a vertical column of "X's" instead of a plain line? Would he actually hallucinate the missing "X's"? What if we used a column of smiling faces? Would he fill in the scotoma with smiling faces?

So we put the vertical column "X's" on the computer screen and asked Josh to look to the immediate right of this column so that the middle three "X's" fell on the scotoma.

"What do you see?" I asked.

"I see 'X's' on top, 'X's' on the bottom, and there's a big gap in the middle."

I told him to keep looking at it since we had already established that filling in takes time.

"Look, doctor, I'm staring at it and I know you want me to see an 'X' there, but I don't see it. No 'X's.' Sorry." He stared at it for three minutes, four minutes, five minutes, and then we both gave up.

Then I tried a long vertical row of tiny 'x's,' one set above and one below the scotoma. "Now what do you see?"

"Oh, yeah, it's a continuous column of 'x's,' little 'x's.' " Josh turned to me and said, "I know you're really tricking me. There are no 'x's' really there. Are there?"

"I'm not going to tell you. But I want to know one more thing. Do the 'x's' on the left side of where you're looking (which I knew were in his scotoma) appear any different from the ones above and below?"

Josh replied, "It looks like a continuous column of 'x's.' I don't see any difference."

Josh was filling in the little "x's" but not the big "X's." This difference is important for two reasons. First it rules out the possibility of confabulation. Often in neurology tests, patients will make up a story, putting on a show for the physician's benefit. Knowing there were "x's" above and below, Josh could have guessed that he "saw" them in between without really doing so. But why would he only engage in such guesswork for the little "x's" and not the big ones? Since he did not fill in the missing large "X's," we can assume that in the case of the little "x's" we're dealing with a genuine perceptual completion process, not with guesswork or confabulation.

Why did the genuine perceptual completion occur only for the little "x's" and not the large ones? Perhaps the brain treats the tiny "x's" as forming a continuous texture and therefore completes it, but when confronted with large "x's" it switches to a different mode of operation and "sees" that some of the "X's" were missing. My hunch is that the tiny letters activated a different part of Josh's visual pathway, one that deals with continuity of textures and surfaces, whereas the large letters would be processed in the pathway in his temporal lobes that is concerned with objects (discussed in the last chapter) rather than surfaces. It makes sense that the brain should be especially skilled at completing gaps when dealing with continuous surface textures and colors but not when dealing with objects. The reason is that surfaces in the real world are usually composed of uniform "stuff" or surface texture—like a block of grainy wood or a sandstone cliff—but there is no such thing as a natural surface made up of large alphabetical letters or faces. (Of course man-made surfaces like wallpaper can be made of smiling faces, but the brain didn't originally evolve in a man-made world.)

To test the notion that completion of textures and "stuff" across a gap can occur much more easily than completion of objects or letters, I was tempted to try something a bit outlandish. I put up the numerals 1, 2 and 3 above the scotoma and 7, 8 and 9 below. Would Josh perceptually complete the sequence? What would he see in the middle? Of course, I used tiny numerals to ensure that the brain would treat them as a "texture."

"Hmmm," said Josh, "I see a continuous column of numbers, vertically aligned numbers."

"Can you see a gap in the middle?"

"No."

"Can you read them out loud for me?"

"Um, one, two, three, um, seven, eight, nine. Hey, that's very strange. I can see the numbers in the middle, but I can't read them. They look like numbers, but I don't know what they are."

"Do they look blurred?"

"No, they don't look blurred. They kind of look strange. I can't tell what they are—like hieroglyphics or something."

We had induced a curious form of temporary dyslexia in Josh. Those middle numbers did not exist, were not flashed before his eyes, yet his brain was making up the textural attributes of the number string and completing it. This is another striking demonstration of division of labor in the visual pathways. The system in his brain that deals with surfaces and edges is saying, "There is numberlike stuff in this region—that's what you should see in the middle," but since there are no actual numbers, his object pathway remains silent and the net result is illegible "hieroglyphics"!

It has been known for over two decades now that what we call the visual system is actually several systems; that there are multiple specialized cortical areas concerned with different visual attributes such as motion, color and other dimensions. Does filling in occur separately in each of these areas, or does it occur all at once in just one single area? To find out, we asked Josh to look at the center of a blank screen on the computer monitor, and then we suddenly switched on a pattern of twinkling black dots on a red background.

Josh whistled, apparently taking as much delight in all this as I was. "My God, doctor," he said, "I can actually see my scotoma for the first time." He yanked a felt pen from my hand and much to my dismay proceeded to start drawing on the monitor, producing what appeared to be an outline of the irregular margins of the scotoma (Josh's ophthalmologist, Dr. Lilian Levinson, had earlier mapped out his scotoma using a sophisticated technique called perimetry and I could therefore compare his drawing with hers; they were identical).

"But Josh, what do you see inside the scotoma?" I asked.

"Well, it's very strange, doctor. For the first few seconds, I saw only the red color bleeding into this part of the screen, but the twinkling black dots did not fill in. Then after a few seconds, the dots filled in, but they weren't twinkling. And last, the actual twinkle—the motion sensation—filled in as well." He turned around, rubbed his eye, looked at me and said, "What does all this mean?"[11]

The answer is that filling in seems to occur at different speeds for different perceptual attributes like color, motion (twinkle) and texture. Motion takes longer to fill in than color, and so on. Indeed, such differential filling in provides additional evidence that such specialized areas do exist in the human brain. For if perception were just one process happening in a single location in the brain, it should happen all at once, not in stages.

Finally, we tested Josh's ability to fill in more sophisticated shapes, like the corners of squares. Remember when you tried aiming your blind spot on a corner, it was chopped off—your brain apparently couldn't fill it in. When we tried the same experiment on Josh, we got the opposite result. He had no difficulty in seeing the missing corner, proving that very sophisticated types of completion were taking place in his brain.

By now, Josh was feeling tired, but we had succeeded in making him as intensely curious about the filling-in process as we were. Having heard the King Charles story from me, he decided to try to aim his scotoma at my graduate student's head. Would his brain prefer to complete her head (contrary to what happened in your blind spot) to prevent such a horrendous spectacle? The answer is no. Josh always saw this person with a head missing. Thus he could fill in parts of simple geometric shapes but not complex objects like faces or things of that nature. This experiment again shows that filling in is not simply a matter of guesswork, for there is no reason Josh shouldn't have been able to "guess" that my student's head was still there.

An important distinction must be made between perceptual and conceptual completion. To understand the difference, just think of the space behind your head now as you are sitting on your chair reading this book. You can let your mind wander, thinking about the kinds of objects that might be behind your head or body. Is there a window? A Martian? A gaggle of geese? With your imagination, you can "fill in" this missing space with just about anything, but since you can change your mind about the content, I call this process conceptual filling in.

Perceptual filling in is very different. When you fill in your blind spot with a carpet design, you don't have such choices about what fills that spot; you can't change your mind about it. Perceptual filling in is carried out by visual neurons. Their decisions, once made, are irreversible: Once they signal to higher brain centers "Yes, this is a repetitive texture" or "yes, this is a straight line," what you perceive is irrevocable. We will return to this distinction between perceptual and conceptual filling in, which philosophers are very interested in, later when we talk about consciousness and whether Martians see red in Chapter 12. For now, it suffices to emphasize that we're dealing with true perceptual completion across the scotomas, not just guesswork or deduction.

This phenomenon is far more important that one might imagine from the parlor games I've just described. Decapitating department chairmen is amusing, but why should the brain engage in perceptual completion? The answer lies in a Darwinian explanation of how the visual system evolved. One of the most important principles in vision is that it tries to get away with as little processing as it can to get the job done. To economize on visual processing, the brain takes advantage of statistical regularities in the world—such as the fact that contours are generally continuous or that table surfaces are uniform—and these regularities are captured and wired into the machinery of the visual pathways early in visual processing. When you look at your desk, for instance, it seems likely that the visual system extracts information about its edges and creates a mental representation that resembles a cartoon sketch of the table (again, this initial extraction of edges occurs because your brain is mainly interested in regions of change, of abrupt discontinuity, at the edge of desk, which is where the information is). The visual system might then apply surface interpolation to "fill in" the color and texture of the table, saying in effect, "Well, there's this grainy stuff here; it must be the same grainy stuff all over." This act of interpolation saves an enormous amount of computation; your brain can avoid the burden of scrutinizing every little section of the desk and can simply employ loose guesswork instead (bearing in mind the distinction between conceptual guesswork and perceptual guesswork).

•

What has all of this got to do with James Thurber and other patients with Charles Bonnet syndrome? Might the findings that we have discussed so far about the brain's capacity for "filling in" blind spots and scotomas also help us understand the extraordinary visual hallucinations they experience?

Medical syndromes are named after their discoverers, not the patients who suffer from them, and this one was named after a Swiss naturalist, Charles Bonnet, who lived from 1720 to 1773. Even though he suffered from precarious health and was always on the brink of losing his own eyesight and hearing, Bonnet was a shrewd observer of the natural world. He was the first person to observe parthenogenesis—the production of offspring by an unfertilized female—and that led him to propose an absurd theory known as preformationism, the idea that each egg carried by a female must contain an entire preformed individual, presumably with miniature eggs of its own, each of which in turn contains even tinier individuals with eggs, and so on, ad infinitum. As luck would have it, many physicians remember Charles Bonnet as the gullible chap who hallucinated little people in eggs and not as the insightful biologist who discovered parthenogenesis.

Fortunately, Bonnet was more perceptive when he observed and reported on an unusual medical situation in his own family. His maternal grandfather, Charles Lullin, had successfully undergone what in those days was dangerous and traumatic surgery—the removal of cataracts at age seventy-seven. Eleven years after the operation, the grandfather began suffering vivid hallucinations. People and objects would appear and disappear without warning, grow in size and then recede. When he stared at the tapestries in his apartment, he saw bizarre transformations involving people with strange gazes and animals that were, he realized, flowing from his brain and not the weaver's loom.

This phenomenon, as I mentioned earlier, is fairly common in elderly people with visual handicaps like macular degeneration, diabetic retinopathy, corneal damage and cataracts. A recent study in the *Lancet,* a British medical journal, reported that many older men and women with poor vision hide the fact that they "see things which aren't really there." Out of five hundred visually handicapped people, sixty admitted that they hallucinated, sometimes only once or twice a year, but others experienced visual fantasies at least twice a day. For the most part the content of their imaginary world is mundane, perhaps involving an unfamiliar person, a bottle or a hat, but the hallucinations can also be quite funny. One woman saw two miniature policemen guiding a midget villain to a tiny prison van. Others saw ghostly translucent figures floating in the hallway, dragons, people wearing flowers on their heads and even beautiful shining angels, little circus animals, clowns and elves. A surprising number of them report seeing children. Peter Halligan, John Marshall and I once saw a patient at Oxford who not only "saw" children in her left visual field but could actually hear their laughter, only to turn her head and realize no one was there. The images can be in black and white or color, stationary or in motion, and just as clear as, less clear than or more clear than reality. At times the objects blend into actual surroundings so that an imaginary person sits in a real chair, ready to speak. The images are rarely threatening—no slavering monsters or scenes of brutal carnage.

Patients were always easily corrected by others while hallucinating. A woman said that she once sat at her window watching cows in a neighboring meadow. It was actually very cold and the middle of winter, and she complained to her maid about the cruelty of the farmer. The astonished maid looked, saw no cows and said, "What are you talking about? What cows?" The woman flushed with embarrassment. "My eyes are tricking me. I can't trust them anymore."

Another woman said, "In my dreams I experience things which affect me, which are related to my life. These hallucinations, however, have nothing to do with me." Others are not so sure. An elderly childless man was intrigued by recurrent hallucinations of a little girl and boy and wondered whether these hallucinations reflected his unfulfilled wish to become a father. There's even a report of a woman who saw her recently deceased husband three times a week.

Given how common this syndrome is, I am tempted to wonder whether the occasional reports of "true" sightings of ghosts, UFOs and angels by otherwise sane intelligent people may merely be examples of Charles Bonnet hallucinations. Is it any surprise that roughly one third of Americans claim to have seen angels? I'm not asserting that angels don't exist (I have no idea whether they do or not) but simply that many of the sightings may be due to ocular pathology.

Poor lighting and the changing tones at dusk favor such hallucinations. If the patients blink, nod their heads or turn on a light, the visions often cease. Nevertheless, they have no voluntary control over the apparitions, which usually appear without warning. Most of us can imagine the scenes these people describe—a miniature police van with miniature criminals running about—but we exert conscious control over such imaginations. With Charles Bonnet syndrome, on the other hand, the images appear completely unbidden as if they are real objects.

•

This sudden appearance of intrusive images was apparent in the case of Larry MacDonald, a twenty-seven-year-old agronomist who suffered a terrible automobile accident. Larry's head smashed into the windshield, fracturing the frontal bones above his eyes and the orbital plates that protected his optic nerves. Comatose for two weeks, he could neither walk nor talk when he regained consciousness. But that wasn't the worst of his problems. As Larry recalls, "The world was filled with hallucinations, both visual and auditory. I couldn't distinguish what was real from what was fake. Doctors and nurses standing next to my bed were surrounded by football players and Hawaiian dancers. Voices came at me from everywhere and I couldn't tell who was talking." Larry felt panic and confusion.

Gradually, however, his condition improved as his brain struggled to repair itself after the trauma. He regained control over his bodily functions and learned to walk. He could talk, with difficulty, and learned to distinguish real voices from imagined ones—a feat that helped him suppress the auditory hallucinations.

I met Larry five years after his accident because he had heard about my interest in visual hallucinations. He talked slowly, with effort, but was otherwise intelligent and perceptive. His life was normal except for one astonishing problem. His visual hallucinations, which used to occur anywhere and everywhere in his visual field with brilliant colors and spinning motions, had retreated into the lower half of his field of vision, where he was completely blind. That is, he would only see imaginary objects below a center line extending from his nose outward. Everything above the line was completely normal; he would always see what was really out there. Below the line, he had intermittent recurrent hallucinations.

"Back in the hospital, colors used to be a lot more vivid," Larry said.

"What did you see?" I asked.

"I saw animals and cars and boats, you know. I saw dogs and elephants and all kinds of things."

"You can still see them?"

"Oh, yeah, I see them right now here in the room."

"You are seeing them now as we speak?"

"Oh, yeah!" said Larry.

I was intrigued. "Larry, you said that when you see them ordinarily, they tend to cover other objects in the room. But right now you're looking straight at me. It's not like you see something covering me right now, right?"

"As I look at you, there is a monkey sitting on your lap," Larry announced.

"A monkey?"

"Yes, right there on your lap."

I thought he was joking. "Tell me how you know you're hallucinating."

"I don't know. But it's unlikely there would be a professor here with a monkey sitting in his lap so I think there probably isn't one." He smiled cheerfully. "But it looks extremely vivid and real." I must have looked shocked, for Larry continued, "For one thing they fade after a few seconds or minutes, so I know they're not real. And even though the image sometimes blends quite well into the rest of the scene around it, like the monkey on your lap," he continued, "I realize that it is highly improbable and usually don't tell people about it." Speechless, I glanced down at my lap while Larry just smiled. "Also, there is something odd about the images—they often look too good to be true. The colors are vibrant, extraordinarily vivid, and the images actually look more real than real objects, if you see what I mean."

I was not sure. What does he mean by "more real than real"? There is a school of art called superrealism in which the paintings of things like

Campbell's soup cans are created with the kind of fine detail you only get through a magnifying glass. These objects are strange to look at, but maybe that was how Larry saw images in his scotoma.

"Does this bother you, Larry?"

"Well, it kind of does because it makes me curious about why I experience them, but it really doesn't get in my way. I'm much more worried about the fact that I'm blind than about the fact that I see hallucinations. In fact, sometimes they are fun to watch because I never know what I'm going to see next."

"Are the images you see, like this monkey in my lap, things you've seen before in your life or can the hallucinations be completely new?"

Larry thought a moment and said, "I think they can be completely new images, but how can that be? I always thought that hallucinations were limited to things you've already seen elsewhere in your life. But then lots of times the images are rather ordinary. Sometimes, when I'm looking for my shoes in the morning, the whole floor suddenly is covered with shoes. It's hard to find my own shoes! More often the visions come and go, as if they have a life of their own, even though they are unconnected to what I'm doing or thinking about at the time."

Not long after my conversations with Larry, I met another Charles Bonnet patient, whose world was stranger yet. She was plagued by cartoons! Nancy was a nurse from Colorado who had an arteriovenous malformation or AVM—basically a cluster of swollen and fused arteries and veins in the back of her brain. If it were to rupture, she could die from a brain hemorrhage, so her doctors zapped the AVM with a laser to reduce it in size and "seal it off." In so doing they left scar tissue on parts of her visual cortex. Like Josh, she had a small scotoma and hers was immediately to the left of where she was looking, covering about ten degrees of space. (If she stretched her arm out in front of her and looked at her hand, the scotoma would be about twice the size of her palm.)

"Well, the most extraordinary thing is that I see images inside this scotoma," Nancy said, sitting in the same chair that Larry had occupied earlier. "I see them dozens of times a day, not continuously, but at different times lasting several seconds each time."

"What do you see?"

"Cartoons."

"What?"

"Cartoons."

"What do you mean by cartoons? You mean Mickey Mouse?"

"On some occasions I see Disney cartoons. But most commonly not. Mostly what I see is just people and animals and objects. But these are always line drawings, filled in with uniform color like comic books. It's most amusing. They remind me of Roy Lichtenstein drawings."

"What else can you tell me? Do they move?"

"No. They are absolutely stationary. The other thing is that my cartoons have no depth, no shading, no curvature."

So that's what she meant when she said they were like comic books. "Are they familiar people or are they people you've never seen?" I asked.

"They can be either," Nancy said. "I never know what's coming next."

Here is a woman whose brain creates Walt Disney cartoons in defiance of copyright. What is going on? And how could any sane person see a monkey on my lap and accept it as normal?

To understand these bizarre symptoms, we are going to have to revise our models of how the visual system and perception operate from day to day. In the not too distant past, physiologists drew diagrams of visual areas with arrows pointing up. An image would be processed at one level, sent on up to the next level and so on, until the "gestalt" eventually emerged in some mysterious manner. This is the so-called bottom-up view of vision, championed by artificial intelligence researchers over the last three decades, even though many anatomists have long emphasized that there are massive feedback pathways projecting from the so-called higher areas to lower visual areas. To pacify these anatomists, textbook diagrams usually also included arrows pointing backward, but, by and large, the notion of back projections was given more lip service than functional meaning.

A newer view of perception—championed by Dr. Gerald Edelman of the Neurosciences Institute in La Jolla, California—suggests that the brain's information flow resembles the images in a funhouse full of mirrors, continually reflected back and forth, and continually changed by the process of reflection.[12] Like separate light beams in a funhouse, visual information can take many different paths, sometimes diverging, sometimes reinforcing itself, sometimes traveling in opposite directions.

If this sounds confusing, let's return to the distinction I made earlier between seeing a cat and imagining a cat. When we see a cat, its shape, color, texture and other visible attributes will impinge upon our retina and travel through the thalamus (a relay station in the middle of the brain) and up into the primary visual cortex for processing into two streams or pathways. As discussed in the previous chapter, one pathway goes to regions dealing with depth and motion—allowing you to grab or dodge objects and to move around the world—and the other to regions dealing with shape, color and object recognition (these are the how and what vision pathways). Eventually, all the information is combined to tell us that this is a cat—say, Felix—and to enable us to recall everything we've ever learned or felt about cats in general and Felix in particular. Or at least that's what the textbooks tell us.

Now think of what's going on in your brain when you imagine a cat.[13] There's good evidence to suggest that we are actually running our visual machinery in reverse! Our memories of all cats and of this particular cat flow from top to bottom—from higher regions to the primary visual cortex—and the combined activities of all these areas lead to the perception of an imaginary cat by the mind's eye. Indeed, the activity in the primary visual cortex may be almost as strong as if you really did see a cat, but in fact the cat is not there. This means that the primary visual cortex, far from being a mere sorting office for information coming in from the retina, is more like a war room where information is constantly being sent back from scouts, enacting all sorts of scenarios, and then information is sent back up again to those same higher areas where the scouts are working. There's a dynamic interplay between the brain's so-called early visual areas and the higher visual centers, culminating in a sort of virtual reality simulation of the cat. (All this was discovered mainly from animal experiments and neuroimaging studies in humans.)

It's not yet clear exactly how this "interplay" occurs or what its function might be. But it may explain what is happening in the Charles Bonnet patients like Larry and Nancy or the senior citizens sitting in a darkened room at the nursing home. I suggest that they are filling in missing information in much the same way that Josh did except that they are using high-level stored memories.[14] So, in Bonnet syndrome, the images are based on a sort of "conceptual completion" rather than perceptual completion; the images being "filled in" are coming from memory (top down)—not from the outside (bottom up). Clowns, water lilies, monkeys and cartoons populate the blind region rather than just the information immediately surrounding the scotoma such as lines and small "x's." Of course, when Larry sees a monkey in my lap he isn't duped; he knows perfectly well it's not real because he realizes it's highly improbable that there should be a monkey in my office.

But if this argument is correct—if the early visual areas are activated each time you imagine something—then why don't you and I hallucinate all the time or at least occasionally confuse our internally generated images with real objects? Why don't you see a monkey in the chair when you simply think of one? The reason is that even if you close your eyes, cells in your retina and in early sensory pathways are constantly active—producing a flat, baseline signal. This baseline signal informs your higher visual centers that there is no object (monkey) hitting the retina—thereby vetoing the activity evoked by top-down imagery. But if the early visual pathways are damaged, this baseline signal is removed and so you hallucinate.[15]

It makes good evolutionary sense that even though your internal images can be very realistic, they can never actually substitute for the real thing. You cannot, as Shakespeare said, "cloy the hungry edge of appetite by bare imagination of a feast." A good thing, too, because if you could satisfy your hunger by thinking about a feast, you wouldn't bother to eat and would quickly become extinct. Likewise, any creature that could imagine orgasms is unlikely to transmit its genes to the next generation. (Of course, we can do so to a limited extent as when our hearts pound when imagining an amorous encounter—the basis of what is sometimes called visualization therapy.)

Additional support for this interaction between top-down imagery and bottom-up sensory signals in perception comes from what we saw in phantom limb patients who have vivid impressions of clenching their nonexistent fingers and digging imaginary fingernails into their phantom palms, generating unbearable pain. Why do these patients actually *feel* clenching, "nails digging" and pain, whereas you or I can imagine the same finger position but feel nothing? The answer is that you and I have real input coming in from our hands telling us that there is no pain, even though we have memory traces in our brain linking the act of clenching with nails digging (especially if you don't often cut your nails). But in an amputee, these fleeting associations and preexisting pain memories can now emerge without contradiction from ongoing sensory input. The same sort of thing might be happening in Charles Bonnet syndrome.

But why did Nancy always see cartoons in her scotoma? One possibility is that in her brain the feedback comes mainly from the what pathway in the temporal lobe, which, you will recall, has cells specialized for color and shapes but not for motion and depth, which are handled by the how pathway. Therefore, her scotoma is filled with images that lack depth and motion, having only outlines and shapes, as do cartoons.

If I'm right, all these bizarre visual hallucinations are simply an exaggerated version of the processes that occur in your brain and mine every time we let our imagination run free. Somewhere in the confused welter of interconnecting forward and backward pathways is the interface between vision and imagination We don't have clear ideas yet about where this interface is or how it works (or even whether there is a single interface), but these patients provide some tantalizing clues about what might be going on. The evidence from them suggests that what we call perception is really the end result of a dynamic interplay between sensory signals and high-level stored information about visual images from the past. Each time any one of us encounters an object, the visual system begins a constant questioning process. Fragmentary evidence comes in and the higher centers say, "Hmmmmm, maybe this is an animal." Our brains then pose a series of visual questions: as in a twenty-questions game. Is it a mammal? A cat? What kind of cat? Tame? Wild? Big? Small? Black or white or tabby? The higher visual centers then project partial "best fit" answers back to lower visual areas including the primary visual cortex. In this manner, the impoverished image is progressively worked on and refined (with bits "filled in," when appropriate). I think that these massive feed forward and feedback projections are in the business of conducting successive iterations that enable us to home in on the closest approximation to the truth.[16] To overstate the argument deliberately, perhaps we are hallucinating all the time and what we call perception is arrived at by simply determining which hallucination best conforms to the current sensory input. But if, as happens in Charles Bonnet syndrome, the brain does not receive confirming visual stimuli, it is free simply to make up its own reality. And, as James Thurber was well aware, there is apparently no limit to its creativity.

CHAPTER 6

Through the Looking Glass

The world is not only queerer than we imagine;
it is queerer than we can imagine.

—J.B.S. HALDANE

Who was this rolling out of the bedroom in a wheelchair? Sam couldn't believe his eyes. His mother, Ellen, had just returned home the night before, having spent two weeks at the Kaiser Permanente hospital recuperating from a stroke. Mom had always been fastidious about her looks. Clothes and makeup were Martha Stewart perfect, with beautifully coiffed hair and fingernails painted in tasteful shades of pink or red. But today something was seriously wrong. The naturally curly hair on the left side of Ellen's head was uncombed, so that it stuck out in little nestlike clumps, whereas the rest of her hair was neatly styled. Her green shawl was hanging entirely over her right shoulder and dragging on the floor. She had applied rather bright red lipstick to her upper right and lower right lips, leaving the rest of her mouth bare. Likewise, there was a trace of eyeliner and mascara on her right eye but the left eye was unadorned. The final touch was a spot of rouge on her right cheek—

very carefully applied so as not to appear as if she were trying to hide her ill health but enough to demonstrate that she still cared about her looks. It was almost as though someone had used a wet towel to erase all the makeup on the left side of his mother's face!

"Good grief!" cried Sam. "What did you do to your makeup?"

Ellen raised her eyebrow in surprise. What was her son talking about? She had spent half an hour getting ready this morning and felt she looked as good as she possibly could, given the circumstances.

Ten minutes later, as they sat eating breakfast, Ellen ignored all the food on the left side of her plate, including the fresh-squeezed orange juice she so loved.

Sam raced for the phone and called me, as one of the physicians who had spent time with his mother at the hospital. Sam and I had gotten to know one another while I had been seeing a stroke patient who shared a room with his mother. "It's all right," I said, "don't be alarmed. Your mother is suffering from a common neurological syndrome called hemineglect, a condition that often follows strokes in the right brain, especially in the right parietal lobe. Neglect patients are profoundly indifferent to objects and events in the left side of the world, sometimes including the left side of their own bodies."

"You mean she's blind on the left side?"

"No, not blind. She just doesn't pay attention to what's on her left. That's why we call it neglect."

The next day I was able to demonstrate this to Sam's satisfaction by doing a simple clinical test on Ellen. I sat directly in front of her and said, "Fixate steadily on my nose and try not to move your eyes." When her gaze was fixed, I held my index finger up near her face, just to the left of her nose, and wiggled it vigorously.

"Ellen, what do you see?"

"I see a finger wiggling," she replied.

"Okay," I said. "Keep your eyes fixed on the same spot on my nose." Then, very slowly and casually, I raised the same finger to the same position, just left of her nose. But this time I was careful not to move it abruptly. "Now what do you see?"

Ellen looked blank. Without having her attention drawn to the finger—via motion or other strong cues—she was oblivious. Sam began to understand the nature of his mother's problem, the important distinction between blindness and neglect. His mother would ignore him completely if he stood on her left side and did nothing. But if he jumped up and down and waved his arms, she would sometimes turn around and look.

For the same reason, Ellen fails to notice the left side of her face in a mirror, forgets to apply makeup on the left side of her face, and doesn't comb her hair or brush her teeth on that side. And, not surprisingly, she even ignores all the food on the left side of her plate. But when her son points to things in the neglected area, forcing her to pay attention, Ellen might say, "Ah, how nice. Fresh-squeezed orange juice!" or "How embarrassing. My lipstick is crooked and my hair unkempt."

Sam was baffled. Would he have to assist Ellen for the rest of her life with simple day-to-day chores like applying makeup? Would his mother remain like this forever, or could I do something to help her?

I assured Sam that I'd try to help. Neglect is a fairly common problem[1] and I've always been intrigued by it. Beyond its immediate relevance to a patient's ability to care for herself, it has profound implications for understanding how the brain creates a spatial representation of the world, how it deals with left and right and how we are able—at a moment's notice—to pay attention to different portions of the visual scene. The great German philosopher Immanuel Kant became so obsessed with our "innate" concepts of space and time that he spent thirty years pacing up and down his veranda thinking about this problem. (Some of his ideas later inspired Mach and Einstein.) If we could somehow transport Ellen back in a time machine to visit him, I'm sure he'd be just as fascinated by her symptoms as you or I and would wonder whether we modern scientists had any inkling of what causes this strange condition.

When you glance at any visual scene, the image excites receptors in your retina and sets in motion a complex cascade of events that culminate in your perception of the world. As we noted in earlier chapters, the message from the eye is first mapped onto an area in the back of brain called the primary visual cortex. From there it is relayed along two pathways, the how pathway to the parietal lobe and the what pathway to the temporal lobe (see Figure 4.5, Chapter 4). The temporal lobes are concerned with recognizing and naming individual objects and responding to them with the appropriate emotions. The parietal lobes, on the other hand, are concerned with discerning the spatial layout of the external world, allowing you to navigate through space, reach out for objects, dodge missiles and otherwise know where you are. This division of labor between temporal and parietal lobes can explain almost all of the peculiar constellation of symptoms one sees in neglect patients in whom one parietal lobe—especially the right—is damaged, as is the case with Ellen. If you let her wander around by herself, she will not pay attention to the left side of space and anything that happens in it. She will even bump into objects on her left side or stub her left toe on a raised pavement. (I'll later explain why this doesn't happen with left parietal damage.) However, because Ellen's temporal lobes are still intact, she has no difficulty recognizing objects and events as long as her attention is drawn to them.

But "attention" is a loaded word, and we know even less about it than we do about neglect. So the statement that the neglect arises from a "failure to pay attention" doesn't really tell us very much unless we have a clear notion of what the underlying neural mechanisms might be. (It's a bit like saying that illness results from a failure of health.) In particular, one would like to know how a normal person—you or I—is able to attend selectively to a single sensory input, whether you are trying to listen to a single voice amid the background din of voices at a cocktail party or just trying to spot a familiar face in a baseball stadium. Why do we have this vivid sense of having an internal searchlight, one that we can direct at different objects and events around us?[2]

We now know that even so basic a skill as attention requires the participation of many far-flung regions of the brain. We've already talked about the visual, auditory and somatosensory systems, but other special brain regions carry out equally important tasks. The reticular activating system—a tangle of neurons in the brain stem that projects widely to vast regions of the brain—activates the entire cerebral cortex, leading to arousal and wakefulness, or—when needed—a small portion of the cortex, leading to selective attention. The limbic system is concerned with emotional behavior and evaluation of the emotional significance and potential value of events in the external world. The frontal lobes are concerned with more abstract processes like judgment, foresight and planning. All of these areas are interconnected in a positive feedback loop—a recursive, echolike reverberation—that takes a stimulus from the outside world, extracts its salient features and then bounces it from region to region, before eventually figuring out what it is and how to respond to it.[3] Should I fight, flee, eat or kiss? The simultaneous deployment of all these mechanisms culminates in perception.

When a large, threatening stimulus—say, an image of a menacing figure, perhaps a mugger looming toward me on the street in Boston—first comes into my brain, I haven't the slightest idea of what it is. Before I can determine, aha, perhaps that's a dangerous person, the visual information is evaluated by both the frontal lobes and the limbic system for relevance and sent on to a small portion of the parietal cortex, which, in conjunction with appropriate neural connections in the reticular formation, enables me to direct my attention to the looming figure. It forces my brain to swivel my eyeballs toward something important out there in the visual scene, pay selective attention to it and say, "Aha!"

But imagine what would happen if any part of this positive feedback loop were interrupted so that the whole process was compromised. You would then no longer notice what was happening on one side of the world. You would be a neglect patient.

But we still have to explain why neglect occurs primarily after injury to the right parietal lobe and not to the left. Why the asymmetry? Though the real reason continues to elude us, Marcel Mesulam of Harvard University has proposed an ingenious theory. We know that the left hemisphere is specialized for many aspects of language and the right hemisphere for emotions and "global" or holistic aspects of sensory processing. But Mesulam suggests there is another fundamental difference. Given its role in holistic aspects of vision, the right hemisphere has a broad "searchlight" of attention that encompasses both the entire left and entire right visual fields. The left hemisphere, on the other hand, has a much smaller searchlight, which is confined entirely to the right side of the world (perhaps because it is so busy with other things, such as language). As a result of this rather odd arrangement, if the left hemisphere is damaged, it loses its searchlight, but the right can compensate because it casts a searchlight on the entire world. When the right hemisphere is damaged, on the other hand, the global searchlight is gone but the left hemisphere cannot fully compensate for the loss because its searchlight is confined only to the right side. This would explain why neglect is only seen in patients whose right hemisphere is damaged.

So neglect is not blindness, but rather a general indifference to objects and events on the left. But how profound is this indifference? After all, even you and I, when driving home from work ignoring familiar terrain, will perk up immediately if we see an accident. This suggests that at some level the unattended visual information from the road must have been getting through. Is Ellen's indifference an extreme version of the same phenomenon? Is it possible that even though she doesn't notice things consciously, some of the information "leaks" through? Do these patients at some level "see" what they don't see? This is not an easy question to answer, but in 1988 two Oxford researchers, Peter Haligan and John Marshall,[4] took up the challenge. They devised a clever way to demonstrate that neglect patients are subconsciously aware of some of the things that are going on on their left side, even though they appear not to be. They showed patients drawings of two houses, one below the other, that were completely identical except for one salient feature—the house on the top had flames and smoke spewing from windows on the left. They then asked the patient whether the houses looked the same or different. The first neglect patient whom they studied said, not surprisingly, that the houses looked identical, since he did not pay attention to the left side of either drawing. But when forced to choose—"Come on, now, which house would you rather live in?"—he picked the bottom house, the one not on fire. For reasons he could not express, he said that he "preferred" that house. A form of blindsight, perhaps? Could it be that even though he is not paying attention to the left side of the house, some of the information about the flames and smoke leaks through to his right hemisphere through some alternate pathway and alerts him to danger? The experiment implies once again that there is no blindness in the left visual field, for if there were, how could he process this level of detail about the left side of the house under any circumstances?

Neglect stories are very popular with medical students. Oliver Sacks[5] tells the strange tale of a woman who, like many left hemineglect patients, ate food only from the right side of her plate. But she knew what was up and realized that if she wanted all her dinner, she had to shift her head, so as to see the food on the left. But given her general indifference to the left and reluctance even to look to the left she adopted a comically ingenious solution. She rolled her wheelchair in a huge circle to the right, traveling 340 degrees or so until finally her eyes would fall on the uneaten food. That consumed, she'd make another rotation, to eat the remaining half of the food on her plate, and so on, round and round, until it was gone. It never occurred to her that she could just turn left because—for her—the left simply didn't exist.

•

One morning not long ago while I was fixing the sprinkler system in our yard, my wife brought me an interesting-looking letter. I receive many letters each week, but this one was postmarked from Panama and had an exotic stamp and curious lettering. I wiped my hands on a towel and started to read a rather eloquent description of what it feels like to suffer from hemineglect.

"When I came to, other than having a severe headache, I perceived absolutely no adverse effects of my mishap," wrote Steve, a former Navy captain who had heard about my interest in neglect and wanted to see me in San Diego for a consultation. "In fact, other than a headache, I felt good. Not wanting to worry my wife—knowing full well I'd had a heart attack and that the head pain was subsiding—I told her that she should not worry; I was fine.

"She responded, 'No, you're not, Steve. You've had a stroke!'

"A stroke? This statement left me both surprised and slightly amused. I'd seen stroke victims on television and in real life, people who either stared into nothingness or showed clear signs of paralysis in a limb or in the face. Since I perceived none of these symptoms, I could not believe my wife was anywhere near correct.

"Actually, I was completely paralyzed on the left side of my body. Both my left arm and left leg were affected as well as my face. Thus began my odyssey into a strange warped world.

"To my mind, I was fully aware of all parts of my body on the right side. The left side simply did not exist! You might feel I'm exaggerating. Someone looking at me would see a person with limbs that, though paralyzed, obviously exist and are just as obviously connected to my body.

"When I shaved, I neglected the left side of my face. When I dressed, I would incessantly leave the left arm outside its sleeve. I would incorrectly button the right button side of my clothing to the left buttonholes, even though I had to complete this operation with my right hand.

"There is no way," Steve concluded, "that you can have any idea of what happens in Wonderland unless a denizen describes it to you."

Neglect is clinically important for two reasons. First, although a majority of patients recover completely after a few weeks, there is a subset in whom the disorder can persist indefinitely. For them, neglect remains a genuine nuisance even though it may not be a life-threatening disorder. Second, even those patients who seem to recover from neglect quickly can be seriously handicapped because their indifference to the left during the first few days hinders rehabilitation. When a physical therapist urges them to exercise the left arm, they don't see the point in doing so because they don't notice that it is not performing well. This is a problem because in stroke rehabilitation most recovery from paralysis occurs in the first few weeks and after this "window of plasticity," the left hand tends not to regain function. Physicians, therefore, do their utmost to coax people into using their left hands and legs in the first few weeks—a task frustrated by the neglect syndrome.

Is there some trick you could use to make the patient accept the left side of the world and start noticing that her arm was not moving? What would happen if you put a mirror on the patient's right side at right angles to her shoulder? (If she were sitting in a phone booth, this would correspond to the right wall of the booth.) If she now looks in the mirror, she will see the *reflection* of everything on her left side, including people, events and objects, as well as her own left arm. But since the reflection itself is on the right—in her nonneglected field—would she suddenly start paying attention to these things? Would she realize that these people, events and objects were on her left even though the reflection of them is on the right? If it worked, a trick of this kind would be nothing short of a miracle. Efforts to treat neglect have frustrated patients and physicians alike ever since the condition was first clinically described more than sixty years ago.

I telephoned Sam and asked whether his mother, Ellen, might be interested in trying out the mirror idea. It might help Ellen recover more quickly and it was easy enough to try.

The manner in which the brain deals with mirror reflections has long fascinated psychologists, philosophers and magicians alike. Many a child has asked the question "Why does a mirror reverse things left to right but not reverse them upside down? How does the mirror 'know' which way it should reverse?"—a question that most parents find embarrassingly difficult to answer. The correct answer to this question comes from the physicist Richard Feynman (as quoted by Richard Gregory, who has written a delightful book on this topic).[6]

Normal adults rarely confuse a mirror reflection for a real object. When you spot a car fast approaching you in your rearview mirror, you don't jam on your brakes. You accelerate forward even though it appears that the image of the car is approaching rapidly from the front. Likewise, if a burglar opened the door behind you as you were shaving in the bathroom, you'd spin around to confront him—not attack the reflection in the mirror. Some part of your brain must be making the needed correction: The real object is behind me even though the image is in front of me.[7]

But like Alice in Wonderland, patients like Ellen and Steve seem to inhabit a strange no-man's-land between illusion and reality—a "warped world," as Steve called it, and there is no easy way to predict how they will react to a mirror. Even though all of us, neglect patients and normal people alike, are familiar with mirrors and take them for granted, there is something inherently surrealistic about mirror images. The optics are simple enough, but no one has any inkling of what brain mechanisms are activated when we look at a mirror reflection, of what brain processes are involved in our special ability to comprehend the paradoxical juxtaposition of a real object and its optical "twin." Given the right parietal lobe's important role in dealing with spatial relationships and "holistic" aspects of vision, would a neglect patient have special problems dealing with mirror reflections?

When Ellen came to my lab, I first conducted a series of simple clinical tests to confirm the diagnosis of hemineglect. She flunked every one of them. First, I asked her to sit on a chair facing me and to look at my nose. I then took a pen, held it up to her right ear and began to move it slowly, in a sweeping arc, all the way to her left ear. I asked Ellen to follow the pen with her eyes, and she did so with no trouble until I reached her nose. At that point her eyes began to wander off, and soon she was looking at me, having "lost sight of" the pen near her nose. Paradoxically, a person who is really blind in her left visual field wouldn't display this behavior. If anything, she would try to move her eyes ahead of the pen in an effort to compensate for her blindness.

Next, I showed Ellen a horizontal line drawn on a sheet of paper and asked her to bisect it with a vertical mark. Ellen pursed her lips, took the pen and confidently placed a mark to the far right of the line because for her only half a line existed—the right half—and she was presumably marking the center of that half.[8]

When I asked her to draw a clock, Ellen made a full circle instead of just a half circle. This is a fairly common response because circle drawing is a highly overlearned motor response and the stroke did not compromise it. But when it came time for Ellen to fill in the numbers, she stopped, stared hard at the circle and then proceeded to write the numbers 1 to 12, cramped entirely on the right side of the circle!

Finally, I took a sheet of paper, put it in front of Ellen and asked her to draw a flower.

"What kind of flower?" she said.

"Any kind. Just an ordinary flower."

Again, Ellen paused, as if the task were difficult, and finally drew another circle. So far so good. Then she painstakingly drew a series of little petals—it was a daisy—all scrunched on the right side of the flower (Figure 6.1).

"That's fine, Ellen," I said. "Now I want you to do something different. I want you to close your eyes and draw a flower."

Ellen's inability to draw the left half of objects was to be expected, since she ignores the left when her eyes are open. But what would happen with them closed? Would the mental representation of a flower—the daisy in her mind's eye—be a whole flower or just half of one? In other words, how deep does the neglect reverberate into her brain?

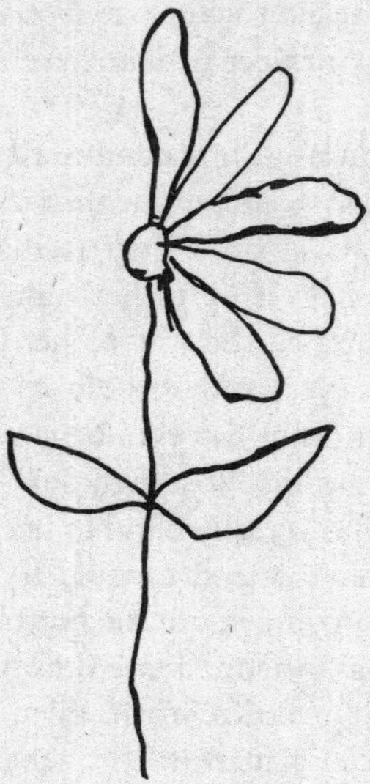

Figure 6.1 *Drawing made by a neglect patient. Notice that the left half of the flower is missing.*

Many neglect patients will also draw only half the flower when drawing from memory—even with their eyes closed. This implies that the patient has also lost the ability to "scan" the left side of the internal mental picture of the flower.

Ellen closed her eyes and drew another circle. Then, furrowing her brow in concentration, she daintily drew five petals—all on the right side of the daisy! It was as though the internal template she used to produce the drawing was only half preserved and therefore the left side of the flower simply drops out, even when she's just imagining it.

After a half-hour break, we returned to the lab to try out the mirror. She sat in her wheelchair, fluffing up her hair with her good hand, and smiled sweetly. I stood on her right holding a mirror on my chest so that when Ellen faced straight forward in the chair, the mirror was parallel to the right arm of the wheelchair (and her profile) and about two feet away from her nose. I then asked her to turn her head about sixty degrees and look into the mirror.

From this vantage point Ellen can clearly see the neglected side of the world reflected in the mirror. She is looking to her right, into her good side, so to speak, and she knows perfectly well what a mirror is, so she knows that it is reflecting objects on her left side. Since the information about the left side of the world is now coming from the right side—the nonneglected side—would the mirror help her "overcome" her neglect so that she correctly reached for the objects on the left, just as a normal person might? Or would she say to herself, "Oops, that object is really in my neglected field, so let me ignore it." The answer, as so often happens in science, was that she did neither. In fact, she did something completely outlandish.

Ellen looked in the mirror and blinked, curious about what we were up to. It ought to have been obvious to her that it was a mirror since it had a wooden frame and dust on its surface, but to be absolutely sure, I asked, "What is this I am holding?" (Remember I was behind the mirror, holding it.)

She replied without hesitating, "A mirror."

I asked her to describe her eyeglasses, lipstick and clothing while looking straight into the mirror. She did so with no trouble. On receiving a cue, one of my students standing on Ellen's left side held out a pen so that it was well within the reach of her good right hand but entirely within the neglected left visual field. (This turned out to be about eight inches below and to the left of her nose.) Ellen could see my student's arm as well as the pen clearly in the mirror, as there was no intent to deceive her about the presence of a mirror.

"Do you see the pen?"

"Yes."

"Okay, please reach out and grab it and write your name on this pad of paper I've placed in your lap."

Imagine my astonishment when Ellen lifted her right hand and without hesitation went straight for the mirror and began banging on it repeatedly. She literally clawed at it for about twenty seconds and said, obviously frustrated, "It's not in my reach."

When I repeated the same process ten minutes later, she said, "It's behind the mirror," and reached around and began groping with my belt buckle.

A little later she even tried peeking over the edge of the mirror to look for the pen.

So Ellen was behaving as though the reflection were a real object that she could reach out and grab. In my fifteen-year career, I'd never seen anything like this—a perfectly intelligent, levelheaded adult making the absurd blunder of thinking that an object was actually inside the mirror.

We wanted to make sure that Ellen's behavior did not arise from some clumsiness of her arm movements or a failure to understand what mirrors are. So we simply tried placing the mirror at arm's length in front of her, just like a bathroom mirror at home. This time the pen appeared just behind and above her right shoulder (but just outside her visual field). She saw it in the mirror and her hand went straight back behind her to grab it. So her failure in the earlier task could not be explained by claiming that she was disoriented, clumsy or confused as a result of her stroke.

We decided to give a name to Ellen's condition—"mirror agnosia" or "the looking glass syndrome" in honor of Lewis Carroll. Indeed, Lewis Carroll is known to have suffered from migraine attacks caused by arterial spasms. If they affected his right parietal lobe, he may have suffered momentary confusion with mirrors that might not only have inspired him to write *Through the Looking Glass* but may help explain his general obsession with mirrors, mirror writing and left-right reversal. One wonders whether Leonardo da Vinci's preoccupation with left-right reversed writing had a similar origin.

The looking glass syndrome was intriguing to watch, but it was also frustrating because I had initially hoped for the exact opposite reaction—that the mirror would make Ellen more aware of the left side of the world and help with rehabilitation.

The next step was to find out how widespread this syndrome is. Do all neglect patients behave like Ellen? In testing another twenty patients, I found that many had the same kind of mirror agnosia. They would reach into the mirror for the pen or a piece of candy when it was held in the neglected field. They knew perfectly well they were looking into a mirror and yet they made the same mistake as Ellen.

Not all of the patients made this error, however. Some of them initially looked perplexed, but upon seeing the reflection of the pen or candy in the mirror, they chuckled, and—with a conspiratorial air—reached correctly for the object on the left just as you or I might. One patient even turned his head to the left—something he was ordinarily reluctant to do—and beamed triumphantly as he snatched the reward. These few patients were clearly paying attention to objects they had previously ignored, raising a fascinating therapeutic possibility. Will repeated exposure to the mirror help some people overcome neglect, gradually becoming more aware of the left side of the world?[9] We are hoping to try this someday in the clinic.

Therapy aside, the scientist in me is equally intrigued by mirror agnosia—the patient's *failure* to reach correctly for the real object. Even my two-year-old son, when shown candy only visible in the mirror, giggled, turned around and snatched the sweet. Yet the much older and wiser Ellen could not do this.

I can think of at least two interpretations of why she might lack this ability. First, it's possible that the syndrome is caused by her neglect. It's as though the patient was saying to herself, unconsciously, "Since the reflection is in the mirror, the object must be on my left. But the left does not exist on my planet—therefore, the object must be inside the mirror." However absurd this interpretation may seem to us with our intact brains, it's the only one that would make any sense to Ellen, given her "reality."

Second, the looking glass syndrome may not be a direct consequence of neglect, even though it is usually accompanied by neglect. We know that when the right parietal lobe is damaged, patients have all kinds of difficulties with spatial tasks, and the looking glass syndrome may simply be an especially florid manifestation of such deficits. Responding correctly to a mirror image requires you simultaneously to hold in your mind the reflection as well as the object that is producing it and then perform the required mental gymnastics to locate correctly the object that produced the reflection. This very subtle ability may be compromised by lesions in the right parietal lobe, given the important role of that structure in dealing with spatial attributes of the world. If so, mirror agnosia might provide a new bedside test for detecting right parietal lesions.[10] In an age of escalating costs of brain imaging, any simple new test would be a useful addition to the neurologist's diagnostic kit.

The strangest aspect of the looking glass syndrome, however, is listening to patients' reactions.

"Doctor, why can't I reach the pen?"

"The darn mirror is in the way."

"The pen is inside the mirror and I can't reach it!"

"Ellen, I want you to grab the real object, not the reflection. Where is the real object?" She replied, "The real object is out there behind the mirror, doctor."

It's astonishing that the mere confrontation with a mirror flips these patients into the twilight zone so that they are unable—or reluctant—to draw the simple logical inference that since the reflection is on the right, the object producing it must be on the left. It's as though for these patients even the laws of optics have changed, at least for this small corner of their universe. We ordinarily think of our intellect and "high-level" knowledge—such as laws concerning geometrical optics—as being immune to the vagaries of sensory input. But these patients teach us that this is not always true. Indeed, for them it's the other way around. Not only is their sensory world warped, but their knowledge base is twisted to accommodate the strange new world they inhabit.[11] Their attention deficits seem to permeate their whole outlook, rendering them unable to tell whether a mirror reflection is a real object or not, even though they can carry on normal conversations on other topics—politics, sports or chess—just as well as you or I. Asking these patients what is the "true location" of the object they see in the mirror is like asking a normal person what is north of the North Pole. Or whether an irrational number (like the square root of 2 or π with a never-ending string of decimals) *really* exists or not. This raises profound philosophical questions about how sure we can be that our own grasp on reality is all that secure. An alien four-dimensional creature watching us from his four-dimensional world might regard our behavior to be just as perverse, inept and absurdly comical as we regard the bumblings of neglect patients trapped in their strange looking-glass world.

CHAPTER 7

The Sound of One Hand Clapping

Man is made by his belief. As he believes, so he is.

—Bhagavad Gita, *500 B.C.*

The social scientists have a long way to go to catch up, but they may be up to the most important scientific business of all, if and when they finally get to the right questions. Our behavior toward each other is the strangest, most unpredictable, and almost entirely unaccountable of the phenomena with which we are obliged to live.

—*Lewis Thomas*

Mrs. Dodds was beginning to lose patience. Why was everyone around her—doctors, therapists, even her son—insisting that her left arm was paralyzed when she knew perfectly well it was working fine? Why, just ten minutes ago she had used it to wash her face.

She knew, of course, that she had had a stroke two weeks ago and that was why she was here, at the University of California Medical Center in Hillcrest. Except for a small headache, she was feeling better now and wished she could go home to clip her rose bushes and resume her daily morning walks along the beach near Point Loma, where she lived. She had seen her granddaughter Becky just yesterday and was thinking how nice it would be to show off to her the garden now that it was in full bloom.

Mrs. Dodds was in fact completely paralyzed on the left side of her body after a stroke that damaged the right hemisphere of her brain. I see many such patients every month. Usually they have many questions about their paralysis. When will I walk again, doctor? Will I be able to wiggle my fingers again? When I yawned this morning, my left arm started to move a little—does that mean I'm starting to recover?

But there is a small subset of patients with right hemisphere damage who, like Mrs. Dodds, seem blissfully indifferent to their predicament—apparently unaware of the fact that the entire left side of their body is paralyzed—even though they are quite mentally lucid in all other respects. This curious disorder—the tendency to ignore or sometimes even to deny the fact that one's left arm or leg is paralyzed—was termed anosognosia ("unaware of illness") by the French neurologist Joseph François Babinski who first observed it clinically in 1908.

"Mrs. Dodds, how are you feeling today?"

"Well, doctor, I have a headache. You know they brought me to the hospital."

"Why did you come to the hospital, Mrs. Dodds?"

"Oh, well," she said, "I had a stroke."

"How do you know?"

"I fell down in the bathroom two weeks ago and my daughter brought me here. They did some brain scans and took X rays and told me I had a stroke." Obviously Mrs. Dodds knew what had occurred and was aware of her surroundings.

"Okay," I said. "And how are you feeling now?"

"Fine."

"Can you walk?"

"Sure I can walk." Mrs. Dodds had been lying in her bed or sitting propped up in a wheelchair for the past two weeks. She had not taken a single step since her fall in the bathroom.

"What about your hands? Hold out your hands. Can you move them?"

Mrs. Dodds seemed mildly annoyed by my questions. "Of course I can use my hands," she said.

"Can you use your right hand?"

"Yes."

"Can you use your left hand?"

"Yes, I can use my left hand."

"Are both hands equally strong?"

"Yes, they are both equally strong."

Now this raises an interesting question: How far can you push this line of questioning in these patients? Physicians are generally reluctant to keep on prodding for fear of precipitating what the neurologist Kurt Goldstein called a "catastrophic reaction," which is simply medical jargon for "the patient starts sobbing" because her defenses crumble. But I thought, if I took her gently, one step at a time, before actually confronting her with her paralysis, perhaps I could prevent such a reaction.[1]

"Mrs. Dodds, can you touch my nose with your right hand?"

She did so with no trouble.

"Can you touch my nose with your left hand?"

Her hand lay paralyzed in front of her.

"Mrs. Dodds, are you touching my nose?"

"Yes, of course I'm touching your nose."

"Can you actually see yourself touching my nose?"

"Yes, I can see it. It's less than an inch from your face."

At this point Mrs. Dodds produced a frank confabulation, almost a hallucination, that her finger was nearly touching my nose. Her vision was fine. She could see her arm perfectly clearly, yet she was insisting that she could see the arm move.

I decided to ask just one more question. "Mrs. Dodds, can you clap?"

With resigned patience she said, "Of course I can clap."

"Will you clap for me?"

Mrs. Dodds glanced up at me and proceeded to make clapping movements with her right hand, as if clapping with an imaginary hand near the midline.

"Are you clapping?"

"Yes, I'm clapping," she replied.

I didn't have the heart to ask her whether she actually heard herself clapping, but, had I done so, we might have found the answer to the Zen master's eternal koan or riddle—what is the sound of one hand clapping?

One doesn't need to invoke Zen koans, however, to realize that Mrs. Dodds presents us with a puzzle every bit as enigmatic as the struggle to understand the nondual nature of reality. Why does this woman, who is apparently sane, intelligent and articulate, deny that she's paralyzed? After all, she's been confined to a wheelchair for nearly two weeks. There must have been scores of occasions when she tried to grab something or just reach out with her left hand, yet all the while it lay lifeless in her lap. How can she possibly insist that she "sees" herself touching my nose?

Actually, Mrs. Dodd's confabulation is on the extreme end of the scale. Denial patients more commonly concoct inane excuses or rationalizations why their left arms do not move when asked to demonstrate the use of that arm. Most don't claim that they can actually see the limp arm moving.

For example, when I asked a woman named Cecilia why she was not touching my nose, she replied with a hint of exasperation, "Well, doctor, I mean these medical students, they've been prodding and poking at me all day. I'm sick of it. I don't want to move my arm."

Another patient, Esmerelda, took a different strategy.

"Esmerelda, how are you doing?"

"I'm fine."

"Can you walk?"

"Yes."

"Can you use your arms?"

"Yes."

"Can you use your right arm?"

"Yes."

"Can you use your left arm?"

"Yes, I can use my left arm."

"Can you point to me with your right hand?"

She pointed straight at me with her good right hand.

"Can you point to me with your left?"

Her left hand lay motionless in front of her.

"Esmerelda, are you pointing?"

"I have severe arthritis in my shoulder; you know that, doctor. It hurts. I can't move my arm now."

On other occasions she employed other excuses: "Well, I've never been very ambidextrous, doctor."

Watching these patients is like observing human nature through a magnifying lens; I'm reminded of all aspects of human folly and of how prone to self-deception we all are. For here, embodied in one elderly woman in a wheelchair, is a comically exaggerated version of all those psychological defense mechanisms that Sigmund and Anna Freud talked about at the beginning of the twentieth century—mechanisms used by you, me and everyone else when we are confronted with disturbing facts about ourselves. Freud claimed that our minds use these various psychological tricks to "defend the ego." His ideas have such intuitive appeal that many of the words he used have infiltrated popular parlance, although no one thinks of them as science because he never did any experiments. (We shall return to Freud later in this chapter to see how anosognosia may give us an experimental handle on these elusive aspects of the mind.)

In the most extreme cases, a patient will not only deny that the arm (or leg) is paralyzed, but assert that the arm lying in the bed next to him, his own paralyzed arm, doesn't belong to him! There's an unbridled willingness to accept absurd ideas.

Not long ago, at the Rivermead Rehabilitation Center in Oxford, England, I gripped a woman's lifeless left hand and, raising it, held it in front of her eyes. "Whose arm is this?"

She looked me in the eye and huffed, "What's that arm doing in my bed?"

"Well, whose arm is it?"

"That's my brother's arm," she said flatly. But her brother was nowhere in the hospital. He lives somewhere in Texas. The woman displayed what we call somatoparaphrenia—the denial of ownership of one's own body parts—which is occasionally seen in conjunction with anosognosia. Needless to say, both conditions are quite rare.

"Why do you think it's your brother's arm?"

"Because it's big and hairy, doctor, and I don't have hairy arms."

•

Anosognosia is an extraordinary syndrome about which almost nothing is known. The patient is obviously sane in most respects yet claims to see her lifeless limb springing into action—clapping or touching my nose—and fails to realize the absurdity of it all. What causes this curious disorder? Not surprisingly, there have been dozens of theories[2] to explain anosognosia. Most can be classified into two main categories. One is a Freudian view, that the patient simply doesn't want to confront the unpleasantness of his or her paralysis. The second is a neurological view, that denial is a direct consequence of the neglect syndrome, discussed in the previous chapter—the general indifference to everything on the left side of the world. Both categories of explanation have many problems, but they also contain nuggets of insight that we can use to build a new theory of denial.

One problem with the Freudian view is that it doesn't explain the difference in magnitude of psychological defense mechanisms between patients with anosognosia and what is seen in normal people—why they are generally subtle in you and me and wildly exaggerated in denial patients. For example, if I were to fracture my left arm and damage certain nerves and you asked me whether I could beat you in a game of tennis, I might tend to play down my injury a little, asserting, "Oh, yes, I can beat you. My arm is getting much better now, you know." But I certainly wouldn't take a bet that I could arm wrestle you. Or if my arm were completely paralyzed, hanging limp at my side, I would not say, "Oh, I can see it touching your nose" or "It belongs to my brother."

The second problem with the Freudian view is that it doesn't explain the asymmetry of this syndrome. The kind of denial seen in Mrs. Dodds and others is almost always associated with damage to the right hemisphere of the brain, resulting in paralysis of the body's left side. When people suffer damage to the left brain hemisphere, with paralysis on the body's right side, they almost never experience denial. Why not? They are as disabled and frustrated as people with right hemisphere damage, and presumably there is just as much "need" for psychological defense, but in fact they are not only aware of the paralysis, but constantly talk about it. Such asymmetry implies that we must look not to psychology but to neurology for an answer, particularly in the details of how the brain's two hemispheres are specialized for different tasks. Indeed, the syndrome seems to straddle the border between the two disciplines, one reason it is so fascinating.

Neurological theories of denial reject the Freudian view completely. They argue instead that denial is a direct consequence of neglect, which also occurs after right hemisphere damage and leaves patients profoundly indifferent to everything that goes on within the left side of the world, including the left side of their own bodies. Perhaps the patient with anosognosia simply doesn't notice that her left arm is not moving in response to her commands, and hence the delusion.

I find two main problems with this approach. One is that neglect and denial can occur independently—some patients with neglect do not experience denial and vice versa. Second, neglect does not account for why denial usually persists even when the patient's attention is drawn to the paralysis. For instance, if I were to force a patient to turn his head and focus on his left arm, to demonstrate to him that it's not obeying his command, he may adamantly continue to deny that it's paralyzed—or even that it belongs to him. It is this vehemence of the denial—not a mere indifference to paralysis—that cries out for an explanation. Indeed, the reason anosognosia is so puzzling is that we have come to regard the "intellect" as primarily propositional in character—that is, certain conclusions follow incontrovertibly from certain premises—and one ordinarily expects propositional logic to be internally consistent. To listen to a patient deny ownership of her arm and yet, in the same breath, admit that it is attached to her shoulder is one of the most perplexing phenomena that one can encounter as a neurologist.

So neither the Freudian view nor the neglect theory provides an adequate explanation for the spectrum of deficits that one sees in anosognosia. The correct way to approach the problem, I realized, is to ask two questions: First, why do normal people engage in all these psychological defense mechanisms? Second, why are the same mechanisms so exaggerated in these patients? Psychological defenses in normal people are especially puzzling because at first glance they seem detrimental to survival.[3] Why would it enhance my survival to cling tenaciously to false beliefs about myself and the world? If I were a puny weakling who believed that I was as strong as Hercules, I'd soon get into serious trouble with the "alpha male" in my social group—my chairman, the president of my company or even my next-door neighbor. But, as Charles Darwin pointed out, if one sees something apparently maladaptive in biology, then look more deeply, because there is often a hidden agenda.

The key to the whole puzzle, I suggest, lies in the division of labor between our two cerebral hemispheres and in our need to create a sense of coherence and continuity in our lives. Most people are familiar with the fact that the human brain consists of two mirror image halves—like the two halves of a walnut—with each half, or cerebral hemisphere, controlling movements on the opposite side of the body. A century of clinical neurology has shown clearly that the two hemispheres are specialized for different mental capacities and that the most striking asymmetry involves language. The left hemisphere is specialized not only for the actual production of speech sounds but also for the imposition of syntactic structure on speech and for much of what is called semantics—comprehension of meaning. The right hemisphere, on the other hand, doesn't govern spoken words but seems to be concerned with more subtle aspects of language such as nuances of metaphor, allegory and ambiguity—skills that are inadequately emphasized in our elementary schools but that are vital for the advance of civilizations through poetry, myth and drama. We tend to call the left hemisphere the major or "dominant" hemisphere because it, like a chauvinist, does all the talking (and maybe much of the internal thinking as well), claiming to be the repository of humanity's highest attribute, language. Unfortunately, the mute right hemisphere can do nothing to protest.

Other obvious specializations involve vision and emotion. The right hemisphere is concerned with holistic aspects of vision such as seeing the forest for the trees, reading facial expressions and responding with the appropriate emotion to evocative situations. Consequently, after right hemisphere strokes, patients tend to be blissfully unconcerned about their predicament, even mildly euphoric, because without the "emotional right hemisphere" they simply don't comprehend the magnitude of their loss. (This is true even of those patients who are aware of their paralysis.)

In addition to these obvious divisions of labor, I want to suggest an even more fundamental difference between the cognitive styles of the two hemispheres,[4] one that not only helps explain the amplified defense mechanisms of anosognosia but may also help account for the more mundane forms of denial that people use in daily life—such as when an alcoholic refuses to acknowledge his drinking problem or when you deny your forbidden attraction to a married colleague.

•

At any given moment in our waking lives, our brains are flooded with a bewildering array of sensory inputs, all of which must be incorporated into a coherent perspective that's based on what stored memories already tell us is true about ourselves and the world. In order to generate coherent actions, the brain must have some way of sifting through this superabundance of detail and of ordering it into a stable and internally consistent "belief system"—a story that makes sense of the available evidence. Each time a new item of information comes in we fold it seamlessly into our preexisting worldview. I suggest that this is mainly done by the left hemisphere.

But now suppose something comes along that does not quite fit the plot. What do you do? One option is to tear up the entire script and start from scratch: completely revise your story to create a new model about the world and about yourself. The problem is that if you did this for every little piece of threatening information, your behavior would soon become chaotic and unstable; you would go mad.

What your left hemisphere does instead is either ignore the anomaly completely or distort it to squeeze it into your preexisting framework, to preserve stability. And this, I suggest, is the essential rationale behind all the so-called Freudian defenses—the denials, repressions, confabulations and other forms of self-delusion that govern our daily lives. Far from being maladaptive, such everyday defense mechanisms prevent the brain from being hounded into directionless indecision by the "combinatorial explosion" of possible stories that might be written from the material available to the senses. The penalty, of course, is that you are "lying" to yourself, but it's a small price to pay for the coherence and stability conferred on the system as a whole.

Imagine, for example, a military general about to wage war on the enemy. It is late at night and he is in the war room planning strategies for the next day. Scouts keep coming into the room to give him information about the lay of the land, terrain, light level and so forth. They also tell him that the enemy has five hundred tanks and that he has six hundred tanks, a fact that prompts the general to decide to wage war. He positions all of his troops in strategic locations and decides to launch battle exactly at 6:00 A.M. with sunrise.

Imagine further that at 5:55 A.M. one little scout comes running into the war room and says, "General! I have bad news." With minutes to go until battle, the general asks, "What is that?" and the scout replies, "I just looked through binoculars and saw that the enemy has seven hundred tanks, not five hundred!"

What does the general—the left hemisphere—do? Time is of the essence and he simply can't afford the luxury of revising all his battle plans. So he orders the scout to shut up and tell no one about what he saw. Denial! Indeed, he may even shoot the scout and hide the report in a drawer labeled "top secret" (repression). In doing so, he relies on the high probability that the majority opinion—the previous information by all the scouts—was correct and that this single new item of information coming from one source is probably wrong. So the general sticks to his original position. Not only that, but for fear of mutiny, he might order the scout actually to lie to the other generals and tell them that he only saw five hundred tanks (confabulation). The purpose of all of this is to impose stability on behavior and to prevent vacillation because indecisiveness doesn't serve any purpose. Any decision, so long as it is *probably* correct, is better than no decision at all. A perpetually fickle general will never win a war!

In this analogy, the general is the left hemisphere[5] (Freud's "ego," perhaps?), and his behavior is analogous to the kinds of denials and repressions you see in both healthy people and patients with anosognosia. But why are these defense mechanisms so grossly exaggerated in the patients? Enter the right hemisphere, which I like to call the Devil's Advocate. To see how this works, we need to push the analogy a step further. Supposing the single scout comes running in, and instead of saying the enemy has more tanks, he declares, "General, I just looked through my telescope and the enemy has nuclear weapons." The general would be very foolish indeed to adhere to his original plan. He must quickly formulate a new one, for if the scout were correct, the consequences would be devastating.

Thus the coping strategies of the two hemispheres are fundamentally different. The left hemisphere's job is to create a belief system or model and to fold new experiences into that belief system. If confronted with some new information that doesn't fit the model, it relies on Freudian defense mechanisms to deny, repress or confabulate—anything to preserve the status quo. The right hemisphere's strategy, on the other hand, is to play "Devil's Advocate," to question the status quo and look for global inconsistencies. When the anomalous information reaches a certain threshold, the right hemisphere decides that it is time to force a complete revision of the entire model and start from scratch. The right hemisphere thus forces a "Kuhnian paradigm shift" in response to anomalies, whereas the left hemisphere always tries to cling tenaciously to the way things were.

Now consider what happens if the right hemisphere is damaged.[6] The left hemisphere is then given free rein to pursue its denials, confabulations and other strategies, as it normally does. It says, "I am Mrs. Dodds, a person with two normal arms that I have commanded to move." But her brain is insensitive to the contrary visual feedback that would ordinarily tell her that her arm is paralyzed and that she's in a wheelchair. Thus Mrs. Dodds is caught in a delusional cul-de-sac. She cannot revise her model of reality because her right hemisphere, with its mechanisms for detecting discrepancies, is out of order. And in the absence of the counterbalance or "reality check" provided by the right hemisphere, there is literally no limit to how far she will wander along the delusional path. Patients will say, "Yes, I'm touching your nose, Dr. Ramachandran," or "All of the medical students have been prodding me and that's why I don't want to move my arm." Or even, "What is my brother's hand doing in my bed, doctor?"

The idea that the right hemisphere is a left-wing revolutionary that generates paradigm shifts, whereas the left hemisphere is a die-hard conservative that clings to the status quo, is almost certainly a gross oversimplification, but, even if it turns out to be wrong, it does suggest new ways of doing experiments and goads us into asking novel questions about the denial syndrome. How deep is the denial? Does the patient really believe he's not paralyzed? What if you were to confront patients directly: Could you then force them to admit the paralysis? Would they deny only their paralysis, or would they deny other aspects of their illness as well? Given that people often think of their car as part of their extended "body image"(especially here in California), what would happen if the front left fender of their car were damaged? Would they deny that?

Anosognosia has been known for almost a century, yet there have been very few attempts to answer these questions. Any light we could shed on this strange syndrome would be clinically important, of course, because the patients' indifference to their predicament not only is an impediment to rehabilitation of the weak arm or leg, but often leads them to unrealistic future goals. (For example, when I asked one man whether he could go back to his old occupation of repairing telephone lines—a job that requires two hands for climbing poles and splicing wires—he said, "Oh, yes, I don't see a problem there.") What I didn't realize, though, when I began these experiments, was that they would take me right into the heart of human nature. For denial is something we do all our lives, whether we are temporarily ignoring the bills accumulating in our "to do" tray or defiantly denying the finality and humiliation of death.

•

Talking to denial patients can be an uncanny experience. They bring us face to face with some of the most fundamental questions one can ask as a conscious human being: What is the self? What brings about the unity of my conscious experience? What does it mean to will an action? Neuroscientists tend to shy away from such questions, but anosognosia patients afford a unique opportunity for experimentally approaching these seemingly intractable philosophical riddles.

Relatives are often bewildered by their loved ones' behavior. "Does Mom really believe she's not paralyzed?" asked one young man. "Surely, there must be some recess of her mind that knows what's happened. Or has she gone totally bonkers?"

Our first and most obvious question, therefore, is, How deeply does the patient believe his own denials or confabulations? Could it be some sort of surface facade or even an attempt at malingering? To answer this question, I devised a simple experiment. Instead of directly confronting the patient by asking him to respond verbally (can you touch my nose with your left hand?), what if I were to "trick" him by asking him to perform a spontaneous motor task that requires two hands—before he has had a chance to think about it. How would he respond?

To find out, I placed a large cocktail tray supporting six plastic glasses half filled with water in front of patients with denial syndrome. Now if I asked you to reach out and grab such a tray, you would place one hand under either side of the tray and proceed to raise it. But if you had one hand tied behind your back, you would naturally go for the middle of the tray—its center of gravity—and lift from there. When I tested stroke patients who were paralyzed on one side of their body but did not suffer from denial, their nonparalyzed hand went straight for the middle of the tray, as expected.

When I tried the same experiment on denial patients, their right hands went straight to the right side of the tray while the left side of the tray remained unsupported. Naturally, when the right hand lifted only the right side of the tray, the glasses toppled, but the patients often attributed this to momentary clumsiness rather than a failure to lift the left side of the tray ("Ooops! How silly of me!"). One woman even denied that she had failed to lift the tray. When I asked her whether she had lifted the tray successfully, she was surprised. "Yes, of course," she replied, her lap all soggy.

The logic of a second experiment was somewhat different. What if one were actually to reward the patient for honesty? To investigate this, I gave our patients a choice between a simple task that can be done with one hand and an equally simple task that requires the use of two hands. Specifically, patients were told that they could earn five dollars if they threaded a light bulb into a bare socket on a heavy table lamp or ten dollars if they could tie a pair of shoelaces. You or I would naturally go for the shoelaces, but most paralyzed stroke patients—who do not suffer from denial—choose the light bulb, knowing their limitations. Obviously five dollars is better than nothing. Remarkably, when we tested four stroke patients who had denial, they opted for the shoelace task every time and spent minutes fiddling with the laces without showing any signs of frustration. Even when the patients were given the same choice ten minutes later they unhesitatingly went for the bimanual task. One woman repeated this bumbling behavior five times in a row, as though she had no memory of her previous failed attempts. A Freudian repression perhaps?

On one occasion, Mrs. Dodds kept on fumbling with the shoelaces using one hand, oblivious to her predicament, until finally I had to pull the shoe away. The next day my student asked her, "Do you remember Dr. Ramachandran?"

She was very pleasant. "Oh, yes, I remember. He's that Indian doctor."

"What did he do?"

"He gave me a child's shoe with blue dots on it and asked me to tie the shoelaces."

"Did you do it?"

"Oh, yes, I tied it successfully with both my hands," she replied.

Something odd was afoot. What normal person would say, "I tied the shoelace *with both my hands*"? It was almost as though inside Mrs. Dodds there lurked another human being—a phantom within—who knows perfectly well that she's paralyzed, and her strange remark was an attempt to mask this knowledge. Another intriguing example was a patient who volunteered, while I was examining him, "I can't wait to get back to two-fisted beer drinking." These peculiar remarks are striking examples of what Freud called a "reaction formation"—a subconscious attempt to disguise something that is threatening to your self-esteem by asserting the opposite. The classic illustration of a reaction formation, of course, comes from *Hamlet*, "Methinks the lady doth protest too much." Is not the very vehemence of her protest itself a betrayal of guilt?

•

Let us return now to the most widely accepted neurological explanation of denial—the idea that it has something to do with neglect, the general indifference that patients often display toward events and objects on the left side of the world. Perhaps when asked to perform an action with her left hand, Mrs. Dodds sends motor commands to the paralyzed arm and copies of these commands are simultaneously sent to her body image centers (in the parietal lobes), where they are monitored and experienced as felt movements. The parietal lobes are thus tipped off about what the intended actions are, but since she's ignoring events on the left side of her body, she also fails to notice that the arm did not obey her command. Although, as I argued earlier, this account is implausible, we did two simple experiments to test the neglect theory of denial directly.[7]

In the first experiment, I tested the idea that the patient is simply monitoring motor signals that are being sent to the arm. Larry Cooper is an intelligent fifty-six-year-old denial patient who had suffered a stroke one week before I went to visit him in the hospital. He lay under a blue and purple quilt his wife had brought to the room, with his arms flopped outside the covers—one paralyzed, one normal. We chatted for ten minutes and then I left the room, only to return five minutes later. "Mr. Cooper!" I exclaimed, approaching his bed. "Why did you just now move your left arm?" Both arms were dead still, in the same position as when I had left the room. I've tried this on normal people and the usual response is utter bewilderment. "What do you mean? I wasn't doing anything with my left arm" or "I don't understand; did I move my left arm?" Mr. Cooper looked at me calmly and said, "I was gesticulating to make a point!" When I repeated the experiment the next day, he said, "It hurts, so I moved it to relieve the pain."

Since there is no possibility that Mr. Cooper could have sent a motor command to his left arm at the exact moment I questioned him, the result suggests that denial stems not merely from a sensory motor deficit. On the contrary, his whole system of beliefs about himself is so profoundly deranged that there's apparently no limit to what he will do to protect these beliefs. Instead of acting befuddled, as a normal person might, he happily goes along with my deception because it makes perfect sense to him, given his worldview.

The second experiment was almost diabolical. What would happen, I wondered, if one were temporarily to "paralyze" the right arm of a denial patient whose left arm, of course, really is paralyzed. Would the denial now encompass his right arm as well? The neglect theory makes a very specific prediction—because he only neglects the left side of his body and not the right side, he should notice that the right arm isn't moving and say, "That's very odd, doctor; my arm isn't moving." (My theory, on the other hand, makes the opposite prediction: He should be insensitive to this "anomaly" since the discrepancy detector in his right hemisphere is damaged.)

To "paralyze" a denial patient's right arm, I devised a new version of the virtual reality box we had used in our phantom limb experiments. Again, it was a simple cardboard box with holes and mirrors, but they were positioned very differently. Our first subject was Betty Ward, a seventy-one-year-old retired schoolteacher who was mentally alert and happy to cooperate in the experiment. When Betty was comfortably seated, I asked her to put a long gray glove on her right hand (her good one) and insert it through a hole in front of the box. I then asked her to lean forward and peek into the box through a hole in the top to look at her gloved hand.

Next, I started a metronome and asked Betty to move her hand up and down in time with the ticking sounds.

"Can you see your hand moving, Betty?"

"Yes, sure," she said. "It's got the right rhythm."

Then I asked Betty to close her eyes. Without her knowledge, a mirror in the box flipped into position and an undergraduate stooge, who was hiding under the table, slipped his gray gloved hand into the box from a hole in the back. I asked Betty to open her eyes and look back into the box. She thought she was looking at her own right hand again, but, because of the mirror, she actually saw the student's hand. Previously I had told the stooge to keep his hand absolutely still.

"Okay, Betty. Keep looking. I'm going to start the metronome again and I want you to move your hand in time with it."

Tick, tock, tick, tock. Betty moved her hand but what she saw in the box was a perfectly still hand, a "paralyzed" hand. Now when you do this experiment with normal people, they jump out of their seat: "Hey, what's going on here?" Never in their wildest dreams would they imagine that an undergraduate was hiding under the table.

"Betty, what do you see?"

"Why, I see my right hand moving up and down, just like before," she replied.[8]

This suggests to me that Betty's denial crossed over to the right side of her body—the normal side with no neglect—for why else would she say that she could see a motionless hand in motion? This simple experiment demolishes the neglect theory of anosognosia and also gives us a clue for understanding what really causes the syndrome. What is damaged in these patients is the manner in which the brain deals with a discrepancy in sensory inputs concerning the body image; it's not critical whether the discrepancy arises from the left or right side of the body.

What we observed in Betty and in the other patients we've discussed so far supports the idea that the left hemisphere is a conformist, largely indifferent to discrepancies, whereas the right hemisphere is the opposite: highly sensitive to perturbation. But our experiments only provide circumstantial evidence for this theory. We needed direct proof.

Even a decade ago, an idea of this kind would have been impossible to test, but the advent of modern imaging techniques such as functional magnetic resonance (fMR) and positron emission tomography (PET) has tremendously accelerated the pace of research by allowing us to watch the living brain in action. Very recently, Ray Dolan, Chris Frith and their colleagues at the Queen Square Neurological Hospital for Neurological Diseases in London performed a beautiful experiment using the virtual reality box that we had used on our phantom limb patients. (Recall this is simply a vertical mirror propped in a box, perpendicular to the person's chest.) Each person inserted his left arm into the box and looked into the left side of the mirror at the reflection of his left arm so that it was optically superimposed on the felt location of his right arm. He was then asked to move both hands synchronously up and down, so that there was no discrepancy between the visual appearance of his moving right hand (actually the reflection of his left) and the kinesthetic movement sensations—from joints and muscles—emerging from his right hand. But if he now moved the two hands out of sync—as when doing the dog paddle—then there was a profound discrepancy between what the right hand appeared to be doing visually and what it *felt* it was doing. By doing a PET scan during this procedure, Dr. Frith was able to locate the center in the brain that monitors discrepancies; it is a small region of the right hemisphere that receives information from the right parietal lobe. Dr. Frith then did a second PET scan with the subject looking into the right side of the mirror at the reflection of his right hand (and moving his left hand out of sync) so the discrepancy in his body image now appeared to come from his *left* side rather than the right. Imagine my delight when I heard from Dr. Frith that once again the right hemisphere "lit up" in the scanner. It didn't seem to matter which side of the body the discrepancy arose from—right or left—it always activated the right hemisphere. This is welcome proof that my "speculative" ideas on hemispheric specialization are on the right track.

•

When I conduct clinical Grand Rounds—presenting a denial patient to medical students—one of the most common questions I am asked is "Do the patients only deny paralysis of body parts or do they deny other disabilities as well? If the patient stubbed her toe, would she deny the pain and swelling in that toe? Do they deny that they are seriously ill? If they suddenly had a migraine attack would they deny it?" Many neurologists have explored this in their patients, and the usual answer is that they don't deny other problems—like my patient Grace who, when I offered her candy if she could tie shoelaces, shot back at me, "You know I'm diabetic, doctor. I can't eat candy!"[9]

Almost all the patients I have tested are well aware of the fact that they've had a stroke and none of them suffers from what you might call "global denial." Yet there are gradations in their belief systems—and accompanying denials—that correlate with the location of their brain lesions. When the injury is confined to the right parietal lobe, confabulations and denials tend to be confined to body image. But when the damage occurs closer to the front of the right hemisphere (a part called the ventromedial frontal lobe), the denial is broader, more varied and oddly self-protective. I remember an especially striking example of this—a patient named Bill who came to see me six months after he had been diagnosed with a malignant brain tumor. The tumor had been growing rapidly and compressing his right frontal lobe, until it was eventually excised by the neurosurgeon. Unfortunately, by then it had already spread and Bill was told that he probably had less than a year to live. Now, Bill was a highly educated man and ought to have grasped the gravity of his situation, yet he seemed nonchalant about it and kept drawing my attention to a little blister on his cheek instead. He bitterly complained that the other doctors hadn't done anything about the blister and asked whether I could help him get rid of it. When I would return to the topic of the brain tumor, he avoided talking about it, saying things like "Well, you know how these doctors sometimes incorrectly diagnose things." So here was an intelligent person flatly contradicting the evidence provided by his physicians and glibly playing down the fact that he had terminal brain cancer. To avoid being hounded by a free-floating anxiety, he adopted the convenient strategy of attributing it to *something* tangible—and the blister was the most convenient target. Indeed, his obsession with the blister is what Freud would call a displacement mechanism—a disguised attempt to deflect his own attention from his impending death. Curiously, it is sometimes easier to deflect than to deny.[10]

The most extreme delusion I've ever heard of is one described by Oliver Sacks, about a man who kept falling out of bed at night. Each time he crashed to the floor, the ward staff would hoist him back up, only to hear a resounding thud a few moments later. After this happened several times, Dr. Sacks asked the man why he kept toppling out of bed. He looked frightened. "Doctor," he said, "these medical students have been putting a cadaver's arm in my bed and I've been trying to get rid of it all night!" Not admitting ownership of his paralyzed limb, the man was dragged to the floor each time he tried to push it away.

•

The experiments we discussed earlier suggest that a denial patient is not just trying to save face; the denial is anchored deep in her psyche.[11] But does this imply that the information about her paralysis is locked away somewhere—repressed? Or does it imply that the information doesn't exist anywhere in her brain? The latter view seems unlikely. If the knowledge doesn't exist, why does the patient say things like "I tied my shoelaces with *both my hands*" or "I can't wait to get back to two-fisted beer drinking"? And why evasive remarks like "I'm not ambidextrous"? Comments like these imply that "somebody" in there knows she is paralyzed, but that the information is not available to the conscious mind. If so, is there some way to access that forbidden knowledge?

To find out, we took advantage of an ingenious experiment performed in 1987 by an Italian neurologist, Eduardo Bisiach, on a patient with neglect and denial. Bisiach took a syringe filled with ice-cold water and irrigated the patient's left ear canal—a procedure that tests vestibular nerve function. Within a few seconds the patient's eyes started to move vigorously in a process called nystagmus. The cold water sets up a convection current in the ear canals, thereby fooling the brain into thinking the head is moving and into making involuntary correctional eye movements that we call nystagmus. When Bisiach then asked the denial patient whether she could use her arms, she calmly replied that she had no use of her left arm! Amazingly, the cold water irrigation of the left ear had brought about a complete (though temporary) remission from the anosognosia.

When I read about this experiment, I jumped out of my seat. Here was a neurological syndrome produced by a right parietal lesion that had been reversed by the simple act of squirting water into the ear. Why hadn't this amazing experiment made headlines in *The New York Times*? Indeed, I discovered that most of my professional colleagues had not even heard of the experiment. I therefore decided to try the same procedure on the next patient I saw with anosognosia.

This turned out to be Mrs. Macken, an elderly woman who three weeks earlier had suffered a right parietal stroke that resulted in left side paralysis. My purpose was not only to confirm Bisiach's observation but also to ask questions specifically to test her memory—something that hadn't been done systematically. If the patient suddenly started admitting that she was paralyzed, what would she say about her earlier denials? Would she deny her denials? If she admitted them, how would she account for them? Could she possibly tell us *why* she had been denying them, or is that an absurd question?

I had been seeing Mrs. Macken every three or four days for two weeks, and each time we had gone through the same rigmarole.

"Mrs. Macken, can you walk?"

"Yes, I can walk."

"Can you use both arms?"

"Yes."

"Are they equally strong?"

"Yes."

"Can you move your left hand?"

"Yes."

"Can you move your right hand?"

"Yes."

"Are they equally strong?"

"Yes."

After going through the questions, I filled a syringe with ice-cold water and squirted it into her ear canal. As expected, her eyes started moving in the characteristic way. After about a minute, I began to question her.

"How are you feeling, Mrs. Macken?"

"Well, my ear hurts. It's cold."

"Anything else? What about your arms? Can you move your arms?"

"Sure," she said.

"Can you walk?"

"Yes, I can walk."

"Can you use both your arms? Are they equally strong?"

"Yes, they are equally strong."

I wondered what these Italian scientists were talking about. But as I was driving home, I realized that I had squirted the water into the wrong ear! (Cold water in the left ear or warm water in the right ear causes the eyes to drift repetitively to the left and jump to the right. And the opposite is true. It's one of those things that many physicians get confused about, or at least I do. So I had inadvertently done the control experiment first!)

The next day we repeated the experiment on the other ear.

"Mrs. Macken, how are you doing?"

"Fine."

"Can you walk?"

"Sure."

"Can you use your right hand?"

"Yes."

"Can you use your left hand?"

"Yes."

"Are they equally strong?"

"Yes."

After the nystagmus, I asked again, "How are you feeling?"

"My ear's cold."

"What about your arms? Can you use your arms?"

"No," she replied, "my left arm is paralyzed."

That was the first time she had used that word in the three weeks since her stroke.

"Mrs. Macken, how long have you been paralyzed?"

She said, "Oh, continuously, all these days."

This was an extraordinary remark, for it implies that even though she had been denying her paralysis each time I had seen her over these last few weeks, the memories of her failed attempts had been registering somewhere in her brain, yet access to them had been blocked. The cold water acted as a "truth serum" that brought her repressed memories about her paralysis to the surface.

Half an hour later I went back to her and asked, "Can you use your arms?"

"No, my left arm is paralyzed." Even though the nystagmus had long since ceased, she still admitted she was paralyzed.

Twelve hours later, a student of mine visited her and asked, "Do you remember Dr. Ramachandran?"

"Oh, yes, he was that Indian doctor."

"And what did he do?"

"He took some ice-cold water and he put it into my left ear and it hurt."

"Anything else?"

"Well, he was wearing that tie with a brain scan on it." True, I was wearing a tie with a PET scan on it. Her memory for details was fine.

"What did he ask you?"

"He asked me if I could use both my arms."

"And what did you tell him?"

"I told him I was fine."

So now she was denying her earlier admission of paralysis, as though she were completely rewriting her "script." Indeed, it was almost as if we had created two separate conscious human beings who were mutually amnesic: the "cold water" Mrs. Macken, who is intellectually honest, who acknowledges her paralysis, and the Mrs. Macken without the cold water, who has the denial syndrome and adamantly denies her paralysis!

Watching the two Mrs. Mackens reminded me of the controversial clinical syndrome known as multiple personalities immortalized in fiction as Dr. Jekyll and Mr. Hyde. I say controversial because most of my more hard-nosed colleagues refuse to believe that the syndrome even exists and would probably argue that it is simply an elaborate form of "play-acting." What we have seen in Mrs. Macken, however, implies that such partial insulation of one personality from the other can indeed occur, even though they occupy a single body.

To understand what is going on here, let us return to our general in the war room. I used this analogy to illustrate that there is a sort of coherence-producing mechanism in the left hemisphere—the general—that prohibits anomalies, allows the emergence of a unified belief system and is largely responsible for the integrity and stability of self. But what if a person were confronted by several anomalies that were not consistent with his original belief system but were nonetheless consistent with each other? Like soap bubbles, they might coalesce into a new belief system insulated from the previous story line, creating multiple personalities. Perhaps balkanization is better than civil war. I find the reluctance of cognitive psychologists to accept the reality of this phenomenon somewhat puzzling, given that even normal individuals have such experiences from time to time. I am reminded of a dream I once had in which someone had just been telling me a very funny joke that made me laugh heartily—implying that there must have been at least two mutually amnesic personalities inside me during the dream. To my mind, this is an "existence proof" for the plausibility of multiple personalities.[12]

The question remains: How did the cold water produce such apparently miraculous effects on Mrs. Macken? One possibility is that it "arouses" the right hemisphere. There are connections from the vestibular nerve projecting to the vestibular cortex in the right parietal lobe as well as to other parts of the right hemisphere. Activation of these circuits in the right hemisphere makes the patient pay attention to the left side and notice that her left arm is lying lifeless. She then recognizes, for the first time, that she is paralyzed.

This interpretation is probably at least partially correct, but I would like to consider a more speculative alternative hypothesis: the idea that this phenomenon is somehow related to rapid eye movement (REM) or dream sleep. People spend a third of their lives sleeping, and 25 percent of that time their eyes are moving as they experience vivid, emotional dreams. During these dreams we are often confronted with unpleasant, disturbing facts about ourselves. Thus in both the cold-water state and REM sleep there are noticeable eye movements and unpleasant, forbidden memories come to the surface, and this may not be a coincidence. Freud believed that in dreams we dredge up material that is ordinarily censored, and one wonders whether the same sort of thing may be happening during "ice water in the ear" stimulation. At the risk of pushing the analogy too far, let's refer to our general, who is now sitting in his bedroom late the next night, sipping a glass of cognac. He now has time to engage in a leisurely inspection of the report given to him by that one scout at 5:55 A.M. and perhaps this mulling over and interpretation correspond to what we call dreaming. If the material makes sense, he may decide to incorporate it into his battle plan for the next day. If it doesn't make sense or if it is too disturbing for him, he will put it into his desk drawer and try to forget about it; that is probably why we cannot remember most of our dreams. I suggest that the vestibular stimulation caused by the cold water partially activates the same circuitry that generates REM sleep. This allows the patient to uncover unpleasant, disturbing facts about herself—including her paralysis—that are usually repressed when she is awake.

This is obviously a highly speculative conjecture, and I would give it only a 10 percent chance of being correct. (My colleagues would probably give it 1 percent!) But it does lead to a simple, testable prediction. Patients with denial should *dream that they are paralyzed*. Indeed, if they are awakened during a REM episode, they may continue to admit their paralysis for several minutes before reverting to denial again. Recall that the effects of calorically induced nystagmus—Mrs. Macken's confession of paralysis—lasted for at least thirty minutes after the nystagmus had ceased.[13]

Canst thou not minister to a mind diseased,
Pluck from the memory a rooted sorrow,
Raze out the written troubles of the brain,
And with some sweet oblivious antidote
Cleanse the stuffed bosom of that perilous stuff
Which weighs upon the heart?

—WILLIAM SHAKESPEARE

Memory has legitimately been called the Holy Grail of neuroscience. Although many a weighty tome has been written on this topic, in truth we know little about it. Most of the work carried out in recent decades has fallen into two categories. One is the formation of the memory trace itself, sought in the nature of physical changes between synapses and in chemical cascades within nerve cells. The second is based on the study of patients like H.M. (briefly described in Chapter 1), whose hippocampus was removed surgically for epilepsy and who was no longer able to make new memories after the surgery, though he can remember most things that happened before surgery.

Experiments on cells and on patients like H.M. have given us some insights about how new memory traces are formed, but they completely fail to explore equally important narrative or constructive aspects of memory. How is each new item edited and censored (when necessary) before being pigeonholed according to when and where it occurred? How are these memories progressively assimilated into our "autobiographic self," becoming part of who we are? These subtle aspects of memory are notoriously difficult to study in normal people, but I realized that one could explore them in patients like Mrs. Macken who "repress" what happened just a few minutes earlier.

You don't even need ice water to chart this new territory. I found that I could gently prod some patients into eventually admitting that the left arm is "not working" or "weak" or sometimes even "paralyzed" (although they seemed unperturbed by this admission). If I managed to elicit such a statement, left the room and returned ten minutes later, the patient would have no recollection of the "confession," having a sort of selective amnesia for matters concerning his left arm. One woman, who cried for a full ten minutes when she realized that she was paralyzed (a "catastrophic reaction"), couldn't remember this event a few hours later, even though it must have been an emotionally charged and salient experience. This is about as close as one can get to a Freudian repression.

The natural course of the denial syndrome provides us with another means of exploring memory functions. For reasons not understood, most patients tend to recover completely from the denial syndrome after two or three weeks, though their limbs are almost always still paralyzed or extremely weak. (Wouldn't it be wonderful if alcoholics or anorexics who reject the awful truth about their drinking or their body image were able to recover from denial so quickly? I wonder whether ice water in the left ear canal will do the trick!) What if I were to go to a patient after he is "over" the denial of his paralysis and ask, "When I saw you last week and asked you about your left arm, what did you tell me?" Would he admit that he had been in denial?

The first patient whom I asked about this was Mumtaz Shah, who had been denying her paralysis for almost a month after her stroke and then recovered completely from the denial (although not from the paralysis). I began with the obvious question: "Mrs. Shah, do you remember me?"

"Yes, you came to see me at Mercy Hospital. You were always showing up with those two student nurses, Becky and Susan." (All this was true; so far she was right on target.)

"Do you remember I asked you about your arms? What did you say?"

"I told you my left arm was paralyzed."

"Do you remember I saw you several times? What did you say each time?"

"Several times, several times—yes, I said the same thing, that I was paralyzed."

(Actually she had told me each time that her arm was fine.)

"Mumtaz. Think clearly. Do you remember telling me that your left arm was fine, that it wasn't paralyzed?"

"Well, doctor, if I said that, then it implies that I was lying. And I am not a liar."

Mumtaz had apparently repressed the dozens of episodes of denial that she had engaged in during my numerous visits to the hospital.

The same thing happened with another patient, Jean, whom I visited at the San Diego Rehabilitation Center. We went through the usual questions.

"Can you use your right arm?"

"Oh, yes."

"Can you use your left arm?"

"Yes."

But when I came to the question "Are they equally strong?" Jean said, "No, my left arm is stronger."

Trying to hide my surprise, I pointed to a mahogany table at the end of the hall and asked her whether she could lift that with her right hand.

"I guess I could," she said.

"How high could you lift it?"

She assessed the table, which must have weighed eighty pounds, pursed her lips and said, "Oh, I suppose I could lift it about an inch."

"Can you lift a table with your left hand?"

"Oh, sure," Jean replied. "I could lift it an inch and a half!"

She held up her right hand and showed me with her thumb and index finger how high she could hoist a table with her lifeless left hand. Again, this is a "reaction formation."

But the next day, after she had recovered from her denial, Jean repudiated these same words.

"Jean, do you remember I asked you a question yesterday?"

"Yes," she said, removing her eyeglasses with her right hand. "You asked me if I could lift a table with my right hand and I said I could lift it about an inch."

"What did you say about your left hand?"

"I said I couldn't use my left hand." She gave me a puzzled look.[14]

•

The "model" of denial that we considered earlier provides a partial explanation for both the subtle forms of denial that we all engage in, as well as the vehement protests of denial patients. It rests on the notion that the left hemisphere attempts to preserve a coherent worldview at all costs, and, to do that well, it has to sometimes shut out information that is potentially "threatening" to the stability of self.

But what if we could somehow make this "unpleasant" fact more acceptable—more nonthreatening to a patient's belief system? Would he then be willing to accept that his left arm is paralyzed? In other words, can you "cure" his denial by simply tampering with the structure of his beliefs?

I began by conducting an informal neurological workup on the patient, in this instance, a woman named Nancy. I then showed her a syringe full of saline solution and said, "As part of your neurological exam, I would like to inject your left arm with this anesthetic, and as soon as I do it, your left arm will be *temporarily* paralyzed for a few minutes." After making sure that Nancy understood this, I proceeded to "inject" her arm with the salt water. My question was, Would she suddenly admit that she was paralyzed, now that it had been made more acceptable to her, or would she say, "Your injection doesn't work; I can move my left arm just fine?" This is a lovely example of an experiment on a person's belief system, a field of inquiry I have christened *experimental epistemology*, just to annoy philosophers.

Nancy sat quietly for a few moments waiting for the "injection" to "take effect" while her eyes darted around looking at various antique microscopes in my office. I then asked her, "Well, can you move your left arm?" "No," she replied, "it doesn't seem to want to do anything. It's not moving." Apparently my mock injection had worked, for she was now able to accept the fact that her left arm was indeed paralyzed.

But how could I be sure that this was not simply the result of my persuasive charm? Maybe I was just "hypnotizing" Nancy into accepting that her arm was paralyzed. So I did the obvious control: I repeated the same procedure with her right arm. After ten minutes, I went back into the room and, after chatting briefly about various topics, said, "As part of the neurological exam, I'm going to inject your right arm with this local anesthetic, and after I give you the shot, your right arm will be paralyzed for a few minutes." I then gave her the injection, with the same syringe containing saline solution, waited a bit and asked, "Can you move your right arm?" Nancy looked down, lifted her right hand to her chin and said, "Yes, it's moving. See for yourself." I feigned surprise. "How could that be possible? I just injected you with the same anesthetic that we used on your left arm!" She shook her head with disbelief and replied, "Well, I don't know, doctor. I guess it's mind over matter. I have always believed that."[15]

What we call rational grounds for our beliefs are often extremely irrational attempts to justify our instincts.

—THOMAS HENRY HUXLEY

When I began this research about five years ago, I had no interest whatsoever in Sigmund Freud. (He might have said I was in denial.) And like most of my colleagues I was very skeptical of his ideas. The entire neuroscience community is deeply suspicious of him because he touted elusive aspects of human nature that ring true but that cannot be empirically tested. But after I had worked with these patients, it soon became clear to me that even though Freud wrote a great deal of nonsense, there is no denying that he was a genius, especially when you consider the social and intellectual climate of Vienna at the turn of the century. Freud was one of the first people to emphasize that human nature could be subjected to systematic scientific scrutiny, that one could actually look for laws of mental life in much the same way that a cardiologist might study the heart or an astronomer study planetary motion. We take all this for granted now, but at that time it was a revolutionary insight. No wonder his name became a household word.

Freud's most valuable contribution was his discovery that your conscious mind is simply a facade and that you are completely unaware of 90 percent of what really goes on in your brain. (A striking example is the zombie in Chapter 4.) And with regard to psychological defenses, Freud was right on the mark. Can anyone doubt the reality of the "nervous laugh" or "rationalizations"? Remarkably, although you are engaging in these mental tricks all the time, you are completely unaware of doing so and you'd probably deny it if it were pointed out to you. Yet when you watch someone else doing it, it is comically conspicuous—often embarrassingly so. Of course, all this is quite well known to any good playwright or novelist (try reading Shakespeare or Jane Austen), but Freud surely deserves credit for pointing out the pivotal role of psychological defenses in helping us organize our mental life. Unfortunately, the theoretical schemes he constructed to explain them were nebulous and untestable. He relied all too often on an obscure terminology and on an obsession with sex to explain the human condition. Furthermore, he never did any experiments to validate his theories.

But in denial patients you can witness these mechanisms evolving before your very eyes, caught in flagrante delicto. One can make a list of the many kinds of self-deception that Sigmund and Anna Freud described and see clear-cut, amplified examples of each of them in our patients. It was seeing this list that convinced me for the first time of the reality of psychological defenses and the central role that they play in human nature.

- *Denial:* The most obvious one, of course, is outright denial. "My arm is working fine." "I can move my left arm—it's not paralyzed."
- *Repression:* As we have seen, the patient will sometimes admit with repeated questioning that she is in fact paralyzed, only to revert soon afterward to denial—apparently "repressing" the memory of the confession she made just a few minutes earlier. Many cognitive psychologists argue that repressed memories, such as sudden recollections of child abuse, are inherently bogus—the harvest of psychological seeds implanted by the therapist and brought to flower by the patient. But here we have proof that something like repression is going on, albeit on a smaller time scale, with no possibility that the patient's behavior was unduly influenced by the experimenter.
- *Reaction formation:* This is the propensity to assert the exact opposite of what one suspects to be true of oneself. For example, a latent homosexual may drink his beer, strut around in cowboy boots and engage in macho behavior, in an unconscious attempt to assert his presumed masculinity. There is even a recent study showing that, when viewing X-rated film clips of male pornography, men who are overt gay bashers paradoxically get bigger erections than men who are not prejudiced. (If you're wondering how the erections were measured, the researchers used a device called a penile plethysmograph.)

  I am reminded of Jean—the woman who said she could lift a large table an inch off the ground with her right hand and then added, when questioned, that her paralyzed left hand was actually stronger than the right; that she could use it to lift the table an inch and a half. Also recall Mrs. Dodds, who when asked whether she tied her shoelaces, replied, "Yes, I did it with *both* my hands." These are striking examples of reaction formation.

- *Rationalization:* We have seen many examples of this in this chapter. "Oh, doctor, I didn't move my arm because I have arthritis in my shoulder and it hurts." Or this from another patient: "Oh, the medical students have been prodding me all day and I don't really feel like moving my arm just now."

  When asked to raise both hands, one man raised his right hand high into the air and said, when he detected my gaze locked onto his motionless left hand, "Um, as you can see, I'm steadying myself with my left hand in order to raise my right."

  More rarely, we see frank confabulation:

  "I am touching your nose with my left hand."

  "Yes, of course I'm clapping."

- *Humor:* Even humor can come to the rescue—not just in these patients but in all of us—as Freud well knew. Just think of the so-called nervous laugh or of all those times when you've used humor to deflate a tense situation. Can it be a coincidence, moreover, that so many jokes deal with potentially threatening topics like death or sex? Indeed, after seeing these patients, I am convinced that the most effective antidote to the absurdity of the human condition may be humor rather than art.

  I remember asking a patient who was a professor of English literature to move his paralyzed left arm. "Mr. Sinclair, can you touch my nose with your left hand?"

  "Yes."

  "Okay, show me. Please go ahead and touch it."

  "I'm not accustomed to taking orders, doctor."

  Taken aback, I asked him whether he was being humorous or sarcastic.

  "No, I'm perfectly serious. I'm not being humorous. Why do you ask?"

  So it would seem that although the patient's remarks are often tinged with a perverse sense of humor, they themselves are unaware that they're being funny.

  Another example: "Mrs. Franco, can you touch my nose with your left hand?"

  "Yes, but watch out. I might poke your eye out."

- *Projection:* This is a tactic used when, wanting to avoid confronting a malady or disability, we conveniently attribute it to someone else. "This paralyzed arm belongs to my brother, for I know perfectly well that my own arm is fine." I leave it for psychoanalysts to decide whether this is a true case of projection. But as far as I'm concerned, it's close enough.

•

So here we have patients engaging in precisely the same types of Freudian defense mechanisms—denial, rationalization, confabulation, repression, reaction formation and so forth—that all of us use every day of our lives. I've come to realize that they present us with a fantastic opportunity to test Freudian theories scientifically for the first time. The patients are a microcosm of you and me but "better," in that their defense mechanisms occur on a compressed time scale and are amplified tenfold. Thus we can carry out experiments that Freudian analysts have only dreamed of. For example, what determines which particular defense you use in a given situation? Why would you use an outright denial in one case and a rationalization or reaction formation in another? Is it your (or the patient's) personality type that determines which defense mechanisms you use? Or does the social context determine which one you muster? Do you use one strategy with a superior and another with social inferiors? In other words, what are the "laws" of psychological defense mechanisms? We still have a long way to go before we can address these questions,[16] but, for me, it's exciting to contemplate that we scientists can begin encroaching on territory that until now was reserved for novelists and philosophers.

Meanwhile, is it possible that some of these discoveries may have practical implications in the clinic? Using cold water to correct someone's delusion about body image is fascinating to watch, but could it also be useful to the patients? Would repeated irrigation permanently "cure" Mrs. Macken of denial and make her willing to participate in rehabilitation? I also started wondering about anorexia nervosa. These patients have disturbances in appetite but are also delusional about their body image—claiming actually to "see" that they are fat when looking in a mirror, even though they are grotesquely thin. Is the disorder of appetite (linked to feeding and satiety centers in the hypothalamus) primary, or does the body image distortion cause the appetite problem? We saw in the last chapter that some neglect patients actually start believing that the object in the mirror is "real"—their sensory disturbances actually cause changes in their belief system. And in denial or anosognosia patients, you often notice a similar warping of their beliefs to accommodate their distorted body image. Could some such mechanisms be involved in anorexia? We know that certain parts of the limbic system such as the insular cortex are connected to the hypothalamic "appetite" centers and also to parts of the parietal lobes concerned with body image. Is it conceivable that how much you eat over a long period of time, your intellectual beliefs about whether you are too fat or thin, your perception of your body image and your appetite are all more closely linked in your brain than you realize—so that a distortion of one of these systems can lead to a pervasive disturbance in the others as well? This idea can be tested directly by doing the cold-water irrigation on a patient with anorexia (to see whether it would temporarily correct her delusion about her body image). This is a far-fetched possibility but it's still worth trying, given the ease of the procedure and the lack of an effective treatment for anorexia. Indeed, the disorder is fatal in about 10 percent of cases.

•

Freud bashing is a popular intellectual pastime these days (although he still has his fans in New York and London). But, as we have seen in this chapter, he did have some valuable insights into the human condition, and, when talking about psychological defenses, he was right on target, although he had no idea why they evolved or what neural mechanisms might mediate them. A less well known, but equally interesting idea put forward by Freud was his claim that he had discerned the single common denominator of all great scientific revolutions: Rather surprisingly, all of them humiliate or dethrone "man" as the central figure in the cosmos.

The first of these, he said, was the Copernican revolution, in which a geocentric or earth-centered view of the universe was replaced with the idea that earth is just a speck of dust in the cosmos.

The second was the Darwinian revolution, which holds that we are puny, hairless neotenous apes that accidentally evolved certain characteristics that have made us successful, at least temporarily.

The third great scientific revolution, he claimed (modestly), was his own discovery of the unconscious and the corollary notion that the human sense of "being in charge" is illusory. He claimed that everything we do in life is governed by a cauldron of unconscious emotions, drives and motives and that what we call consciousness is just the tip of the iceberg, an elaborate post hoc rationalization of all our actions.

I believe Freud correctly identified the common denominator of great scientific revolutions. But he doesn't explain why this is so—why would human beings actually enjoy being "humiliated" or dethroned? What do they get in return for accepting the new worldview that belittles humankind?

Here we can turn things around and provide a Freudian interpretation of why cosmology, evolution and brain science are so appealing, not just to specialists but to everyone. Unlike other animals, humans are acutely aware of their own mortality and are terrified of death. But the study of cosmology gives us a sense of timelessness, of being part of something much larger. The fact that your own personal life is finite is less frightening when you know you are part of an evolving universe—an ever-unfolding drama. This is probably the closest a scientist can come to having a religious experience.

The same goes for the study of evolution, for it gives you a sense of time and place, allowing you to see yourself as part of a great journey. And likewise for the brain sciences. In this revolution, we have given up the idea that there is a soul separate from our minds and bodies. Far from being terrifying, this idea is very liberating. If you think you're something special in this world, engaging in a lofty inspection of the cosmos from a unique vantage point, your annihilation becomes unacceptable. But if you're really part of the great cosmic dance of Shiva, rather than a mere spectator, then your inevitable death should be seen as a joyous reunion with nature rather than as a tragedy.

> *Brahman is all. From Brahman come appearances, sensations, desires, deeds. But all these are merely name and form. To know Brahman one must experience the identity between him and the Self, or Brahman dwelling within the lotus of the heart. Only by so doing can man escape from sorrow and death and become one with the subtle essence beyond all knowledge.*
>
> —Upanishads, *500* B.C.

CHAPTER 8

"The Unbearable Likeness of Being"

"One can't believe impossible things."

"I daresay you haven't had much practice," said the Queen. "When I was your age I always did it for half an hour a day. Why, sometimes I've believed as many as six impossible things before breakfast."

—LEWIS CARROLL, Through the Looking Glass

"As a rule," said Holmes, "the more bizarre a thing is the less mysterious it proves to be. It is your commonplace, featureless crimes which are really puzzling, just as a commonplace face is the most difficult to identify."

—SHERLOCK HOLMES

I'll never forget the frustration and despair in the voice at the other end of the telephone. The call came early one afternoon as I stood over my desk, riffling through papers looking for a misplaced letter, and it took me a few seconds to register what this man was saying. He introduced himself as a former diplomat from Venezuela whose son was suffering from a terrible, cruel delusion. Could I help?

"What sort of delusion?" I asked.

His reply and the emotional strain in his voice caught me by surprise. "My thirty-year-old son thinks that I am not his father, that I am an impostor. He says the same thing about his mother, that we are not his real parents." He paused to let this sink in. "We just don't know what to do or where to go for help. Your name was given to us by a psychiatrist in Boston. So far no one has been able to help us, to find a way to make

Arthur better." He was almost in tears. "Dr. Ramachandran, we love our son and would go to the ends of the earth to help him. Is there any way you could see him?"

"Of course, I'll see him," I said. "When can you bring him in?"

Two days later, Arthur came to our laboratory for the first time in what would turn into a yearlong study of his condition. He was a good-looking fellow, dressed in jeans, a white T-shirt and moccasins. In his mannerisms, he was shy and almost childlike, often whispering his answers to questions or looking wide-eyed at us. Sometimes I could scarcely hear his voice over the background whir of air conditioners and computers.

The parents explained that Arthur had been in a near-fatal automobile accident while he was attending school in Santa Barbara. His head hit the windshield with such crushing force that he lay in a coma for three weeks, his survival by no means assured. But when he finally awoke and began intensive rehabilitative therapy, everyone's hopes soared. Arthur gradually learned to talk and walk, recalled the past and seemed, to all outward appearances, to be back to normal. He just had this one incredible delusion about his parents—that they were impostors—and nothing could convince him otherwise.

After a brief conversation to warm things up and put Arthur at ease, I asked, "Arthur, who brought you to the hospital?"

"That guy in the waiting room," Arthur replied. "He's the old gentleman who's been taking care of me."

"You mean your father?"

"No, no, doctor. That guy isn't my father. He just looks like him. He's—what do you call it?—an impostor, I guess. But I don't think he means any harm."

"Arthur, why do you think he's an impostor? What gives you that impression?"

He gave me a patient look—as if to say, how could I not see the obvious—and said, "Yes, he looks exactly like my father but he *really* isn't. He's a nice guy, doctor, but he certainly isn't my father!"

"But, Arthur, why is this man pretending to be your father?"

Arthur seemed sad and resigned when he said, "That is what is so surprising, doctor. Why should anyone want to pretend to be my father?" He looked confused as he searched for a plausible explanation. "Maybe my real father employed him to take care of me, paid him some money so that he could pay my bills."

Later, in my office, Arthur's parents added another twist to the mystery. Apparently their son did not treat either of them as impostors when they spoke to him over the telephone. He only claimed they were impostors when they met and spoke face-to-face. This implied that Arthur did not have amnesia with regard to his parents and that he was not simply "crazy." For, if that were true, why would he be normal when listening to them on the telephone and delusional regarding his parents' identities only when he looked at them?

"It's so upsetting," Arthur's father said. "He recognizes all sorts of people he knew in the past, including his college roommates, his best friend from childhood and his former girlfriends. He doesn't say that any of them is an impostor. He seems to have some gripe against his mother and me."

I felt deeply sorry for Arthur's parents. We could probe their son's brain and try to shed light on his condition—and perhaps comfort them with a logical explanation for his curious behavior—but there was scant hope for an effective treatment. This sort of neurological condition is usually permanent. But I was pleasantly surprised one Saturday morning when Arthur's father called me, excited about an idea he'd gotten from watching a television program on phantom limbs in which I demonstrated that the brain can be tricked by simply using a mirror. "Dr. Ramachandran," he said, "if you can trick a person into thinking that his paralyzed phantom can move again, why can't we use a similar trick to help Arthur get rid of his delusion?"

Indeed, why not? The next day, Arthur's father entered his son's bedroom and announced cheerfully, "Arthur, guess what! That man you've been living with all these days is an impostor. He really isn't your father. You were right all along. So I have sent him away to China. I am your real father." He moved over to Arthur's side and clapped him on the shoulder. "It's good to see you, son!"

Arthur blinked hard at the news but seemed to accept it at face value. When he came to our laboratory the next day I said, "Who's that man who brought you in today?"

"That's my real father."

"Who was taking care of you last week?"

"Oh," said Arthur, "that guy has gone back to China. He looks similar to my father, but he's gone now."

When I spoke to Arthur's father on the phone later that afternoon, he confirmed that Arthur now called him "Father," but that Arthur still seemed to feel that something was amiss. "I think he accepts me intellectually, doctor, but not emotionally," he said. "When I hug him, there's no warmth."

Alas, even this intellectual acceptance of his parents did not last. One week later Arthur reverted to his original delusion, claiming that the impostor had returned.

•

Arthur was suffering from Capgras' delusion, one of the rarest and most colorful syndromes in neurology.[1] The patient, who is often mentally quite lucid, comes to regard close acquaintances—usually his parents, children, spouse or siblings—as impostors. As Arthur said over and over, "That man looks identical to my father but he really isn't my father. That woman who claims to be my mother? She's lying. She looks just like my mom but it isn't her." Although such bizarre delusions can crop up in psychotic states, over a third of the documented cases of Capgras' syndrome have occurred in conjunction with traumatic brain lesions, like the head injury that Arthur suffered in his automobile accident. This suggests to me that the syndrome has an organic basis. But because a majority of Capgras' patients appear to develop this delusion "spontaneously," they are usually dispatched to psychiatrists, who tend to favor a Freudian explanation of the disorder.

In this view, all of us so-called normal people as children are sexually attracted to our parents. Thus every male wants to make love to his mother and comes to regard his father as a sexual rival (Oedipus led the way), and every female has lifelong deep-seated sexual obsessions over her father (the Electra complex). Although these forbidden feelings become fully repressed by adulthood, they remain dormant, like deeply buried embers after a fire has been extinguished. Then, many psychiatrists argue, along comes a blow to the head (or some other unrecognized release mechanism) and the repressed sexuality toward a mother or father comes flaming to the surface. The patient finds himself suddenly and inexplicably sexually attracted to his parents and therefore says to himself, "My God! If this is my mother, how come I'm attracted to her?" Perhaps the only way he can preserve some semblance of sanity is to say to himself, "This must be some other, strange woman." Likewise, "I could never feel this kind of sexual jealousy toward my real dad, so this man must be an impostor."

This explanation is ingenious, as indeed most Freudian explanations are, but then I came across a Capgras' patient who had similar delusions about his pet poodle: The Fifi before him was an impostor; the real Fifi was living in Brooklyn. In my view that case demolished the Freudian explanation for Capgras' syndrome. There may be some latent bestiality in all of us, but I suspect this is not Arthur's problem.

A better approach for studying Capgras' syndrome involves taking a closer look at neuroanatomy, specifically at pathways concerned with visual recognition and emotions in the brain. Recall that the temporal lobes contain regions that specialize in face and object recognition (the what pathway described in Chapter 4). We know this because when specific portions of the what pathway are damaged, patients lose the ability to recognize faces,[2] even those of close friends and relatives—as immortalized by Oliver Sacks in his book *The Man Who Mistook His Wife for a Hat*. In a normal brain, these face recognition areas (found on both sides of the brain) relay information to the limbic system, found deep in the middle of the brain, which then helps generate emotional responses to particular faces (Figure 8.1). I may feel love when I see my mother's face, anger when I see the face of a boss or a sexual rival or deliberate indifference upon seeing the visage of a friend who has betrayed me and has not yet earned my forgiveness. In each instance, when I look at the face, my temporal cortex recognizes the image—mother, boss, friend—and passes on the information to my amygdala (a gateway to the limbic system) to discern the emotional significance of that face. When this activation is then relayed to the rest of my limbic system, I start experiencing the nuances of emotion—love, anger, disappointment—appropriate to that particular face. The actual sequence of events is undoubtedly much more complex, but this caricature captures the gist of it.

After thinking about Arthur's symptoms, it occurred to me that his strange behavior might have resulted from a disconnection between these two areas (one concerned with recognition and the other with emotions). Maybe Arthur's face recognition pathway was still completely normal, and that was why he could identify everyone, including his mother and father, but the connections between this "face region" and his amygdala had been selectively damaged. If that were the case, Arthur would recognize his parents but would not experience any emotions when looking at their faces. He would not feel a "warm glow" when looking at his beloved mother, so when he sees her he says to himself, "If this is my mother, why doesn't her presence make me *feel* like I'm with my mother?" Perhaps his only escape from this dilemma—the only sensible interpretation he could make given the peculiar disconnection between the two regions of his brain—is to assume that this woman merely resembles Mom. She must be an impostor.[3]

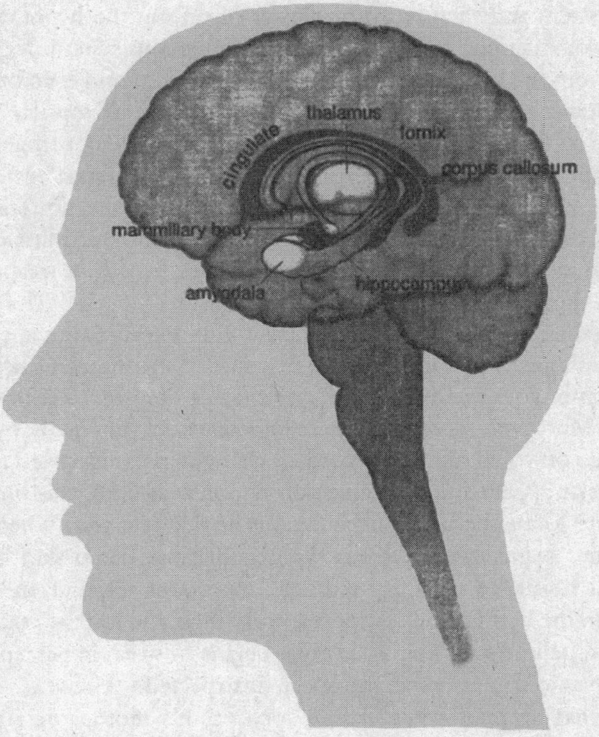

Figure 8.1 *The limbic system is concerned with emotions. It consists of a number of nuclei (cell clusters) interconnected by long* C*-shaped fiber tracts. The amygdala—in the front pole of the temporal lobe—receives input from the sensory areas and sends messages to the rest of the limbic system to produce emotional arousal. Eventually, this activity cascades into the hypothalamus and from there to the autonomic nervous system, preparing the animal (or person) for action.*

Now, this is an intriguing idea, but how does one go about testing it? As complex as the challenge seems, psychologists have found a rather simple way to measure emotional responses to faces, objects, scenes and events encountered in daily life. To understand how this works, you need to know something about the autonomic nervous system—a part of your brain that controls the involuntary, seemingly automatic activities of organs, blood vessels, glands and many other tissues in your body. When you are emotionally aroused—say, by a menacing or sexually alluring face—the information travels from your face recognition region to your limbic system and then to a tiny cluster of cells in the hypothalamus, a kind of command center for the autonomic nervous system. Nerve fibers extend from the hypothalamus to the heart, muscles and even other parts of the brain, helping to prepare your body to take appropriate action in response to that particular face. Whether you are going to fight, flee or mate, your blood pressure will rise and your heart will start beating faster to deliver more oxygen to your tissues. At the same time, you start sweating, not only to dissipate the heat building up in your muscles but to give your sweaty palms a better grip on a tree branch, a weapon or an enemy's throat.

From the experimenter's point of view, your sweaty palms are the most important aspect of your emotional response to the threatening face. The dampness of your hands is a sure giveaway of how you feel toward that person. Moreover, we can measure this reaction very easily by placing electrodes on your palm and recording changes in the electrical resistance of your skin. (Called the galvanic skin response or GSR, this simple little procedure forms the basis of the famous lie detector test. When you tell a fib, your palms sweat ever so slightly. Because damp skin has lower electrical resistance than dry skin, the electrodes respond and you are caught in the lie.) For our purposes, every time you look at your mother or father, believe it or not, your body begins to sweat imperceptibly and your galvanic skin response shoots up as expected.

So, what happens when Arthur looks at his mother or father? My hypothesis predicts that even though he sees them as resembling his parents (remember, the face recognition area of his brain is normal), he should *not* register a change in skin conductance. The disconnection in his brain will prevent his palms from sweating.

With the family's permission, we began testing Arthur on a rainy winter day in our basement laboratory on campus. Arthur sat in a comfortable chair, joking about the weather and how he expected his father's car to float away before we finished the morning's experiments. Sipping hot tea to take the chill from his bones, Arthur gazed at a video screen saver while we affixed two electrodes to his left index finger. Any tiny increase in sweat on his finger would change his skin resistance and show up as a blip on the screen.

Next I showed him a sequence of photos of his mother, father and grandfather interleaved with pictures of strangers, and I compared his galvanic skin responses to that of six college undergraduates who were shown an identical sequence of photos and who served as controls for comparison. Before the experiment, subjects were told that they would be shown pictures of faces, some of which would be familiar and some unfamiliar. After the electrodes were attached, they were shown each photograph for two seconds with a fifteen- to twenty-five-second delay between pictures so skin conductance could return to baseline.

In the undergraduates, I found that there was a big jolt in the GSR in response to photos of their parents—as expected—but not to photos of strangers. In Arthur, on the other hand, the skin response was uniformly low. There was no increased response to his parents, or at times there would be a tiny blip on the screen after a long delay, as if he were doing a double take. This result provided direct proof that our theory was correct. Clearly Arthur was not responding emotionally to his parents, and this may be what led to the loss of his galvanic skin response.

But how could we be sure that Arthur was even seeing the faces? Maybe his head injury had damaged the cells in the temporal lobes that would help him distinguish between faces, resulting in a flat GSR whether he looks at his mother or at a stranger. This seemed unlikely, however, since he readily acknowledged that the people who took him to the hospital—his mother and father—looked like his parents. He also had no difficulty in recognizing the faces of famous people like Bill Clinton and Albert Einstein. Still, we needed to test his recognition abilities more directly.

To obtain direct proof, I did the obvious thing. I showed Arthur sixteen pairs of photographs of strangers, each pair consisting of either two slightly different pictures of the same person or snapshots of two different people. We asked him, Do the photographs depict the same person or not? Putting his nose close to each photo and gazing hard at the details, Arthur got fourteen out of sixteen trials correct.

We were now sure that Arthur had no problem in recognizing faces and telling them apart. But could his failure to produce a strong galvanic skin response to his parents be part of a more global disturbance in his emotional abilities? How could we be certain that the head injury had not also damaged his limbic system? Maybe he had no emotions, period.

This seemed improbable because throughout the months I spent with Arthur, he showed a full range of human emotions. He laughed at my jokes and offered his own funny stories in return. He expressed frustration, fear and anger, and on rare occasions I saw him cry. Whatever the situation, his emotions were appropriate. Arthur's problem, then, was neither his ability to recognize faces nor his ability to experience emotions; what was lost was his ability to *link* the two.

So far so good, but why is the phenomenon specific to close relatives? Why not call the mailman an impostor, since his, too, is a familiar face?

It may be that when any normal person (including Arthur, prior to his accident) encounters someone who is emotionally very close to him—a parent, spouse or sibling—he expects an emotional "glow," a warm fuzzy feeling, to arise even though it may sometimes be experienced only very dimly. The absence of this glow is therefore surprising and Arthur's only recourse then is to generate an absurd delusion—to rationalize it or to explain it away. On the other hand, when one sees the mailman, one doesn't expect a warm glow and consequently there is no incentive for Arthur to generate a delusion to explain his lack of "warm fuzzy" response. A mailman is simply a mailman (unless the relationship has taken an amorous turn).

Although the most common delusion among Capgras' patients is the assertion that a parent is an impostor, even more bizarre examples can be found in the older medical literature. Indeed, in a case on record the patient was convinced that his stepfather was a robot, proceeded to decapitate him and opened his skull to look for microchips. Perhaps in this patient, the dissociation from emotions was so extreme that he was forced into an even more absurd delusion than Arthur's: that his stepfather was not even a human being, but was a mindless android![4]

About a year ago, when I gave a lecture on Arthur at the Veterans Administration Hospital in La Jolla, a neurology resident raised an astute objection to my theory. What about people who are born with a disease in which their amygdalas (the gateway to the limbic system) calcify and atrophy or those who lose their amygdalas (we each have two of them) completely in surgery or through an accident? Such people do exist, but they do not develop Capgras' syndrome, even though their GSRs are flat to all emotionally evocative stimuli. Likewise, patients with damage to their frontal lobes (which receive and process information from the limbic system for making elaborate future plans) also often lack a GSR. Yet they, too, do not display Capgras' syndrome.

Why not? The answer may be that these patients experience a general blunting of all their emotional responses and therefore do not have a baseline for comparison. Like a purebred Vulcan or Data on *Star Trek,* one could legitimately argue, they don't even know what an emotion is, whereas Capgras' patients like Arthur enjoy a normal emotional life in all other respects.

This idea teaches us an important principle about brain function, namely, that all our perceptions—indeed, maybe all aspects of our minds—are governed by comparisons and not by absolute values. This appears to be true whether you are talking about something as obvious as judging the brightness of print in a newspaper or something as subtle as detecting a blip in your internal emotional landscape. This is a far-reaching conclusion, and it also helps illustrate the power of our approach—indeed of the whole discipline that now goes by the name cognitive neuroscience. You can discover important general principles about how the brain works and begin to address deep philosophical questions by doing relatively simple experiments on the right patients. We started with a bizarre condition, proposed an outlandish theory, tested it in the lab and—in meeting objections to it—learned more about how the healthy brain actually works.

Taking these speculations even further, consider the extraordinary disorder called Cotard's syndrome, in which a patient will assert that he is dead, claiming to smell rotten flesh or worms crawling all over his skin. Again, most people, even neurologists, would jump to the conclusion that the patient was insane. But that wouldn't explain why the delusion takes this highly specific form. I would argue instead that Cotard's is simply an exaggerated form of Capgras' syndrome and probably has a similar origin. In Capgras', the face recognition area alone is disconnected from the amygdala, whereas in Cotard's perhaps all the sensory areas are disconnected from the limbic system, leading to a complete lack of emotional contact with the world. Here is another instance in which an outlandish brain disorder that most people regard as a psychiatric problem can be explained in terms of known brain circuitry. And once again, these ideas can be tested in the laboratory. I would predict that Cotard's syndrome patients will have a complete loss of GSR for all external stimuli—not just faces—and this leaves them stranded on an island of emotional desolation, as close as anyone can come to experiencing death.

Arthur seemed to enjoy his visits to our laboratory. His parents were pleased that there was a logical explanation for his predicament, that he wasn't just "crazy." I never revealed the details to Arthur because I wasn't sure how he'd react.

Arthur's father was an intelligent man, and at one point, when Arthur wasn't around, he asked me, "If your theory is correct, doctor—if the information doesn't get to his amygdala—then how do you explain how he has no problems recognizing us over the phone? Does that make sense to you?"

"Well," I replied, "there is a separate pathway from the auditory cortex, the hearing area of the temporal lobes, to the amygdala. One possibility is that this hearing route has not been affected by the accident—only the visual centers have been disconnected from Arthur's amygdala."

This conversation got me wondering about the other well-known functions of the amygdala and the visual centers that project to it. In particular, scientists recording cell responses in the amygdala found that, in addition to responding to facial expression and emotions, the cells also respond to the direction of eye gaze. For instance, one cell might fire if another person is looking directly at you, whereas a neighboring cell will fire only if that person's gaze is averted by a fraction of an inch. Still other cells fire when the gaze is way off to the left or the right.

This phenomenon is not surprising, given the important role that gaze direction[5] plays in primate social communications—the averted gaze of guilt, shame or embarrassment; the intense, direct gaze of a lover or the threatening stare of an enemy. We tend to forget that emotions, even though they are privately experienced, often involve interactions with other people and that one way we interact is through eye contact. Given the links among gaze direction, familiarity and emotions, I wondered whether Arthur's ability to judge the direction of gaze, say, by looking at photographs of faces, would be impaired.

To find out, I prepared a series of images, each showing the same model looking either directly at the camera lens or at a point an inch or two to the right or left of the lens. Arthur's task was simply to let us know whether the model was looking straight at him or not. Whereas you or I can detect tiny shifts in gaze with uncanny accuracy, Arthur was hopeless at the task. Only when the model's eyes were looking way off to one side was he able to discern correctly that she wasn't looking at him.

This finding in itself is interesting but not altogether unexpected, given the known role of amygdala and temporal lobes in detecting gaze direction. But on the eighth trial of looking at these photos, Arthur did something completely unexpected. In his soft, almost apologetic voice, he exclaimed that the model's identity had changed. He was now looking at a new person!

This meant that a mere change in direction of gaze had been sufficient to provoke Capgras' delusion. For Arthur, the "second" model was apparently a new person who merely resembled the "first."

"This one is older," Arthur said firmly. He stared hard at both images. "This is a lady; the other one is a girl." Later in the sequence, Arthur made another duplication—one model was old, one young and a third even younger. At the end of the test session he continued to insist that he had seen three different people. Two weeks later he did it again on a retest using images of a completely new face.

How could Arthur look at the face of what was obviously one person and claim that she was actually three different people? Why did simply changing the direction of gaze lead to this profound inability to link successive images?

Answers lie in the mechanics of how we form memories, in particular our ability to create enduring representations of faces. For example, suppose you go to the grocery store one day and a friend introduces you to a new person—Joe. You form a memory of that episode and tuck it away in your brain. Two weeks go by and you run into Joe in the library. He tells you a story about your mutual friend, you share a laugh and your brain files a memory about this second episode. Another few weeks pass and you meet Joe again in his office—he's a medical researcher and he's wearing a white lab coat—but you recognize him instantly from earlier encounters. More memories of Joe are created during this time so that you now have in your mind a "category" called Joe. This mental picture becomes progressively refined and enriched each time you meet Joe, aided by an increasing sense of familiarity that creates an incentive to link the images and the episodes. Eventually you develop a robust concept of Joe—he tells great stories, works in a lab, makes you laugh, knows a lot about gardening, and so forth.

Now consider what happens to someone with a rare and specific form of amnesia, caused by damage to the hippocampus (another important brain structure in the temporal lobes). These patients have a complete inability to form new memories, even though they have perfect recollection of all events in their lives that took place before the hippocampus was injured. The logical conclusion to be drawn from the syndrome is not that memories are actually stored in the hippocampus (hence the preservation of old memories), but that the hippocampus is vital for the acquisition of new memory traces in the brain. When such a patient meets a new person (Joe) on three consecutive occasions—in the supermarket, the library and the office—he will not remember ever having met Joe before. He will simply not recognize him. He will insist each time that Joe is a complete stranger, no matter how many times they have interacted, talked, exchanged stories and so forth.

But is Joe really a complete stranger? Rather surprisingly, experiments show that such amnesia patients actually retain the ability to form new categories that transcend successive Joe episodes. If our patient met Joe ten times and each time Joe made him laugh, he'd tend to feel vaguely jovial or happy on the next encounter but still would not know who Joe is. There would be no sense of familiarity whatsoever—no memory of each Joe episode—and yet the patient would acknowledge that Joe makes him happy. This means that the amnesia patient, unlike Arthur, can link successive episodes to create a new concept (an unconscious expectation of joy) even though he forgets each episode, whereas Arthur remembers each episode but fails to link them.

Thus Arthur is in some respects the mirror image of our amnesia patient. When he meets a total stranger like Joe, his brain creates a file for Joe and the associated experiences he has with Joe. But if Joe leaves the room for thirty minutes and returns, Arthur's brain—instead of retrieving the old file and adding to it—sometimes creates a completely new one.

Why does this happen in Capgras' syndrome? It may be that to link successive episodes the brain relies on signals from the limbic system—the "glow" or sense of familiarity associated with a known face and set of memories—and if this activation is missing, the brain cannot form an enduring category through time. In the absence of this glow, the brain simply sets up separate categories each time; that is why Arthur asserts that he is meeting a new person who simply resembles the person he met thirty minutes ago. Cognitive psychologists and philosophers often make a distinction between tokens and types—that all our experiences can be classified into general categories or types (people or cars) versus specific exemplars or tokens (Joe or my car). Our experiments with Arthur suggest that this distinction is not merely academic; it is embedded deep in the architecture of the brain.

As we continued testing Arthur, we noticed that he had certain other quirks and eccentricities. For instance, Arthur sometimes seemed to have a general problem with visual categories. All of us make mental taxonomies or groupings of events and objects: Ducks and geese are birds but rabbits are not. Our brains set up these categories even without formal education in zoology, presumably to facilitate memory storage and to enhance our ability to access these memories at a moment's notice.

Arthur, on the other hand, often made remarks hinting that he was confused about categories. For example, he had an almost obsessive preoccupation with Jews and Catholics, and he tended to label a disproportionate number of recently encountered people as Jews. This propensity reminded me of another rare syndrome called Fregoli, in which a patient keeps seeing the same person everywhere. In walking down the street, nearly every woman's face might look like his mother's or every young man might resemble his brother. (I would predict that instead of having severed connections from face recognition areas to the amygdala, the Fregoli patient may have an excess of such connections. Every face would be imbued with familiarity and "glow," causing him to see the same face over and over again.)

Might such Fregoli-like confusion occur in otherwise normal brains? Could this be a basis for forming racist stereotypes? Racism is so often directed at a single physical type (Blacks, Asians, Whites and so forth). Perhaps a single unpleasant episode with one member of a visual category sets up a limbic connection that is inappropriately generalized to include all members of that class and is notoriously impervious to "intellectual correction" based on information stored in higher brain centers. Indeed one's intellectual views may be colored (no pun intended) by this emotional knee-jerk reaction; hence the notorious tenacity of racism.

•

We began our journey with Arthur trying to explain his strange delusions about impostors and uncovered some new insights into how memories are stored and retrieved in the human brain. His story offers insights into how each of us constructs narratives about our life and the people who inhabit it. In a sense your life—your autobiography—is a long sequence of highly personal episodic memories about your first kiss, prom night, wedding, birth of a child, fishing trips and so on. But it is also much more than that. Clearly, there is a personal identity, a sense of a unified "self" that runs like a golden thread through the whole fabric of our existence. The Scottish philosopher David Hume drew an analogy between the human personality and a river—the water in the river is ever-changing and yet the river itself remains constant. What would happen, he asked, if a person were to dip his foot into a river and then dip it in again after half an hour—would it be the same river or a different one? If you think this is a silly semantic riddle, you're right, for the answer depends on your definition of "same" and "river."

But silly or not, one point is clear. For Arthur, given his difficulty with linking successive episodic memories, there may indeed be two rivers! To be sure, this tendency to make copies of events and objects was most pronounced when he encountered faces—Arthur did not often duplicate objects. Yet there were occasions when he would run his fingers through his hair and call it a "wig," partly because his scalp felt unfamiliar as a result of scars from the neurosurgery he had undergone. On rare occasions, Arthur even duplicated countries, claiming at one point that there were two Panamas (he had recently visited that country during a family reunion).

Most remarkable of all, Arthur sometimes duplicated himself! The first time this happened, I was showing Arthur pictures of himself from a family photo album and I pointed to a snapshot of him taken two years before the accident.

"Whose picture is this?" I asked.

"That's another Arthur," he replied. "He looks just like me but it isn't me." I couldn't believe my ears. Arthur may have detected my surprise since he then reinforced his point by saying, "You see? He has a mustache. I don't."

This delusion, however, did not occur when Arthur looked at himself in a mirror. Perhaps he was sensible enough to realize that the face in the mirror could not be anyone else's. But Arthur's tendency to "duplicate" himself—to regard himself as a distinct person from a former Arthur—also sometimes emerged spontaneously during conversation. To my surprise, he once volunteered, "Yes, my parents sent a check, but they sent it to the other Arthur."

Arthur's most serious problem, however, was his inability to make emotional contact with people who matter to him most—his parents—and this caused him great anguish. I can imagine a voice inside his head saying, "The reason I don't experience warmth must be because I'm not the real Arthur." One day Arthur turned to his mother and said, "Mom, if the real Arthur ever returns, do you promise that you will still treat me as a friend and love me?" How can a sane human being who is perfectly intelligent in other respects come to regard himself as two people? There seems to be something inherently contradictory about splitting the Self, which by its very nature is unitary. If I started to regard myself as several people, which one would I plan for? Which one is the "real" me? This is a real and painful dilemma for Arthur.

Philosophers have argued for centuries that if there is any one thing about our existence that is completely beyond question, it is the simple fact that "I" exist as a single human being who endures in space and time. But even this basic axiomatic foundation of human existence is called into question by Arthur.

CHAPTER 9

God and the Limbic System

It is very difficult to elucidate this [cosmic religious] feeling to anyone who is entirely without it. . . . The religious geniuses of all ages have been distinguished by this kind of religious feeling, which knows no dogma. . . . In my view, it is the most important function of art and science to awaken this feeling and keep it alive in those who are receptive to it.

—ALBERT EINSTEIN

[God] is the greatest democrat the world knows, for He leaves us "unfettered" to make our own choice between evil and good. He is the greatest tyrant ever known, for He often dashes the cup from our lips and under cover of free will leaves us a margin so wholly inadequate as to provide only mirth for Himself at our expense. Therefore it is that Hinduism calls it all His sport (Lila), or calls it all an illusion (Maya). . . . Let us dance to the tune of his bansi (flute), and all would be well.

—MOHANDAS K. GANDHI

Imagine you had a machine, a helmet of sorts that you could simply put on your head and stimulate any small region of your brain without causing permanent damage. What would you use the device for?

This is not science fiction. Such a device, called a transcranial magnetic stimulator, already exists and is relatively easy to construct. When applied to the scalp, it shoots a rapidly fluctuating and extremely powerful magnetic field onto a small patch of brain tissue, thereby activating it and providing hints about its function. For example, if you were to stimulate certain parts of your motor cortex, different muscles would contract. Your finger might twitch or you'd feel a sudden involuntary, puppetlike shrugging of one shoulder.

So, if you had access to this device, what part of your brain would you stimulate? If you happened to be familiar with reports from the early days of neurosurgery about the septum—a cluster of cells located near the front of the thalamus in the middle of your brain—you might be tempted to apply the magnet there.[1] Patients "zapped" in this region claim to experience intense pleasure, "like a thousand orgasms rolled into one." If you were blind from birth and the visual areas in your brain had not degenerated, you might stimulate bits of your own visual cortex to find out what people mean by color or "seeing." Or, given the well-known clinical observation that the left frontal lobe seems to be involved in feeling "good," maybe you'd want to stimulate a region over your left eye to see whether you could induce a natural high.

When the Canadian psychologist Dr. Michael Persinger got hold of a similar device a few years ago, he chose instead to stimulate parts of his temporal lobes. And he found to his amazement that he experienced God for the first time in his life.

I first heard about Dr. Persinger's strange experiment from my colleague, Patricia Churchland, who spotted an account of it in a popular Canadian science magazine. She phoned me right away. "Rama, you're not going to believe this. There's a man in Canada who stimulated his temporal lobe and experienced God. What do you make of it?"

"Does he have temporal lobe seizures?" I asked.

"No, not at all. He's a normal guy."

"But he stimulated his own temporal lobes?"

"That's what the article said."

"Hmmmm, I wonder what would happen if you tried stimulating an atheist's brain. Would he experience God?" I smiled to myself and said, "Hey, maybe we should try the device on Francis Crick."

Dr. Persinger's observation was not a complete surprise as I've always suspected that the temporal lobes, especially the left lobe, are somehow involved in religious experience. Every medical student is taught that patients with epileptic seizures originating in this part of the brain can have intense, spiritual experiences during the seizures and sometimes become preoccupied with religious and moral issues even during the seizure-free or interictal periods.

But does this syndrome imply that our brains contain some sort of circuitry that is actually specialized for religious experience? Is there a "God module" in our heads? And if such a circuit exists, where did it come from? Could it be a product of natural selection, a human trait as natural in the biological sense as language or stereoscopic vision? Or is there a deeper mystery at play, as a philosopher, epistemologist or theologian might argue?

Many traits make us uniquely human, but none is more enigmatic than religion—our propensity to believe in God or in some higher power that transcends mere appearances. It seems very unlikely that any creature other than humans can ponder the infinite or wonder about "the meaning of it all." Listen to John Milton in *Paradise Lost:*

For who would lose, though full of pain
This intellectual being
Those thoughts that wander through eternity to be swallowed up
and lost
In the wide womb of uncreated night.

But where do such feelings come from? It may be that any intelligent sentient being that can look into its own future and confront its own mortality will sooner or later begin to engage in such disquieting ruminations. Does my little life have any real significance in the grand scheme of things? If my father's sperm had not fertilized that particular egg on that fateful night, would I not have existed, and in what real sense then would the universe have existed? Would it not then, as Erwin Schrödinger said, have been a mere "play before empty benches"? What if my dad had coughed at that critical moment so that a different sperm had fertilized the ovum? Our minds start reeling when pondering such possibilities. We are bedeviled by paradox: On the one hand our lives seem so important—with all those cherished highly personal memories—and yet we know that in the cosmic scheme of things, our brief existence amounts to nothing at all. So how do people make sense of this dilemma? For many the answer is straightforward: They seek solace in religion.

But surely there's more to it than that. If religious beliefs are merely the combined result of wishful thinking and a longing for immortality, how do you explain the flights of intense religious ecstasy experienced by patients with temporal lobe seizures or their claim that God speaks directly to them? Many a patient has told me of a "divine light that illuminates all things," or of an "ultimate truth that lies completely beyond the reach of ordinary minds who are too immersed in the hustle and bustle of daily life to notice the beauty and grandeur of it all." Of course, they might simply be suffering from hallucinations and delusions of the kind that a schizophrenic might experience, but if that's the case, why do such hallucinations occur mainly when the temporal lobes are involved? Even more puzzling, why do they take this particular form? Why don't these patients hallucinate pigs or donkeys?

•

In 1935, the anatomist James Papez noticed that patients who died of rabies often experienced fits of extreme rage and terror in the hours before death. He knew that the disease was transmitted by dog bites and reasoned that something in the dog's saliva—the rabies virus—traveled along the victim's peripheral nerves located next to the bite, up the spinal cord and into the brain. Upon dissecting victims' brains, Papez found the destination of the virus—clusters of nerve cells or nuclei connected by large C-shaped fiber tracts deep in the brain (Figure 9.1). A century earlier, the famous French neurologist Pierre Paul Broca had named this structure the limbic system. Because rabies patients suffered violent emotional fits, Papez reasoned that these limbic structures must be intimately involved in human emotional behavior.[2]

The limbic system gets its input from all sensory systems—vision, touch, hearing, taste and smell. The latter sense is in fact directly wired to the limbic system, going straight to the amygdala (an almond-shaped structure that serves as a gateway into the limbic system). This is hardly surprising given that in lower mammals, smell is intimately linked with emotion, territorial behavior, aggression and sexuality.

The limbic system's output, as Papez realized, is geared mainly toward the experience and expression of emotions. The experience of emotions is mediated by back-and-forth connections with the frontal lobes, and much of the richness of your inner emotional life probably depends on these interactions. The outward expression of these emotions, on the other hand, requires the participation of a small cluster of densely packed cells called the hypothalamus, a control center with three major outputs of its own. First, hypothalamic nuclei send hormonal and neural signals to the pituitary gland, which is often described as the "conductor" of the endocrine orchestra. Hormones released through this system influence almost every part of the human body, a biological tour de force we shall consider in the analysis of mind-body interactions (Chapter 11). Second, the hypothalamus sends commands to the autonomic nervous system, which controls various vegetative or bodily functions, including the production of tears, saliva and sweat and the control of blood pressure, heart rate, body temperature, respiration, bladder function, defecation and so on. The hypothalamus can be regarded, then, as the "brain" of this archaic, ancillary nervous system. The third output drives

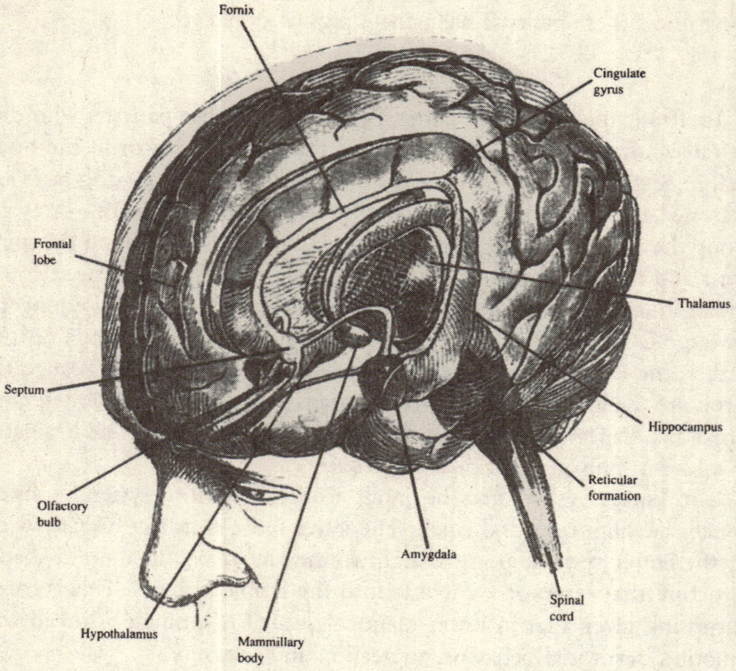

Figure 9.1 *Another view of the limbic system. The limbic system is made up of a series of interconnected structures surrounding a central fluid-filled ventricle of the forebrain and forming an inner border of the cerebral cortex. The structures include the hippocampus, amygdala, septum, anterior thalamic nuclei, mammillary bodies and cingulate cortex. The fornix is a long fiber bundle joining the hippocampus to the mammillary bodies. Pictured also are the corpus callosum, a fiber tract joining right and left neocortex, the cerebellum, a structure involved in modulating movement, and the brain stem. The limbic system is neither directly sensory nor motor but constitutes a central core processing system of the brain that deals with information derived from events, memories of events and emotional associations to these events. This processing is essential if experience is to guide future behavior (Winson, 1985).* Reprinted from *Brain, Mind and Behavior* by Bloom and Laserson (1988) by Educational Broadcasting Corporation. Used with permission from W. H. Freeman and Company.

actual behaviors, often remembered by the mnemonic the "four F's"—fighting, fleeing, feeding and sexual behavior. In short, the hypothalamus is the body's "survival center," preparing the body for dire emergencies or, sometimes, for the passing on of its genes.

Much of our knowledge about the functions of the limbic system comes from patients who have epileptic seizures originating in this part of the brain. When you hear the word "epilepsy," you usually think of someone having fits or a seizure—the powerful involuntary contraction of all muscles of the body—and falling to the ground. Indeed, these symptoms characterize the most well-known form of epilepsy, called a grand mal seizure. Such seizures usually arise because a tiny cluster of neurons somewhere in the brain is misbehaving, firing chaotically until activity spreads like wildfire to engulf the entire brain. But seizures can also be "focal"; that is, they can remain confined largely to a single small patch of the brain. If such focal seizures are mainly in the motor cortex, the result is a sequential march of muscle twitching—or the so-called jacksonian seizures. But if they happen to be in the limbic system, then the most striking symptoms are emotional. Patients say that their "feelings are on fire," ranging from intense ecstasy to profound despair, a sense of impending doom or even fits of extreme rage and terror. Women sometimes experience orgasms during seizures, although for some obscure reason men never do. But most remarkable of all are those patients who have deeply moving spiritual experiences, including a feeling of divine presence and the sense that they are in direct communion with God. Everything around them is imbued with cosmic significance. They may say, "I finally understand what it's all about. This is the moment I've been waiting for all my life. Suddenly it all makes sense." Or, "Finally I have insight into the true nature of the cosmos." I find it ironic that this sense of enlightenment, this absolute conviction that Truth is revealed at last, should derive from limbic structures concerned with emotions rather than from the thinking, rational parts of the brain that take so much pride in their ability to discern truth and falsehood.

God has vouchsafed for us "normal" people only occasional glimpses of a deeper truth (for me they can occur when listening to some especially moving passage of music or when I look at Jupiter's moon through a telescope), but these patients enjoy the unique privilege of gazing directly into God's eyes every time they have a seizure. Who is to say whether such experiences are "genuine" (whatever that might mean) or "pathological"? Would you, the physician, really want to medicate such a patient and deny visitation rights to the Almighty?

The seizures—and visitations—last usually only for a few seconds each time. But these brief temporal lobe storms can sometimes permanently alter the patient's personality so that even between seizures he is different from other people.[3] No one knows why this happens, but it's as though the repeated electrical bursts inside the patient's brain (the frequent passage of massive volleys of nerve impulses within the limbic system) permanently "facilitate" certain pathways or may even open new channels, much as water from a storm might pour downhill, opening new rivulets, furrows and passages along the hillside. This process, called kindling, might permanently alter—and sometimes enrich—the patient's inner emotional life.

These changes give rise to what some neurologists have called "temporal lobe personality." Patients have heightened emotions and see cosmic significance in trivial events. It is claimed that they tend to be humorless, full of self-importance, and to maintain elaborate diaries that record quotidian events in elaborate detail—a trait called hypergraphia. Patients have on occasion given me hundreds of pages of written text filled with mystical symbols and notations. Some of these patients are sticky in conversation, argumentative, pedantic and egocentric (although less so than many of my scientific colleagues), and they are obsessively preoccupied with philosophical and theological issues.

Every medical student is taught that he shouldn't ever expect to see a "textbook case" in the wards, for these are merely composites concocted by the authors of medical tomes. But when Paul, the thirty-two-year-old assistant manager of a local Goodwill store, walked into our lab not long ago, I felt that he had strolled straight out of *Brain's Textbook of Neurology*—the Bible of all practicing neurologists. Dressed in a green Nehru shirt and white duck trousers, he held himself in a regal posture and wore a magnificent jeweled cross at his neck.

There is a soft armchair in our laboratory, but Paul seemed unwilling to relax. Many patients I interview are initially uneasy, but Paul was not nervous in that sense—rather, he seemed to see himself as an expert witness called to offer testimony about himself and his relationship with God. He was intense and self-absorbed and had the arrogance of a believer but none of the humility of the deeply religious. With very little prompting, he launched into his tale.

"I had my first seizure when I was eight years old," he began. "I remember seeing a bright light before I fell on the ground and wondering where it came from." A few years later, he had several additional seizures that transformed his whole life. "Suddenly, it was all crystal clear to me, doctor," he continued. "There was no longer any doubt anymore." He experienced a rapture beside which everything else paled. In the rapture was a clarity, an apprehension of the divine—no categories, no boundaries, just a Oneness with the Creator. All of this he recounted in elaborate detail and with great persistence, apparently determined to leave nothing out.

Intrigued by all this, I asked him to continue. "Can you be a little more specific?"

"Well, it's not easy, doctor. It's like trying to explain the rapture of sex to a child who has not yet reached puberty. Does that make any sense to you?"

I nodded. "What do you think of the rapture of sex?"

"Well, to be honest," he said, "I'm not interested in it anymore. It doesn't mean much to me. It pales completely beside the divine light that I have seen." But later that afternoon, Paul flirted shamelessly with two of my female graduate students and tried to get their home telephone numbers. This paradoxical combination of loss of libido and a preoccupation with sexual rituals is not unusual in patients with temporal lobe epilepsy.

The next day Paul returned to my office carrying an enormous manuscript bound in an ornate green dust jacket—a project he had been working on for several months. It set out his views on philosophy, mysticism and religion; the nature of the trinity; the iconography of the Star of David; elaborate drawings depicting spiritual themes, strange mystical symbols and maps. I was fascinated, but baffled. This was not the kind of material I usually referee.

When I finally looked up, there was a strange light in Paul's eyes. He clasped his hands and stroked his chin with his index fingers. "There's one other thing I should mention," he said. "I have these amazing flashbacks."

"What kind of flashbacks?"

"Well, the other day, during a seizure, I could remember every little detail from a book I read many years ago. Line after line, page after page word for word."

"Are you sure of this? Did you get the book and compare your memories with the original?"

"No, I lost the book. But this sort of thing happens to me a lot. It's not just that one book."

I was fascinated by Paul's claim. It corroborated similar assertions I had heard many times before from other patients and physicians. One of these days I plan to conduct an "objective test" of Paul's astonishing mnemonic abilities. Does he simply imagine he's reliving every minute detail? Or, when he has a seizure, does he lack the censoring or editing that occurs in normal memory so that he is forced to record every trivial detail—resulting in a paradoxical improvement in his memory? The only way to be sure would be to retrieve the original book or passage that he was talking about and test him on it. The results could offer important insights about how memory traces are formed in the brain.

Once, when Paul was reminiscing about his flashbacks, I interjected, "Paul, do you believe in God?"

He looked puzzled. "But what else *is* there?" he said.

•

But why do patients like Paul have religious experiences? I can think of four possibilities. One is that God really does visit these people. If that is true, so be it. Who are we to question God's infinite wisdom? Unfortunately, this can be neither proved nor ruled out on empirical grounds.

The second possibility is that because these patients experience all sorts of odd, inexplicable emotions, as if a cauldron had boiled over, perhaps their only recourse is to seek ablution in the calm waters of religious tranquility. Or the emotional hodgepodge may be misinterpreted as mystical messages from another world.

I find the latter explanation unlikely for two reasons. First, there are other neurological and psychiatric disorders such as frontal lobe syndrome, schizophrenia, manic depressive illness or just depression in which the emotions are disturbed, but one rarely sees religious preoccupations in such patients to the same degree. Second, even though schizophrenics may occasionally talk about God, the feelings are usually fleeting; they don't have the same intense fervor or the obsessive and stereotyped quality that one sees in temporal lobe epileptics. Hence emotional changes alone cannot provide a complete explanation for religious preoccupation.[4]

The third explanation invokes connections between sensory centers (vision and hearing) and the amygdala, that part of the limbic system specialized in recognizing the emotional significance of events in the external world. Obviously, not every person or event you encounter throughout a typical day sets off alarm bells; that would be maladaptive and you'd soon go mad. To cope with the world's uncertainties, you need a way of gauging the salience of events before you relay a message to the rest of the limbic system and to the hypothalamus telling them to assist you in fighting or fleeing.

But consider what might happen if spurious signals stemming from limbic seizure activity were to travel these pathways. You'd get the sort of kindling I described earlier. These "salience" pathways would become strengthened, increasing communication between brain structures. Sensory brain areas that see people and events and hear voices and noises would become more closely linked to emotional centers. The result? *Every* object and event—not just salient ones—would become imbued with deep significance, so that the patient would see "the universe in a grain of sand" and "hold[s] infinity in the palm of his hand." He would float on an ocean of religious ecstasy, carried by a universal tide to the shores of Nirvana.

The fourth hypothesis is even more speculative. Could it be that human beings have actually evolved specialized neural circuitry for the sole purpose of mediating religious experience? The human belief in the supernatural is so widespread in all societies all over the world that it's tempting to ask whether the propensity for such beliefs might have a biological basis.[5] If so, you'd have to answer a key question: What sorts of Darwinian selection pressures could lead to such a mechanism? And if there is such a mechanism, is there a gene or set of genes concerned mainly with religiosity and spiritual leanings—a gene that atheists might lack or have learned to circumvent (just kidding!)?

These kinds of arguments are popular within a relatively new discipline called evolutionary psychology. (It used to be called sociobiology, a term that fell into disrepute for political reasons.) According to its central tenets, many human traits and propensities, even ones we might ordinarily be tempted to attribute to "culture," may in fact have been specifically chosen by the guiding hand of natural selection because of their adaptive value.

One good example is the tendency for men to be polygamous and promiscuous whereas women tend to be more monogamous. Of the hundreds of human cultures throughout the world, only one, the Thodas of South India, have officially endorsed polyandry (the practice of having more than one husband or male mate). Indeed, the old adage "Higamous hogamous, women are monogamous; hogamous higamous, men are polygamous" reflects this state of affairs. It all makes good evolutionary sense, since a woman invests a good deal more time and effort—a nine-month-long, risky, arduous pregnancy—in each offspring, so that she has to be very discerning in her choice of sexual partners. For a man, the optimal evolutionary strategy is to disseminate his genes as widely as possible, given his few minutes (or, alas, seconds) of investment in each encounter. These behavioral propensities are unlikely to be cultural. If anything, culture tends to forbid or minimize them rather than encourage them, as we all know.

On the other hand, we must be careful not to carry these "evolutionary psychology" arguments too far. Just because a trait is universal—present in all cultures including cultures that have never been in contact—it doesn't follow that the trait is genetically specified. For instance, almost every culture that we know of has some form of cooking, however primitive. (Yes, even the English.) Yet one would never argue from this that there is a cooking module in the brain specified by cooking genes that were honed by natural selection. The ability to cook is almost certainly an offshoot of a number of other unrelated skills such as a good sense of smell and taste and the ability to follow a recipe step-by-step, as well as a generous dose of patience.

So is religion (or at least the belief in God and spirituality) like cooking—with culture playing by far the dominant role—or is it more like polygamy, for which there appears to be a strong genetic basis? How would an evolutionary psychologist account for the origin of religion? One possibility is that the universal human tendency to seek authority figures—giving rise to an organized priesthood, the participation in rituals, chanting and dancing, sacrificial rites and adherence to a moral code—encourages conformist behavior and contributes to the stability of one's own social group—or "kin"—who share the same genes. Genes that encourage the cultivation of such conformist traits would therefore tend to flourish and multiply, and people who lacked them would be ostracized and punished for their socially deviant behavior. Perhaps the easiest way to ensure such stability and conformity is to believe in some transcendent higher power that controls our destiny. No wonder temporal lobe epilepsy patients experience a sense of omnipotence and grandeur, as if to say, "I am the chosen one. It is my duty and privilege to transmit God's work to you lesser beings."

This is admittedly a speculative argument even by the rather lax standards of evolutionary psychology. But whether or not one believes in religious conformity "genes," it's clear that certain parts of the temporal lobe play a more direct role in the genesis of such experiences than any other part of the brain. And if the personal experiences of Dr. Persinger are anything to go by, then this must be true not just of epileptics but also of you and me.

I hasten to add that as far as the patient is concerned, whatever changes have occurred are authentic—sometimes even desirable—and the physician has no right, really, to attribute a value label to such esoteric embellishments of personality. On what basis does one decide whether a mystical experience is normal or abnormal? There is a common tendency to equate "unusual" or "rare" with abnormal, but this is a logical fallacy. Genius is a rare but highly valued trait, whereas tooth decay is common but obviously undesirable. Which one of these categories does mystical experience fall into? Why is the revealed truth of such transcendent experiences in any way "inferior" to the more mundane truths that we scientists dabble in? Indeed, if you are ever tempted to jump to this conclusion, just bear in mind that one could use exactly the same evidence—the involvement of the temporal lobes in religion—to argue for, rather than against, the existence of God. By way of analogy, consider the fact that most animals don't have the receptors or neural machinery for color vision. Only a privileged few do, yet would you want to conclude from this that color wasn't real? Obviously not, but if not, then why doesn't the same argument apply to God? Perhaps only the "chosen" ones have the required neural connections. (After all, "God works in mysterious ways.") My goal as a scientist, in other words, is to discover how and why religious sentiments originate in the brain, but this has no bearing one way or the other on whether God really exists or not.

So we now have several competing hypotheses of why temporal lobe epileptics have such experiences. Even though all these theories invoke the same neural structures, they postulate very different mechanisms and it would be nice to find a way to distinguish among them. One of the ideas—the notion that kindling has indiscriminately strengthened all connections from the temporal cortex to the amygdala—can be addressed directly by studying the patient's galvanic skin response. Ordinarily an object is recognized by the visual areas of the temporal lobes. Its emotional salience—is it a friendly face or a fierce lion?—is signaled by the amygdala and transmitted to the limbic system so that you become emotionally aroused and start sweating. But if the kindling has strengthened *all* the connections within these pathways, then everything becomes salient. No matter what you look at—a nondescript stranger, a chair or a table—it should activate the limbic system strongly and make you perspire. So unlike you and me, who should display a heightened GSR response only for our moms, dads, spouses or lions, or even a loud thud or bang, the patient with temporal lobe epilepsy should show an increased galvanic skin response to everything under the sun.

To test this possibility, I contacted two of my colleagues who specialize in the diagnosis and treatment of epilepsy—Dr. Vincent Iragui and Dr. Evelyn Tecoma. Given the highly controversial nature of the whole concept of "temporal lobe personality" (not everyone agrees that these personality traits are seen more frequently in epileptics), they were quite intrigued by my ideas. A few days later, they recruited two of their patients who manifested obvious "symptoms" of this syndrome—hypergraphia, spiritual leanings and an obsessive need to talk about their feelings and about religious and metaphysical topics. Would they want to volunteer in a research study?

Both were eager to participate. In what may turn out to be the very first scientific experiment ever done on religion directly, I sat them in comfortable chairs and attached harmless electrodes to their hands. Once settled in front of a computer screen, they were shown random samples of several types of words and images—for example, words for ordinary inanimate objects (a shoe, vase, table and the like), familiar faces (parents, siblings), unfamiliar faces, sexually arousing words and pictures (erotic magazine pinups), four-letter words involving sex, extreme violence and horror (an alligator eating a person alive, a man setting himself afire) and religious words and icons (such as the word "God").

If you and I were to undergo this exercise, we would show huge GSR responses to the scenes of violence and to the sexually explicit words and pictures, a fairly large response to familiar faces and usually nothing at all to other categories (unless you have a shoe fetish, in which case you'd respond to one).

What about the patients? The kindling hypothesis would predict a uniform high response to all categories. But to our amazement what we found in the two patients tested was a heightened response mainly to religious words and icons. Their responses to the other categories, including the sexual words and images, which ordinarily evoke a powerful response, was strangely diminished compared to what is seen in normal individuals.[6]

Thus the results show that there has been no general enhancement of all the connections—indeed, if anything, there has been a decrement. But rather surprisingly, there's been a selective amplification of response to religious words. One wonders whether this technique could be useful as a sort of "piety index" to distinguish religious dabblers or frauds ("closet atheists") from true believers. The absolute zero on the scale could be set by measuring Francis Crick's galvanic skin response.

I want to emphasize that not every temporal lobe epilepsy patient becomes religious. There are many parallel neural connections between the temporal cortex and the amygdala. Depending on which particular ones are involved, some patients may have their personalities skewed in other directions, becoming obsessed with writing, drawing, arguing philosophy or, rarely, being preoccupied with sex. It's likely that their GSR responses would shoot upward in response to these stimuli rather than to religious icons, a possibility that is being studied in our laboratory and others.

Was God talking to us directly through the GSR machine? Did we now have a direct hotline to heaven? Whatever one makes of the selective amplification of responses to religious words and icons, the finding eliminates one of the proposed explanations for these experiences—that these people become spiritual simply because *everything* around them becomes so salient and deeply meaningful. On the contrary, the finding suggests that there has been a selective enhancement of responses to some categories of stimuli—such as religious words and images—and an actual reduction in response to other categories such as sexually loaded ones (as is consistent with the diminished libido that some of these patients report).

So do these findings imply that there are neural structures in the temporal lobes that are specialized for religion or spirituality, that are selectively enhanced by the epileptic process? This is a seductive hypothesis, but other interpretations are possible. For all we know, the changes that have triggered these patients' religious fervor could be occurring anywhere, not necessarily in the temporal lobes. Such activity would still eventually cascade into the limbic system and give you exactly the same result—an enhanced GSR for religious images. So strong GSR itself is no guarantee that the temporal lobes are directly involved in religion.[7]

There is, however, another experiment that could be done to resolve this issue once and for all. The experiment takes advantage of the fact that when seizures become seriously disabling, life-threatening and unresponsive to medication, portions of the temporal lobe are often surgically removed. So we can ask, What would happen to the patient's personality—especially his spiritual leanings—if we removed a chunk of his temporal lobe? Would some of his acquired personality changes be "reversed"? Would he suddenly stop having mystical experiences and become an atheist or an agnostic? Would we have performed a "Godectomy"?

We have yet to conduct such a study, but meanwhile we have already learned something from our GSR studies—that the seizures have permanently altered the patients' inner mental life, often producing interesting and highly selective distortions of their personality. After all, one rarely sees such profound emotional upheavals or religious preoccupations in other neurological disorders. The simplest explanation for what happens in the epileptics is that there have been permanent changes in temporal lobe circuitry caused by selective enhancement of some connections and effacement of others—leading to new peaks and valleys in the patients' emotional landscape.

So what's the bottom line? The one clear conclusion that emerges from all this is that there are circuits in the human brain that are involved in religious experience and these become hyperactive in some epileptics. We still don't know whether these circuits evolved specifically for religion (as evolutionary psychologists might argue) or whether they generate other emotions that are merely conducive to such beliefs (although that cannot explain the fervor with which the beliefs are held by many patients). We are therefore still a long way from showing that there is a "God module" in the brain that might be genetically specified, but to me the exciting idea is that one can even begin to address questions about God and spirituality scientifically.

Then to the rolling Heav'n itself I cried,
Asking, "What Lamp had Destiny to guide
Her little Children stumbling in the Dark?"
And—"A blind Understanding!" Heav'n replied.

—The Rubáiyát of Omar Khayyám

For many of the topics we've discussed in earlier chapters—phantom limbs, neglect syndrome and Capgras' syndrome—we now have reasonable interpretations as a result of our experiments. But in seeking brain centers concerned with religious experience and God, I realized that I had entered the "twilight zone" of neurology. There are some questions about the brain that are so mysterious, so deeply enigmatic, that most serious scientists simply shy away from them, as if to say, "That would be premature to study" and "I'd be a fool if I embarked on such a quest." And yet these are the very issues that fascinate us most of all. The most obvious one, of course, is religion, a quintessentially human trait, but it is only one unsolved mystery of human nature. What about other uniquely human traits—such as our capacity for music, math, humor and poetry? What allowed Mozart to compose an entire symphony in his head or mathematicians like Fermat or Ramanujan to "discover" flawless conjectures and theorems without ever going through step-by-step formal proofs? And what goes on in the brain of a person like Dylan Thomas that allowed him to write such evocative poetry? Is the creative spark simply an expression of the divine spark that exists in all of us? Ironically clues come from a bizarre condition called "idiot savant syndrome" (or, to use the more politically correct phrase, the savant syndrome). These individuals (retarded and yet highly talented) can give us valuable insights about the evolution of human nature—a topic that became an obsession for some of the greatest scientific minds of the last century.

The Victorian era witnessed a vigorous intellectual debate between two brilliant biologists—Charles Darwin and Alfred Russel Wallace. Darwin, of course, is a household name. Everyone associates him with the discovery of natural selection as the main driving force of organic evolution. It is a pity that Wallace is almost completely unknown except among biologists and historians of science, since he was an equally brilliant scholar and independently came up with the same idea. In fact, the very first scientific paper on evolution by natural selection was presented jointly by Darwin and Wallace and communicated to the Linnean Society by Joseph Hooker in 1850. Instead of feuding endlessly over priority, as many of today's scientists do, they cheerfully acknowledged each other's contributions and Wallace even wrote a book called *Darwinism*, championing what he referred to as "Darwin's" theory of natural selection. Upon hearing of this book, Darwin responded, "You should not speak of Darwinism for it can as well be called Wallacism."

What does the theory state? There are three components:[8]

1. Since offspring vastly outnumber the available resources, there must be a constant struggle for existence in the natural world.
2. No two individuals of a species are exactly identical (except in the rare case of identical twins). Indeed, there are always random variations, however minute, in body type that arise from the random shuffling of genes that takes place during cell division—a shuffling that ensures that offspring differ from each other and from their parents, thereby increasing their candidature for evolutionary change.
3. Those fortuitous combinations of genes that cause individuals to be slightly better adapted to a given local environment tend to multiply and propagate within a population since they increase the survival and reproduction of those individuals.

Darwin believed that his principle of natural selection could account not only for the emergence of morphological traits like fingers or noses, but also for the structure of the brain and therefore our mental capacities. In other words, natural selection could explain our talents for music, art, literature and other human intellectual achievements. Wallace disagreed. He conceded that Darwin's principle might explain fingers and toes and maybe even some simple mental traits, but that certain quintessentially human abilities like mathematical and musical talent could not possibly have arisen through the blind workings of chance.

Why not? According to Wallace, as the human brain evolved, it encountered a new and equally powerful force called culture. Once culture, language and writing emerged, he argued, human evolution became Lamarckian—that is, you could pass on the accumulated wisdom of a lifetime to your offspring. These progeny will be much wiser than the offspring of illiterates not because your genes have changed but simply because this knowledge—in the form of culture—has been transferred from your brain to your child's brain. In this way, the brain is symbiotic with culture; the two are as interdependent as the naked hermit crab and its shell or the nucleated cell and its mitochondria. For Wallace, culture propels human evolution, making us absolutely unique in the animal kingdom. Isn't it extraordinary, he said, that we are the only animal in which the mind is vastly more important than any bodily organ, assuming a tremendous significance because of what we call "culture." Moreover, our brain actually helps us avoid the need for further specialization.[9] Most organisms evolve to become more and more specialized as they take up new environmental niches, be it a longer neck for the giraffe or sonar for the bat. Humans, on the other hand, have evolved an organ, a brain, that gives us the capacity to evade specialization. We can colonize the Arctic without evolving a fur coat over millions of years like the polar bear because we can go kill one, take its coat and drape it on ourselves. And then we can give it to our children and grandchildren.

Wallace's second argument against "blind chance giving rise to the talents of a Mozart" involves what might be called potential intelligence (a phrase used by Richard Gregory). Say, you take a barely literate young tribesman from a contemporary aboriginal society (or even use a time machine to garner a Cro-Magnon man) and give him a modern public school education in Rio or New York or Tokyo. He will, of course, be no different from any other child reared in those cities. According to Wallace, this means that the aborigine or Cro-Magnon possesses a potential intelligence that vastly exceeds anything that he might need for coping with his natural environment. This kind of potential intelligence can be contrasted with kinetic intelligence, which is realized through formal education. But why the devil did this potential intelligence evolve? It couldn't have arisen for learning Latin in English schools. It couldn't have evolved for learning the calculus, even though almost anyone who tries hard enough can master it. What was the selection pressure for the emergence of these latent abilities? Natural selection can only explain the emergence of actual abilities that are expressed by the organism—never potential ones. When they are useful and promote survival, they are passed on to the next generation. But what to make of a gene for *latent* mathematical ability? What benefit does that confer on a nonliterate person? It seems like overkill.

Wallace wrote, "The lowest savages with the least copious vocabularies [have] the capacity of uttering a variety of distinct articulate sounds and of applying them to an almost infinite amount of modulation and inflection [which] is not in any way inferior to that of the higher [European] races. An instrument has been developed in advance of the needs of its possessor." And the argument holds, with even greater force, for other esoteric human abilities such as mathematics or musical talent.

There's the rub. *An instrument has been developed in advance of the needs of its possessor,* but we know that evolution has no foresight! Here is an instance in which evolution appears to have foreknowledge. How is this possible?

Wallace wrestled mightily with this paradox. How can improvement in esoteric mathematical skills—in latent form—affect the survival of one race that has this latent ability and the extinction of another that doesn't? "It is a somewhat curious fact," he wrote, "that when all modern writers admit the great antiquity of man, most of them maintain the very recent development of intellect, and will hardly contemplate the possibility of men, equal in mental capacity to ourselves, having existed in prehistoric times."

But we know they did. Both the Neanderthal and Cro-Magnon cranial capacities were actually larger than ours, and it's not inconceivable that their latent potential intelligence may have been equal to or even greater than that of *Homo sapiens.*

So how is it possible that these astonishing, latent abilities emerged in the prehistoric brain but have only been realized in the last one thousand years? Wallace's answer: It was done by God! "Some higher intelligence must have directed the process by which the human nature was developed." Thus human grace is an earthly expression of "divine grace."

This is where Wallace parted company with Darwin, who resolutely maintained that natural selection was the prime force in evolution and could account for the emergence of even the most esoteric mental traits, without the helping hand of a Supreme Being.

How would a modern biologist resolve Wallace's paradox? She would probably argue that esoteric and "advanced" human traits like musical and mathematical ability are specific manifestations of what is usually called "general intelligence"—itself the culmination of a "runaway" brain that exploded in size and complexity within the last three million years.[10] General intelligence evolved, the argument goes, so that one can communicate, hunt game, hoard food in granaries, engage in elaborate social rituals and do the myriad things that humans enjoy and that help them survive. But once this intelligence was in place, you could use it for all sorts of other things, like the calculus, music and the design of scientific instruments to extend the reach of our senses. By way of analogy, consider the human hand: Even though it evolved its amazing versatility for grasping at tree branches, it can now be used to count, write poetry, rock the cradle, wield a scepter and make shadow puppets.

But with respect to the mind, this argument doesn't make much sense to me. I'm not saying it's wrong, but the idea that the ability to spear antelope was then somehow used for the calculus is a bit dubious. I'd like to suggest another explanation, one that takes us back not only to the savant syndrome that I mentioned earlier but also to the more general question of the sporadic emergence of talent and genius in the normal population.

"Savants" are persons whose mental capacity or general intelligence is abysmally low, yet who have islands of astonishing talent. For example, there are savants on record with an IQ of less than 50, barely able to function in normal society, yet they could with ease generate an eight-digit prime number, a feat that most tenured mathematics professors cannot match. One savant could come up with the cube root of a six-figure number in seconds and could double 8,388,628 twenty-four times to obtain 140,737,488,355,328 in several seconds. Such individuals are a living refutation of the argument that specialized talents are merely clever deployments of general intelligence.[11]

The realms of art and music are punctuated with savants whose talents have amazed and delighted audiences through the ages. Oliver Sacks describes Tom, a thirteen-year-old boy who was blind and incapable of tying his own shoes. Although he had never been instructed in music or educated in any way, he learned to play the piano simply by hearing others play. He absorbed arias and tunes from hearing them sung and could play any piece of music on the first try as well as the most accomplished performer. One of his most remarkable feats was to perform three pieces of music all at once. With one hand he played "Fisher's Horn Pipe," with the other he played "Yankee Doodle Dandy" and simultaneously he sang "Dixie." He could also play the piano with his back to the keyboard, his inverted hands racing up and down the ivories. Tom composed his own music, and yet, as a contemporary observer pointed out, "He seems to be an unconscious agent acting as he is acted on and his mind [is] a vacant receptor where nature stores her jewels to recall them at her pleasure."

Nadia, whose IQ measured between 60 and 70, was an artistic genius. At age six, she showed all the signs of severe autism—ritualistic behavior, inability to relate to others and limited language. She could barely put two words together. Yet from this early age, Nadia could draw lifelike pictures of people around her, of horses and even of complex visual scenes unlike the "tadpolelike" drawings of other children her age. Her sketches were so animated that they seemed to leap out from the canvas and were good enough to hang in any Madison Avenue gallery (Figure 9.2).

Other savants have incredibly specific talents. One boy can tell you the time of day, to the exact second, without referring to any timepiece. He can do this even in his sleep, sometimes mumbling the exact time while dreaming. The "clock" inside his head is as accurate as any Rolex. Another can estimate the exact width of an object seen from twenty feet away. You or I would give a ballpark figure. She would say, "That rock is exactly two feet, eleven and three-quarter inches wide." And she'd be right.

These examples show that specialized esoteric talents do not emerge spontaneously from general intelligence, for if that were true, how can an "idiot" display them?

Nor do we have to invoke the extreme pathological example of savants to make this point, for there is an element of this syndrome in every talented person or indeed in every genius. "Genius," contrary to popular misconception, is not synonymous with superhuman intelligence. Most of the geniuses whom I have had the privilege of knowing are more like idiot savants than they would care to admit—extraordinarily talented in a few domains but quite ordinary in other respects.

Consider the oft-told story of the Indian mathematical genius Ramanujan, who at the turn of the century worked as a clerk in the Madras seaport, a few miles from where I was born. He had matriculated to the early part of high school, where he performed badly in all his subjects, and he had no formal education in advanced mathematics. Yet he was astonishingly gifted in math and was obsessed by it. So poor that he couldn't afford paper, he would use discarded envelopes to scribble his

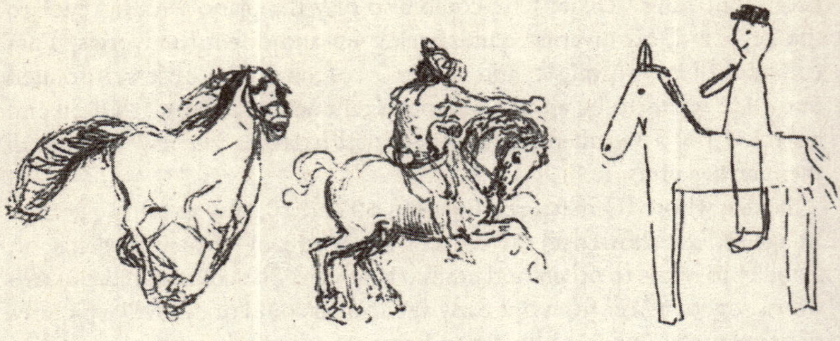

Figure 9.2 *(a) A drawing of a horse made by Nadia, the autistic savant, when she was five years old. (b) A horse drawn by Leonardo da Vinci. (c) A drawing of a horse by a normal eight-year-old. Notice that Nadia's drawing is vastly superior to that of the normal eight-year-old and almost as good as (or perhaps better than!) da Vinci's horse.* (a) and (c) reprinted from *Nadia*, by Lorna Selfe, with permission from Academic Press (New York).

mathematical equations, discovering several new theorems before the age of twenty-two. Since he was not acquainted with any number theorists in India, he decided to communicate his discoveries to several mathematicians in other parts of the world, including Cambridge, England. One of the world's top number theorists of that time, G.H. Hardy, received his scribbles and immediately thought Ramanujan was a crackpot. Having glanced at them, he went out to play tennis. As the game wore on, Ramanujan's equations kept haunting him. He kept seeing the numbers in his mind. "I had never seen anything in the least like them before," Hardy later wrote. "They must be true because no one would have had the imagination to invent them." So he promptly went back and checked the validity of the elaborate equations on backs of envelopes, saw that most of them were correct and immediately sent a note to his colleague J.E. Littlewood, who also went over the manuscripts. Both luminaries quickly realized that Ramanujan was probably a genius of the highest caliber. They invited him to Cambridge, where he worked for many years, eventually surpassing them in the originality and importance of his contributions.

I mention this story because if you were to go out to dinner with Ramanujan you wouldn't think there was anything unusual about him. He was just like any other person except for the fact that his mathematical skills were way off scale—almost supernatural, some have said. Again, if mathematical ability is simply a function of general intelligence, a result of the brain's getting bigger and better overall, then more intelligent people should be better at math, and vice versa. But if you met Ramanujan, you'd know that that just isn't true.

What is the solution? Ramanujan's own "explanation"—that the fully formed equations were whispered to him in dreams by the presiding village deity, Goddess Namagiri—doesn't really help us very much. But I can think of two other possibilities.

The first, more parsimonious, view is that general intelligence is really a number of different mental traits—with both the genes and the traits themselves influencing each other's expression. Since genes combine randomly in the population, every now and then you will get a fortuitous combination of traits—such as vivid visual imagery combined with excellent numerical skills—and such shuffling can throw up all sorts of unexpected interactions. Thus is born that extraordinary flowering of talent we call genius—the gifts of an Albert Einstein who could "visualize" his equations or a Mozart who saw, and did not merely hear, his musical compositions unfold in his mind's eye. Such genius is rare only because the lucky genetic combinations are rare.

But there's a problem with this argument. If genius results from serendipitous genetic combinations, how does one explain the talents of Nadia and Tom, whose general intelligence is abysmal? (Indeed, an autistic savant's social skills may be less than those of a Bonobo ape.) It's difficult, moreover, to see why such unique talent should actually be *more* common among savants than it is among the general population, who, if anything, have a larger number of healthy traits to shuffle around in each generation. (As many as 10 percent of autistic children have perfect pitch, compared with only 1 or 2 percent of the general population.) Furthermore, the traits in that individual would have to "interlock" precisely and interact in such a way that the outcome is something elegant rather than nonsensical, a scenario that is as unlikely as a confederacy of dunces producing a work of artistic or scientific genius.

This brings me to the second explanation for the savant syndrome in particular and for genius in general. How can someone who can't tie shoelaces or carry on a normal conversation calculate prime numbers? The answer might lie in a region of the left hemisphere called the angular gyrus, which, when damaged, leaves some people (like Bill, the Air Force pilot in Chapter 1 who couldn't subtract) with an inability to do simple calculations, such as subtract 7 from 100. This does not mean that the left angular gyrus is the brain's math module, but it's fair to say that this structure is doing something crucial for mathematical computation and is not essential for language, working memory or vision. But you do seem to need the left angular gyrus for math.

Consider the possibility that savants suffer early brain damage before or shortly after birth. Is it possible that their brains undergo some form of remapping as seen in phantom limb patients? Does the prenatal or neonatal injury lead to unusual rewiring? In savants, one part of the brain may for some obscure reason receive a greater than average input or some other equivalent impetus to become denser and larger—a huge angular gyrus, for example. What would be the consequence for mathematical ability? Would this produce a child who can generate eight-digit prime numbers? In truth, we know so little about how neurons perform such abstract operations that it's difficult to predict what the effect of such a change might be. An angular gyrus doubled in size could lead not to a mere doubling of mathematical ability but to a logarithmic or hundredfold increase. You can imagine an explosion of talent resulting from this simple but "anomalous" increase in brain volume. The same argument might hold for drawing, music, language, indeed any human trait.[12]

This argument is zany and unashamedly speculative, but at least it's testable. A math savant should have a large or hypertrophied left angular gyrus, whereas an artistic savant may have a hypertrophied right angular gyrus. Such experiments have not been done, to my knowledge, although we do know that damage to the *right* parietal cortex, where the angular gyrus is located, can profoundly disrupt artistic skills (just as damage to the left disrupts calculation).

A similar argument can be put forth to explain the occasional emergence of genius or extraordinary talent in the normal population, or to answer the especially vexing question of how such abilities cropped up in evolution in the first place. Maybe when the brain reaches a critical mass, new and unforeseen traits, properties that were not specifically chosen by natural selection, emerge. Maybe the brain had to become big for some other more obviously adaptive reason—throwing spears, talking or navigation—and the simplest way to achieve this was to increase one or two growth-related hormones or morphogens (genes that alter size and shape in developing organisms). But since such a hormone- or morphogen-based growth spurt cannot selectively increase the size of some parts while sparing others, the bonus might be an altogether bigger brain, including an enormous angular gyrus and the accompanying tenfold or hundredfold enhancement in mathematical ability. Notice that this argument is very different from the widely held belief that you develop some very "general" ability that is then deployed for a specialized skill.

Taking this speculation even further, is it possible that humans find such esoteric talents—be it music, poetry, drawing or math—to be sexually attractive mainly because they serve as an externally visible signature of a giant brain? Just as the peacock's large, iridescent tail or the size of a majestic bull elephant's tusks constitutes "truth in advertising" for the animal's health, so the human ability to croon a tune or pen a sonnet might be a marker for a superior brain. ("Truth in advertising" may play an important role in mate selection. Indeed, Richard Dawkins has suggested, half seriously, that the size and strength of a human male's erection may be markers for general health.)

This line of reasoning raises some fascinating possibilities. For instance, you could inject hormones or morphogens into a fetal human brain or infant to try to increase brain size artificially. Would this result in a race of geniuses with superhuman talents? Needless to say, the experiment would be unethical to do in humans, but an evil genius might be tempted to try it on the great apes. Is so, would you see a sudden efflorescence of extraordinary mental talents in these apes? Could you accelerate the pace of simian evolution through a combination of genetic engineering, hormonal intervention and artificial selection?

My basic argument about savants—that some specialized brain regions may have become enlarged at the expense of others—may or may not turn out to be correct. But even if it's valid, bear in mind that no savant is going to be a Picasso or an Einstein. To be a true genius, you need other abilities, not just isolated islands of talent. Most savants are not truly creative. If you look at a drawing by Nadia, you do see creative artistic ability,[13] but among mathematical and musical savants, there are no such examples. What seems to be missing is an ineffable quality called creativity, which brings us face to face with the very essence of what it is to be human. There are those who assert that creativity is simply the ability to randomly link seemingly unrelated ideas, but surely that is not enough. The proverbial monkey with a typewriter will eventually produce a Shakespeare play, but it would need a billion lifetimes before it could generate a single intelligible sentence—let alone a sonnet or a play.

Not long ago when I told a colleague about my interest in creativity, he repeated the well-worn argument that we simply toss ideas around in our heads, producing random combinations until we hit on aesthetically pleasing ones. So I challenged him to "toss around" some words and ideas by coming up with a single evocative metaphor for "taking things to ridiculous extremes" or "overdoing things." He scratched his head and after half an hour confessed that he couldn't think of anything all that original (despite his very high verbal IQ, I might add). I pointed out to him that Shakespeare had crammed five such metaphors in a single sentence:

> To gild refined gold, to paint the lily, to throw a perfume on the violet, to smooth the ice, or add another hue unto the rainbow . . . is wasteful and ridiculous excess.

It sounds so simple. But how come Shakespeare thought of it and nobody else? Each of us has the same words at our command. There's nothing complicated or esoteric about the idea that's being conveyed. In fact, it's crystal clear once it is explained and has that universal "why didn't I think of that?" quality that characterizes the most beautiful and creative insights. Yet you and I would never come up with an equally elegant set of metaphors by simply dredging up and randomly shuffling words in our minds. What's missing is the creative spark of genius, a trait that remains as mysterious to us now as it did to Wallace. No wonder he felt impelled to invoke divine intervention.

CHAPTER 10

The Woman Who Died Laughing

God is a comedian performing before an audience that is afraid to laugh.

—FRIEDRICH NIETZSCHE

God is a hacker.

—FRANCIS CRICK

On the morning of his mother's funeral in 1931, Willy Anderson—a twenty-five-year-old plumber from London—donned a new black suit, clean white shirt and nice shoes borrowed from his brother. He had loved his mother very much and his grief was palpable. The family gathered amid tearful hugs and sat silently through an hour-long funeral service in a church that was much too hot and stuffy. Willy was relieved finally to get outdoors into the chilly open air of the cemetery and bow his head with the rest of the family and friends. But just as the gravediggers began lowering his mother's roped casket into the earth, Willy began to laugh. It started as a muffled snorting sound that evolved into a prolonged giggle. Willy bowed his head farther down, dug his chin into his shirt collar and drew his right hand up to his mouth, trying to stifle the unbidden mirth. It was no use. Against his will and to his profound embarrassment, he began to laugh out loud, the sounds exploding rhythmically until he doubled over. Everyone at the funeral stared, mouth agape, as the young man staggered backward, desperately looking for retreat. He walked bent at the waist, as if in supplication for forgiveness for the laughter that would not subside. The mourners could hear him at the far end of the cemetery, his laughter echoing amid the gravestones.

That evening, Willy's cousin took him to the hospital. The laughter had subsided after some hours, but it was so inexplicable, so stunning in its inappropriateness, that everyone in the family felt it should be treated as a medical emergency. Dr. Astley Clark, the physician on duty, examined Willy's pupils and checked his vital signs. Two days later, a nurse found Willy lying unconscious in his bed, having suffered a severe subarachnoid hemorrhage, and he died without regaining consciousness. The postmortem showed a large ruptured aneurysm in an artery at the base of his brain that had compressed part of his hypothalamus, mammillary bodies and other structures on the floor of his brain.

And then there was Ruth Greenough, a fifty-eight-year-old librarian from Philadelphia. Although she had suffered a mild stroke, she was able to keep her small branch library running smoothly. But one morning in 1936, Ruth had a sudden violent headache, and within seconds her eyes turned up and she was seized with a laughing fit. She began shaking with laughter and couldn't stop. Short expirations followed each other in such rapid succession that Ruth's brain grew oxygen-starved and she broke into a sweat, at times holding her hand to her throat as if she were choking. Nothing she did would stop the convulsions of laughter, and even an injection of morphine given by the doctor had no effect. The laughter went on for an hour and a half. All the while, Ruth's eyes remained turned upward and wide open. She was conscious and could follow her doctor's instructions but was not able to utter a single word. At the end of an hour and a half, Ruth lay down completely exhausted. The laughter persisted but was noiseless—little more than a grimace. Suddenly she collapsed and became comatose, and after twenty-four hours Ruth died. I can say that she literally died laughing. The postmortem revealed that a cavity in the middle of her brain (called the third ventricle) was filled with blood. A hemorrhage had occurred, involving the floor of her thalamus and compressing several adjacent structures. The English neurologist Dr. Purdon Martin, who described Ruth's case, said, "The laughter is a mock or sham and it mocks the laughter at the time, but this is the greatest mockery of all, that the patient should be forced to laugh as a portent of his own doom."[1]

More recently, the British journal *Nature* reported a modern case of laughter elicited by direct electrical stimulation of the brain during surgery. The patient was a fifteen-year-old girl named Susan who was being treated for intractable epilepsy. Doctors hoped to excise the tissue at the focal point of her seizures and were exploring nearby areas to make sure they did not remove any critically important functions. When the surgeon stimulated Susan's supplementary motor cortex (close to a region in the frontal lobes that receives input from the brain's emotional centers), he got an unexpected response. Susan started laughing uncontrollably, right on the operating table (she was awake for the procedure). Oddly enough, she ascribed her merriment to everything she saw around her, including a picture of a horse, and added that the people standing near her looked incredibly funny. To the doctors, she said: "You guys are just so *funny* standing around."[2]

•

The kind of pathological laughter seen in Willy and Ruth is rare; only a couple of dozen such cases have been described in the medical literature. But when you gather them together, a striking fact jumps out at you. The abnormal activity or damage that sets people giggling is almost always located in portions of the limbic system, a set of structures including the hypothalamus, mammillary bodies and cingulate gyrus that are involved in emotions (see Figure 8.1). Given the complexity of laughter and its infinite cultural overtones, I find it intriguing that a relatively small cluster of brain structures is behind the phenomenon—a sort of "laughter circuit."

But identifying the location of such a circuit doesn't tell us why laughter exists or what its biological function might be. (You can't say it evolved because it feels good. That would be a circular argument, like saying sex exists because it feels good instead of saying it feels good because it motivates you to spread your genes.) Asking why a given trait evolved (be it yawning, laughing, crying or dancing) is absolutely vital for understanding its biological function, and yet this question is rarely raised by neurologists who study patients with brain lesions. This is astonishing given that the brain was shaped by natural selection just as any other organ in the body, such as the kidney, liver or pancreas, was.

Fortunately, the picture is changing, thanks in part to "evolutionary psychology," the new discipline that I mentioned in the last chapter.[3] The central tenet of this controversial field is that many salient aspects of human behavior are mediated by specialized modules (mental organs) that were specifically shaped by natural selection. As our Pleistocene ancestors romped across ancient savannas in small probands, their brains evolved solutions to their everyday problems—things like recognizing kin, seeking healthy sexual partners or eschewing foul-smelling food.

For example, evolutionary psychologists would argue that your disgust for feces—far from being taught to you by your parents—is probably hard-wired in your brain. Since feces might contain infectious bacteria, eggs and parasites, those ancestral hominids who had "disgust for feces" genes survived and passed on those genes, whereas those who didn't were wiped out (unlike dung beetles, who probably find the bouquet of feces irresistible). This idea may even explain why feces infected with cholera, salmonellosis or shigella are especially foul smelling.[4]

Evolutionary psychology is one of those disciplines that tend to polarize scientists. You are either for it or vehemently against it with much arm waving and trading of raspberries behind backs, much as people are nativists (genes specify everything) or empiricists (the brain is a blank slate whose wiring is subsequently specified by the environment, including culture). The real brain, it turns out, is far messier than what's implied by these simple-minded dichotomies. For some traits—and I'm going to argue that laughter is one of them—the evolutionary perspective is essential and helps explain why a specialized laughter circuit exists. For other traits this way of thinking is a waste of time (as we noted in Chapter 9, the notion that there might be genes or mental organs for cooking is silly, even though cooking is a universal human trait).

The distinction between fact and fiction gets more easily blurred in evolutionary psychology than in any other discipline, a problem that is exacerbated by the fact that most "ev-psych" explanations are completely untestable: You can't run experiments to prove or disprove them. Some of the proposed theories—that we have genetically specified mechanisms to help us detect fertile mates or that women suffer from morning sickness to protect the fetus from poisons in foods—are ingenious. Others are ridiculously far-fetched. One afternoon, in a whimsical mood, I sat down and wrote a spoof of evolutionary psychology just to annoy my colleagues in that field. I wanted to see how far one could go in conjuring up completely arbitrary, ad hoc, untestable evolutionary explanations for aspects of human behavior that most people would regard as "cultural" in origin. The result was a satire titled "Why Do Gentlemen Prefer Blondes?" To my amazement, when I submitted my tongue-in-cheek essay to a medical journal, it was promptly accepted. And to my even greater surprise, many of my colleagues did not find it amusing; to them it was a perfectly plausible argument, not a spoof.[5] (I describe it in the endnotes in case you are curious.)

•

What about laughter? Can we come up with a reasonable evolutionary explanation, or will the true meaning of laughter remain forever elusive?

If an alien ethologist were to land on earth and watch us humans, he would be mystified by many aspects of our behavior, but I'll wager that laughter would be very near the top of the list. As he watches people interacting, he notices that every now and then we suddenly stop what we're doing, grimace and make a loud repetitive sound in response to a wide variety of situations. What function could this mysterious behavior possibly serve? Cultural factors undoubtedly influence humor and what people find funny—the English are thought to have a sophisticated sense of humor, whereas Germans or Swiss, it is said, rarely find anything amusing. But even if this is true, might there still be some sort of "deep structure" underlying all humor? The details of the phenomenon vary from culture to culture and are influenced by the way people are raised, but this doesn't mean there's no genetically specified mechanism for laughter—a common denominator underlying all types of humor. Indeed, many people have suggested that such a mechanism does exist, and theories on the biological origins of humor and laughter have a long history, going all the way to Schopenhauer and Kant, two singularly humorless German philosophers.

Consider the following two jokes. (Not surpisingly, it was difficult to find examples that are not racist, sexist or ethnic. After a diligent search I found one that was and one that wasn't.)

A fellow is sitting in a truck stop café in California, having lunch, when suddenly a giant panda bear walks in and orders a burger with fries and a chocolate milkshake. The bear sits down, eats the food, then stands up, shoots several of the other customers and runs out the door. The fellow is astonished, but the waiter seems completely undisturbed. "What the hell is going on?" the customer asks. "Oh, well, there's nothing surprising about that," says the waiter. "Just go look in the dictionary under 'panda.' " So the guy goes to the library, takes out a dictionary and looks up "panda"—a big furry, black and white animal that lives in the rain forest of China. It eats shoots and leaves.

A guy carrying a brown paper bag goes into a bar and orders a drink. The bartender smiles, pours the drink and then, unable to contain his curiosity, says, "So, what's in the bag?" The man gives a little laugh and says, "You wanna see? Sure, you can see what's in the bag," and he reaches in and pulls out a tiny piano, no more than six inches tall.

"What's that?" asks the bartender. The man doesn't say anything; he just reaches into the bag a second time and pulls out a tiny man, about a foot tall, and sits him down next to the piano. "Wow," says the bartender, absolutely astonished. "I've never in my life seen anything like that." The little man begins to play Chopin. "Holy cow," says the bartender, "where did you ever get him?" The man sighs and says, "Well, you see, I found this magic lamp and it has a genie in it. He can grant you anything you want but only gives one wish." The bartender scowls, "Oh, yeah, sure you do. Who are you trying to kid?" "You don't believe me?" says the man, somewhat offended. He reaches into his coat pocket and pulls out a silver lamp with an ornate curved handle. "Here it is. Here's the lamp with the genie in it. Go ahead and rub it if you don't believe me." So the bartender pulls the lamp over to his side of the counter and, looking at the man skeptically, rubs the lamp. And then POOF, a genie appears over the bar, bows to the bartender and says, "Sire, your wish is my command. I shall grant thee one wish and one wish only." The bartender gasps but quickly gains his composure and says, "Okay, okay, give me a million bucks!" The genie waves his wand and all of a sudden the room is filled with tens of thousands of quacking ducks. They're all over the place, making a terrible noise: Quack, quack, quack! The bartender turns to the man and says, "Hey! What's the matter with this genie? I asked for a million bucks and I get a million ducks. Is he deaf or something?" The man looks at him and replies, " Well, do you really think I asked for a twelve-inch pianist?"

Why are these stories funny? And what do they have in common with other jokes? Despite all their surface diversity, most jokes and funny incidents have the following logical structure: Typically you lead the listener along a garden path of expectation, slowly building up tension. At the very end, you introduce an unexpected twist that entails a complete reinterpretation of all the preceding data, and moreover, it's critical that the new interpretation, though wholly unexpected, makes as much "sense" of the entire set of facts as did the originally "expected" interpretation. In this regard, jokes have much in common with scientific creativity, with what Thomas Kuhn calls a "paradigm shift" in response to a single "anomaly." (It's probably not coincidence that many of the most creative scientists have a great sense of humor.) Of course, the anomaly in the joke is the traditional punch line and the joke is "funny" only if the listener gets the punch line by seeing in a flash of insight how a completely new interpretation of the same set of facts can incorporate the anomalous ending. The longer and more tortuous the garden path of expectation, the "funnier" the punch line when finally delivered. Good comedians make use of this principle by taking their time to build up the tension of the story line, for nothing kills humor more surely than a premature punch line.

But although the introduction of a sudden twist at the end is necessary for the genesis of humor, it is certainly not sufficient. Suppose my plane is about to land in San Diego and I fasten my seat belt and get ready for touchdown. The pilot suddenly announces that the "bumps" that he (and I) had earlier dismissed as air turbulence are really due to engine failure and that we need to empty fuel before landing. A paradigm shift has occurred in my mind, but this certainly does not make me laugh. Rather, it makes me orient toward the anomaly and prepare for action to cope with the anomaly. Or consider the time I was staying at some friends' house in Iowa City. They were away and I was alone in unfamiliar surroundings. It was late at night and just as I was about to doze off, I heard a thump downstairs. "Probably the wind," I thought. After a few minutes there was another thud, louder than the one before. Again I "rationalized" it away and went back to sleep. Twenty minutes later I heard an extremely loud, resounding "bang" and leapt out of bed. What was happening? A burglar perhaps? Naturally, with my limbic system activated, I "oriented," grabbed a flashlight and ran down the stairs. Nothing funny so far. Then, suddenly I noticed a large flower vase in pieces on the floor and a large tabby cat right next to it—the obvious culprit! In contrast to the airplane incident, this time I started laughing because I realized that the "anomaly" I had detected and the subsequent paradigm shift were of trivial consequence. All of the facts could now be explained in terms of the cat theory rather than the ominous burglar theory.

On the basis of this example, we can sharpen our definition of humor and laughter. When a person strolls along a garden path of expectation and there is a sudden twist at the end that entails a complete reinterpretation of the same facts *and* the new interpretation has trivial rather than terrifying implications, laughter ensues.

But why laughter? Why this explosive, repetitive sound? Freud's view that laughter discharges pent-up internal tension does not make much sense without recourse to an elaborate and far-fetched hydraulic metaphor. He argued that water building up in a system of pipes will find its way out of the path of least resistance (the way a safety valve opens when too much pressure builds up in a system), and laughter might provide a similar safety valve to allow the escape of psychic energy (whatever that might mean). This "explanation" really doesn't work for me; it belongs to a class of explanations that Peter Medawar has called "analgesics" that "dull the ache of incomprehension without removing the cause."

To an ethologist, on the other hand, any stereotyped vocalization almost always implies that the organism is trying to *communicate* something to others in the social group. Now what might this be in the case of laughter? I suggest that the main purpose of laughter might be to allow the individual to alert others in the social group (usually kin) that the detected anomaly is trivial, nothing to worry about. The laughing person in effect announces her discovery that there has been a false alarm; that the rest of you chaps need not waste your precious energy and resources responding to a spurious threat.[6] This also explains why laughter is so notoriously contagious, for the value of any such signal would be amplified as it spread through the social group.

This "false alarm theory" of humor may also explain slapstick. You watch a man—preferably one who is portly and self-important—walk down the street when suddenly he slips on a banana peel and falls down. If his head hit the pavement and his skull split open, you would not laugh as you saw blood spill out; you would rush to his aid or to the nearest telephone to call an ambulance. But if he got up casually, wiped the remains of the fruit from his face and continued walking, you would probably burst out laughing, thereby letting others standing nearby know that they need not rush to his aid. Of course, when watching Laurel and Hardy or Mr. Bean, we are more willing to tolerate "real" harm or injury to the hapless victim because we are fully aware that it's only a movie.

Although this model accounts for the evolutionary origin of laughter, it by no means explains all the functions of humor among modern humans. Once the mechanism was in place, however, it could easily be exploited for other purposes. (This is common in evolution. Feathers evolved in birds originally to provide insulation but were later adapted for flying.) The ability to reinterpret events in the light of new information may have been refined through the generations to help people playfully juxtapose larger ideas or concepts—that is, to be creative. This capacity for seeing familiar ideas from novel vantage points (an essential element of humor) could be an antidote to conservative thinking and a catalyst to creativity. Laughter and humor may be a dress rehearsal for creativity, and if so, perhaps jokes, puns and other forms of humor should be introduced very early into our elementary schools as part of the formal curriculum.[7]

Although these suggestions may help explain the logical structure of humor, they do not explain why humor itself is sometimes used as a psychological defense mechanism. Is it a coincidence, for example, that a disproportionate number of jokes deal with potentially disturbing topics, such as death or sex? One possibility is that jokes are an attempt to trivialize genuinely disturbing anomalies by pretending they are of no consequence; you distract yourself from your anxiety by setting off your own false alarm mechanism. Thus a trait that evolved to appease others in a social group now becomes internalized to deal with truly stressful situations and may emerge as so-called nervous laughter. Thus even as mysterious a phenomenon as "nervous laughter" begins to make sense in the light of some of the evolutionary ideas discussed here.

The smile, too, may have similar evolutionary origins, as a "weaker" form of laughter. When one of your ancestral primates encountered another individual coming toward him from a distance, he may have initially bared his canines in a threatening grimace on the fair assumption that most strangers are potential enemies. Upon recognizing the individual as "friend" or "kin," however, he might abort the grimace halfway, thereby producing a smile, which in turn may have evolved into a ritualized human greeting: "I know you pose no threat and I reciprocate."[8] Thus in my scheme, a smile is an *aborted* orienting response in the same way that laughter is.

•

The ideas we have explored so far help explain the biological functions and possible evolutionary origin of humor, laughter and smiling, but they still leave open the question of what the underlying neural mechanisms of laughter might be. What about Willy, who started giggling at his mother's funeral, and Ruth, who literally died laughing? Their strange behavior implies the existence of a laughter circuit found mainly in portions of the limbic system and its targets in the frontal lobes. Given the well-known role of the limbic system in producing an orienting response to a potenial threat or *alarm*, it is not altogether surprising, perhaps, that it is also involved in the aborted orienting reaction in response to a *false alarm*—laughter. Some parts of this circuit handle emotions—the feeling of merriment that accompanies laughter—whereas other parts are involved in the physical act itself, but at present we do not know which parts are doing what.

There is, however, another curious neurological disorder, called pain asymbolia, which offers additional hints about the neurological structures underlying laughter. Patients with this condition do not register pain when they are deliberately jabbed in the finger with a sharp needle. Instead of saying, "Ouch!" they say, "Doctor, I can feel the pain but it doesn't hurt." Apparently they do not experience the aversive emotional impact of pain. And, mysteriously, I have noticed that many of them actually start giggling, as if they were being tickled and not stabbed. For instance, in a hospital in Madras, India, I recently examined a schoolteacher who told me that a pinprick I administered as part of a routine neurology workup felt incredibly funny—although she couldn't explain why.

I became interested in pain asymbolia mainly because it provides additional support for the evolutionary theory of laughter that I've proposed in this chapter. The syndrome is often seen when there is damage to a structure called the insular cortex—buried in the fold between the parietal and temporal lobes (and closely linked to the structures that were damaged in Willy and Ruth). This structure receives sensory input, including pain from the skin and internal organs, and sends its output to parts of the limbic system (such as the cingulate gyrus) so that one begins to experience the strong aversive reaction—the agony—of pain. Now imagine what would happen if the damage were to disconnect the insular cortex from the cingulate gyrus. One part of the person's brain (the insular cortex) tells him, "Here is something painful, a potential threat," while another part (the cingulate gyrus of the limbic system) says a fraction of a second later, "Oh, don't worry; this is no threat after all." Thus the two key ingredients—threat followed by deflation—are present, and the only way for the patient to resolve the paradox is to laugh, just as my theory would predict.

The same line of reasoning may help explain why people laugh when tickled.[9] You approach a child, hand stretched out menacingly. The child wonders, "Will he hurt me or shake me or poke me?" But no, your fingers make light, intermittent contact with her belly. Again, the recipe—threat followed by deflation—is present and the child laughs, as if to inform other children, "He doesn't mean harm. He's only playing!" This, by the way, may help children practice the kind of mental play required for adult humor. In other words, what we call "sophisticated cognitive" humor has the same logical form as tickling and therefore piggybacks on the same neural circuits—the "threatening but harmless" detector that involves the insular cortex, cingulate gyrus and other parts of the limbic system. Such co-opting of mechanisms is the rule rather than the exception in the evolution of mental and physical traits (although in this case, the co-opting occurs for a related, higher-level function rather than for a completely different function).

These ideas have some bearing on a heated debate that has been going on among evolutionary biologists in general and evolutionary psychologists in particular during the last ten years. I get the impression that there are two warring camps. One camp implies (with disclaimers) that every one of our mental traits—or at least 99 percent of them—is specifically selected for by natural selection. The other camp, represented by Stephen Jay Gould, calls members of the first camp "ultra-Darwinists" and argues that other factors must be kept in mind. (Some of the factors pertain to the actual selection process itself and others to the raw material that natural selection can act on. They complement rather than contradict the idea of natural selection.) Every biologist I know has strong views on what these factors might be. Here are some of my favorite examples:

- What you now observe may be a bonus or useful by-product of something else that was selected for a completely different purpose. For example, a nose evolved for smelling and warming and moistening air but can also be used for wearing spectacles. Hands evolved for grasping branches but can now be used for counting as well.
- A trait may represent a further refinement (through natural selection) of another trait that was originally selected for a completely different purpose. Feathers evolved from reptilian scales to keep birds warm but have since been co-opted and transformed into wing feathers for flying; this is called preadaptation.
- Natural selection can only select from what is available, and what is available is often a very limited repertoire, constrained by the organism's previous evolutionary history as well as certain developmental pathways that either are permanently closed or remain open.

I'd be very surprised if these three statements were not true to some extent regarding the many mental traits that constitute human nature. Indeed, there are many other principles of this sort (including plain old Lady Luck or contingency) that are not covered by the phrase "natural selection."[10] Yet ultra-Darwinists steadfastly adhere to the view that almost all traits, other than those obviously learned, are specific products of natural selection. For them, preadaptation, contingency and the like play only a minor role in evolution; they are "exceptions that prove the rule." Moreover, they believe that you can in principle reverse engineer various human mental traits by looking at environmental and social constraints. ("Reverse engineering" is the idea that you can best understand how something works by asking what environmental challenge it evolved *for*. And then, working backward, you consider plausible solutions to that challenge. It is an idea that is popular, not surprisingly, with engineers and computer programmers.) As a biologist, I am inclined to go with Gould; I believe that natural selection is certainly the single most important driving force of evolution, but I also believe that each case needs to be examined individually. In other words, it is an empirical question whether some mental or physical trait that you observe in an animal or person was selected for by natural selection. Furthermore, there are dozens of ways to solve an environmental problem, and unless you know the evolutionary history, taxonomy and paleontology of the animal you are looking at, you cannot figure out the exact route taken by a particular trait (like feathers, laughter or hearing) as it evolved into its present form. This is technically referred to as the "trajectory" taken by the trait "through the fitness landscape."

My favorite example of this phenomenon involves the three little bones in our middle ear—the malleus, incus and stapes. Now used for hearing, two of these bones (the malleus and incus) were originally part of the lower jaw of our reptilian ancestors, who used them for chewing. Reptiles needed flexible, multielement, multihinged jaws so they could swallow giant prey, whereas mammals preferred a single strong bone (the dentary) for cracking nuts and chewing tough substances like grains. So as reptiles evolved into mammals, two of the jawbones were co-opted into the middle ear and used for amplifying sounds (partly because early mammals were nocturnal and relied largely on hearing for survival). This is such an ad hoc, bizarre solution that unless you know your comparative anatomy well or discovered fossil intermediates, you never could have deduced it from simply considering the functional needs of the organism. Contrary to the ultra-Darwinist view, reverse engineering doesn't always work in biology for the simple reason that God is not an engineer; he's a hacker.

What has all this got to do with human traits like smiling? Everything. If my argument concerning the smile is correct, then even though it evolved through natural selection, not *every* feature of a smile is adaptive for its current demand. That is, the smile takes the particular form that it does not because of natural selection alone but because it evolved from *the very opposite*—the threat grimace! There is no way you could deduce this through reverse engineering (or figure out its particular trajectory through the fitness landscape) unless you also know about the existence of canine teeth, knew that nonhuman primates bare their canines as a mock threat or knew that mock threats in turn evolved from real threat displays. (Big canines are genuinely dangerous.)

I find great irony in the fact that every time someone smiles at you she is in fact producing a half threat by flashing her canines. When Darwin published *On the Origin of Species* he delicately hinted in his last chapter that we too may have evolved from apelike ancestors. The English statesman Benjamin Disraeli was outraged by this and at a meeting held in Oxford he asked a famous rhetorical question: "Is man a beast or an angel?" To answer this, he need only have looked at his wife's canines as she smiled at him, and he'd have realized that in this simple universal human gesture of friendliness lies concealed a grim reminder of our savage past.

As Darwin himself concluded in *The Descent of Man:*

> But we are not here concerned with hopes and fears, only with truth. We must acknowledge, as it seems to me, that man with all his noble qualities, with sympathy which he feels for the most debased, with benevolence which extends not only to other men but to the humblest creature, with his God-like intellect which has penetrated into the movements and constitution of the solar system—with all these exalted powers—man still bears in his bodily frame the indelible stamp of his lowly origin.

CHAPTER 11

"You Forgot to Deliver the Twin"

It is an old maxim of mine that when you have excluded the impossible, whatever remains, however improbable, must be the truth.

—SHERLOCK HOLMES

Mary Knight, age thirty-two, bright red hair pinned neatly in a bun, walked into Dr. Monroe's office, sat down and grinned. She was nine months pregnant and so far everything seemed to be going well. This was a long-awaited, much desired pregnancy, but it was also her first visit to Dr. Monroe. The year was 1932 and money was tight. Mary's husband did not have steady work, and so Mary had only talked to a midwife down the street, on an informal basis.

But today was different. Mary had felt the baby kicking for some time and suspected that labor was about to begin. She wanted Dr. Monroe to check her over, to make sure that the baby was in the right position to coach her through this last stage of pregnancy. It was time to prepare for birth.

Dr. Monroe examined the young woman. Her abdomen was vastly

enlarged and low, suggesting that the fetus had dropped. Her breasts were swollen, the nipples mottled.

But something was not right. The stethoscope was not picking up a clear fetal heartbeat. Maybe the baby was turned in a funny way, or perhaps it was in trouble, but, no, that wasn't it. Mary Knight's navel was all wrong. One sure sign of pregnancy is an everted or pushed-out belly button. Mary's was inverted, in the normal fashion. She had an "innie" rather than an "outie."

Dr. Monroe whistled softly. He'd learned about pseudocyesis or false pregnancy in medical school. Some women who desperately want to be pregnant—and occasionally some who deeply dread pregnancy—develop all the signs and symptoms of true pregnancy. Their abdomens swell to enormous proportions, aided by a sway back posture and the mysterious deposition of abdominal fat. Their nipples become pigmented, as happens in pregnant women. They stop menstruating, lactate, have morning sickness and sense fetal movements. Everything seems normal except for one thing: There is no baby.

Dr. Monroe knew that Mary Knight was suffering from pseudocyesis, but how would he tell her? How could he explain that it was all in her head, that the dramatic change in her body was caused by a delusion?

"Mary," he said softly, "the baby is coming now. It will be born this afternoon. I'm going to give you ether so that you won't be in pain. But labor has begun and we can proceed."

Mary was elated and submitted to the anesthesia. Ether was given routinely during labor and she'd expected it.

A little later, as Mary woke up, Dr. Monroe took her hand and stroked it gently. He gave her a few minutes to compose herself and then said, "Mary, I'm so sorry to have to tell you this. It's terrible news. The baby was stillborn. I did everything I could but it was no use. I'm so, so sorry."

Mary broke down crying, but she accepted Dr. Monroe's news. Right there, on the table, her abdomen began to subside. The baby was gone and she was devastated. She'd have to go home and tell her husband and mother. What a terrible disappointment this would be for the entire family.

A week passed. And then, to Dr. Monroe's astonishment, Mary burst into his office with her belly protruding, as huge as ever. "Doctor!" she shouted. "I've come back! You forgot to deliver the twin! I can feel him kicking in there!"[1]

•

About three years ago, I came across Mary Knight's story in a crumbling 1930s medical monograph. The report was by Dr. Silas Weir Mitchell, the same Philadelphia physician who coined the term "phantom limb." Not surprisingly, he referred to Mary's condition as phantom pregnancy and coined the term "pseudocyesis" (false swelling). Had the story come from almost any other person I might have dismissed it as rubbish, but Weir Mitchell was an astute clinical observer, and over the years I have learned to pay careful attention to his writings. I was struck especially by the relevance of his report to contemporary debates on how the mind influences the body, and vice versa.

Because I was born and raised in India, people often ask me whether I believe there are connections between the mind and body that Western cultures don't comprehend. How do yogis exert control over their blood pressure, heart rate and respiration? Is it true that the most skilled among them can reverse their peristalsis (leaving aside the question of why anyone would ever want to)? Does illness result from chronic stress? Will meditation make you live longer?

If you'd asked me those questions five years ago, I'd have conceded grudgingly, "Sure, obviously the mind can affect the body. A cheerful attitude might help accelerate your recovery from an illness by enhancing your immune system. There's also the so-called placebo effect we don't understand completely—merely believing in a therapy seems to improve one's well-being, if not actual physical health."

But as to notions of the mind curing the incurable, I've tended to be deeply skeptical. It's not just my training in Western medicine; I also find many of the empirical claims unconvincing. So what if breast cancer patients with more positive attitudes live, on average, two months longer than patients who deny their illness? To be sure, two months is better than nothing, but compared to the effects of an antibiotic like penicillin in improving the survival rates of pneumonia patients, this is hardly anything to boast about. (I know it's not fashionable to praise antibiotics these days, but one only has to see a single child saved from pneumonia or diphtheria by a few shots of penicillin to be convinced that antibiotics really are wonder drugs.)

But as a student I was also taught that a certain proportion of incurable cancers—a very tiny fraction, to be sure—disappear mysteriously without any treatment and that "many a patient with a tumor pronounced malignant has outlived his physician." I still remember my skepticism when my professor explained to me that such occurrences were known as "spontaneous remissions." For how can *any* phenomenon in science, which is all about cause and effect, occur *spontaneously*—especially something as dramatic as the dissolution of a malignant cancer?

When I raised this objection, I was reminded of the basic fact of "biological variability"—that cumulative effects of small individual differences can account for myriad, unexpected responses. But saying that tumor regression arises from variability is not saying a hell of a lot; it's hardly an explanation. Even if it is due to variability, surely we must ask the question, What is the critical variable that causes the regression in any particular patient? For if we could solve that, then we would have ipso facto discovered a cure for cancer! Of course, it may turn out that the remission is the result of a fortuitous combination of several variables, but that doesn't make the problem insoluble; it merely makes it more difficult. So why isn't much more attention being paid by the cancer establishment to these very cases, instead of regarding them as curiosities? Couldn't one study these rare survivors in detail, looking for clues that confer resistance to virulent agents or reapply the brakes to renegade tumor suppressor genes? This strategy has been applied successfully to acquired immunodeficiency syndrome (AIDS) research. The finding that some long-term survivors carry a gene mutation that prevents the virus from invading their immune cells is now being exploited in the clinic.

But now let us return to mind-body medicine. The observation that some cancers occasionally regress spontaneously doesn't necessarily prove that hypnosis or a positive attitude can induce such remissions. We must not commit the blunder of lumping all mysterious phenomena together simply because they are mysterious, for that may be all they have in common. What I need to be convinced is a single proven example of one's mind's directly influencing one's bodily processes, an example that is clear-cut and repeatable.

When I stumbled across the case of Mary Knight, it occurred to me that pseudocyesis or phantom pregnancy might be an example of the kind of connection I was looking for. If the human mind can conjure up something as complex as pregnancy, what else can the brain do to or for the body? What are the limits to mind-body interactions and what pathways mediate these strange phenomena?

Remarkably, the delusion of phantom pregnancy is associated with a whole gamut of physiological changes associated with pregnancy—cessation of menstruation, breast enlargement, nipple pigmentation, pica (the desire for strange foods), morning sickness and most remarkable of all—progressive abdominal enlargement and "quickening" culminating in actual labor pains! Sometimes, but not always, there is enlargement of the uterus and cervix, but the radiological signs are negative. As a medical student I learned that even experienced obstetricians can be fooled[2] by the clinical picture unless they are careful and that in the past many a C-section was performed on a patient with pseudocyesis. As Dr. Monroe detected in Mary, the telltale diagnostic sign lies in the belly button.

Modern physicians who are familiar with pseudocyesis assume it results from a pituitary or ovarian tumor that causes hormones to be released, mimicking the signs of pregnancy. Tiny, clinically undetectable prolactin-secreting tumors (adenomas) of the pituitary could suppress ovulation and menstruation and lead to the other symptoms. But if that were true, why is the condition sometimes reversible? What kind of tumor could explain what happened to Mary Knight? She goes into "labor" and her abdomen shrinks. Then her abdomen gets big again because of the "twin." If a tumor could do all that, it would present an even greater mystery than pseudocyesis.

So what causes pseudocyesis? Cultural factors undoubtedly play a major role[3] and may explain the decline of pseudocyesis from an incidence of one in two hundred in the late 1700s to about one in ten thousand pregnancies today. In the past, many women felt extreme social pressure to have a baby, and when they felt they were pregnant, there was no ultrasound to disprove the diagnosis. No one could say with certainty, "Look here, there's no fetus." Conversely, pregnant women today submit to round after round of evaluations leaving little room for ambiguity; confronting the patient with physical evidence of an ultrasound is usually sufficient to dispel the delusion and associated physical changes.

The influence of culture on the incidence of pseudocyesis cannot be denied, but what causes the actual physical changes? According to the few studies carried out on this curious affliction of mind and body, the abdominal swelling itself is usually caused by a combination of five factors: an accumulation of intestinal gas, a lowering of the diaphragm, a pushing forward of the pelvic portion of the spine, a dramatic growth of the greater omentum—a pendulous apron of fat that hangs loose in front of the intestines—and in rare cases an actual uterine enlargement. The hypothalamus—a part of the brain that regulates endocrine secretions—may also go awry, producing profound hormonal shifts that mimic nearly all the signs of pregnancy. Furthermore, it's a two-way street: The body's effects on the mind are just as profound as those of the mind on the body, giving rise to complex feedback loops involved in generating and maintaining false pregnancy. For instance, the abdominal distension produced by gas and the woman's "pregnant body posture" might be explained, in part, by classic operant conditioning. When Mary, who wants to be pregnant, sees her abdomen enlarge and feels her diaphragm fall, she learns unconsciously that the lower it falls, the more pregnant she looks. Likewise, a combination of air swallowing (aerophagia) and autonomic constriction of the gastrointestinal sphincters that would increase gas retention could also probably be learned unconsciously. In this manner, Mary's "baby" and its "missing twin" are literally conjured out of thin air through a process of unconscious learning.

So much for the abdominal swelling. But what about the breast, nipple and other changes? The most parsimonious explanation for the whole spectrum of clinical signs you see in pseudocyesis would be that the intense longing for a child and associated depression might reduce levels of dopamine and norepinephrine—the "joy transmitters" in the brain. This in turn could reduce the production of both follicle-stimulating hormone (FSH), which causes ovulation, and a substance called prolactin-inhibition factor.[4] Low levels of these hormones would lead to a cessation of ovulation and menstruation and an elevation of the level of prolactin (the maternal hormone), which causes breast enlargement and lactation, nipple tingling and maternal behavior (although this has yet to be proved in humans), along with an increased production of estrogen and progesterone by the ovaries, contributing to the overall impression of pregnancy. This notion is consistent with the well-known clinical observation that severe depression can stop menstruation—an evolutionary strategy for avoiding a waste of precious resources on ovulation and pregnancy when you are disabled and depressed.

But the cessation of menstruation during depression is common, whereas pseudocyesis is very rare. Perhaps there's something special about the depression of being childless in a child-obsessed culture. If the syndrome occurs only when the depression is associated with fantasies about pregnancy, it raises a fascinating question: How does a highly specific wish or delusion originating in the neocortex get translated by the hypothalamus to induce FSH reduction and prolactin elevation—if that is indeed the cause? And even more puzzling, how do you explain the observation that some patients with pseudocyesis do *not* have an elevated prolactin level or that in many patients labor pains begin at exactly nine months? What triggers the labor contractions if there is no growing fetus?

Whatever the ultimate answer to these questions, pseudocyesis provides a valuable opportunity for exploring the mysterious no-man's-land between mind and body.

False pregnancy and labor in women are surprising enough, but there are even a few recorded instances of pseudocyesis in men! The whole gamut of changes—including abdominal swelling, lactation, craving for strange foods, nausea, even labor pains—can occur as an isolated syndrome in some men. But more commonly it is seen in men who empathize deeply with their pregnant spouse, producing the so-called sympathetic pregnancy or couvade syndrome. I have often wondered whether the man's emotional empathy with the pregnant woman (or perhaps pheromones from her) somehow releases prolactin—a key pregnancy hormone—in her husband's brain, causing some of these changes to emerge. (This hypothesis is not as outlandish as it seems; male tamarin marmosets develop an elevated prolactin level when in close proximity to nursing mothers, and this may encourage paternal or filial affection and reduce infanticide.) I am tempted to interview men participating in Lamaze classes and to measure prolactin levels in those who experience some of these couvadelike signs.

•

Pseudocyesis is dramatic. But is it an isolated, exceptional example of mind-body medicine? I think not. Other stories come to mind, including one I first heard in medical school. A friend said, "Did you know that according to Lewis Thomas you can hypnotize someone and eliminate their warts?"

"Rubbish," I scoffed.

"No, it's true," she said. "There are documented cases.[5] You get hypnotized and the warts disappear in a few days or sometimes overnight."

Now on the face of it this sounds very silly, but if it's true, it would have far-reaching implications for modern science. A wart is essentially a tumor (a benign cancer) produced by the papilloma virus. If that can be eliminated by hypnotic suggestion, why not cancer of the cervix, which is also produced by the papilloma virus (albeit a different strain)? I am not claiming that this will work—perhaps nerve pathways influenced by hypnosis reach the skin but not the lining of the cervix—but unless we do the relevant experiment, we will never know.

Assuming, for the sake of argument, that warts can be eliminated by hypnosis, the question arises, How can a person simply "think away" a tumor? There are at least two possibilities. One involves the autonomic nervous system—the pathways of nerves that help control blood pressure, sweating, heart rate, urine output, erections and other physiological phenomena not under direct control of conscious thought. These nerves form specialized circuits that service distinct functions in various body segments. Thus some nerves control hair standing on end, others cause sweating and some generate the local constriction of blood vessels. Is it possible that the mind, acting through the autonomic nervous system, could literally asphyxiate the wart by constricting blood vessels in its immediate vicinity, making it shrivel up and wither away? This explanation implies an unexpected degree of precise control by the autonomic nervous system and also implies that the hypnotic suggestion can be "understood" by the autonomic nervous system and transferred to the region of the wart.

The second possibility is that the hypnotic suggestion somehow kick starts the immune system, thereby eliminating the virus. But this would not explain at least one recorded case involving a hypnotized person whose warts vanished on just one side of his body. Why or how the immune system could selectively eliminate warts on one side over another is a mystery that invites further flights of speculation.

•

A more common example of mind-body interaction involves the interplay between the immune system and perceptual cues from the world around us. Over three decades ago, medical students were often told that an asthmatic attack could be provoked not only by inhaling pollen from a rose but sometimes by merely seeing a rose, even a plastic rose, prompting a so-called conditioned allergic response. In other words, exposure to a real rose and pollen sets up a "learned" association in the brain between the mere visual appearance of a rose and bronchial constriction. How exactly does this conditioning work? How does the message get from the brain's visual areas all the way down to the mast cells lining the bronchi of the lungs? What are the actual pathways involved? Despite three decades of mind-body medicine, we still have no clear answers.

When I was a medical student in the late 1960s, I asked a visiting professor of physiology from Oxford about this conditioning process and whether the conditioned association could be put to clinical use. "If it's possible to provoke an asthmatic attack through conditioning merely by showing a plastic rose to a patient, then theoretically it ought to be possible to abort or neutralize the attack through conditioning as well.

For example, say you suffer from asthma and I give you a bronchodilator such as norepinephrine (or perhaps an antihistamine or a steroid) every time I show you a plastic sunflower. You might begin associating the sunflower image with relief from asthma. After some time you could simply carry around a sunflower in your pocket and pull it out to look at when you felt an attack coming on."

At the time, this professor (who later became my mentor) thought this was an ingenious but silly idea, and we both had a good laugh. It seemed far-fetched and whimsical. Thus chastised, I kept my thoughts to myself, wondering privately whether you really could condition an immune response and, if so, how selective this conditioning process could be. For instance, we know that if you inject a person with denatured tetanus bacilli he will soon develop immunity to tetanus, but to keep the immunity "alive" the person needs booster shots every few years. But what would happen if you rang a bell or flashed a green light every time these booster shots were administered? Would the brain learn the association? Could you eventually dispense with the boosters and simply ring a bell and flash a light to stimulate the selective proliferation of immunologically competent cells, thereby reviving a person's immunity to tetanus? The implications of such a finding for clinical medicine would be enormous.

To this day I curse myself for not trying this experiment. The ideas remained tucked away in my mind until a few years ago, when, as happens so often in science, someone made an accidental discovery, proving that I had missed the boat. Dr. Ralph Ader of McMaster University was exploring food aversion in mice. To induce nausea in the animals, he gave them a nausea-inducing drug, cyclophosphamide, along with saccharin, wondering whether they would display signs of nausea the next time he gave them the saccharin alone. It worked. As expected, the animals did show food aversion, in this case an aversion to saccharin. But surprisingly, the mice also fell seriously ill, developing all sorts of infections. It is known that the drug cyclophosphamide, in addition to producing nausea, profoundly suppresses the immune system, but why should saccharin alone have this effect? Ader reasoned correctly that the mere pairing of the innocuous saccharin with the immunosuppressive drug caused the mouse immune system to "learn" the association. Once this association is established, every time the mouse encounters the sugar substitute, its immune system will nose-dive, making it vulnerable to infections. Here again is a powerful example of mind affecting body, one that is hailed as a landmark in the history of medicine and immunology.[6]

I mention these examples for three reasons. First, don't listen to your professors—even if they are from Oxford (or as my colleague Semir Zeki would say, *especially* if they are from Oxford). Second, they illustrate our ignorance and illuminate the need for conducting experiments on topics that most people have ignored for no obvious reason; patients who manifest odd clinical phenomena are only one example. Third, perhaps it's time to recognize that the division between mind and body may be no more than a pedagogic device for instructing medical students—and not a useful construct for understanding human health, disease and behavior. Contrary to what many of my colleagues believe, the message preached by physicians like Deepak Chopra and Andrew Weil is not just New Age psychobabble. It contains important insights into the human organism—ones that deserve serious scientific scrutiny.

People have become increasingly impatient with Western medicine's sterility and lack of compassion, and this would explain the current resurgence of "alternative medicine." But unfortunately, even though the remedies touted by New Age gurus have a ring of plausibility, they are rarely subjected to rigorous tests.[7] We have no idea which ones (if any) work and which ones do not, although even the hardened skeptic would agree that there is probably something interesting going on. If we are to make any headway, we need to test these claims carefully and explore the brain mechanisms that underlie such effects. The general principle of immune conditioning has been clearly established, but can you pair different sensory stimuli with different types of immune responses (for example, a bell with a response to typhoid and a whistle to cholera), or is the phenomenon more diffuse—involving only a general boosting of all your immune functions? Does the conditioning affect the immunity itself or only the subsequent inflammatory response to the provoking agent? Does hypnosis tap into the same pathway as placebos?[8] Until we have clear answers to these questions, Western medicine and alternative medicine will always remain parallel enterprises with no points of contact between them.

•

So with all this evidence staring them in the face, why do practitioners of Western medicine continue to ignore the many striking examples of direct links between mind and body?

To understand why, it helps to have a feel for how scientific knowledge progresses. Most of the day-to-day progress of science depends on simply adding another brick to the great edifice—a rather humdrum activity that the late historian Thomas Kuhn called "normal science." This corpus of knowledge, incorporating a number of widely accepted beliefs, is, in each instance, called a "paradigm." Year after year new observations come along and are assimilated into an existing standard model. Most scientists are bricklayers, not architects; they are happy simply adding another stone to the cathedral.

But sometimes the new observation simply doesn't fit. It is an "anomaly," inconsistent with the existing structure. The scientist can then do one of three things. First, he can ignore the anomaly, sweeping it under the carpet—a form of psychological "denial" that is surprisingly common even among eminent researchers.

Second, scientists can make minor adjustments to the paradigm, trying to fit the anomaly into their worldview, and this would still be a form of normal science. Or they can generate ad hoc auxiliary hypotheses that sprout like so many branches from a single tree. But soon these branches become so thick and numerous that they threaten to topple the tree itself.

Finally, they can tear down the edifice and create a completely new one that bears very little resemblance to the original. This is what Kuhn called a "paradigm shift" or scientific revolution.

Now, there are many examples in the history of science of anomalies that were originally ignored as being trivial or even fraudulent but later turned out to be of fundamental importance. This is because the vast majority of scientists are conservative by temperament and when a new fact emerges that threatens to topple the great edifice, the initial reaction is to ignore or deny it. This is not as silly as it seems. Since most anomalies turn out to be false alarms, it is not a bad strategy to play it safe and ignore them. If we tried to accommodate every report of alien abduction or spoon bending into our framework, science would not have evolved into the immensely successful and internally consistent body of beliefs that it is today. Skepticism is as much a vital part of the whole enterprise as the revolutions that make newspaper headlines.

Consider the periodic table of elements, for example. When Mendeleyev arranged elements sequentially according to their atomic weights to create the periodic table, he found that some elements didn't quite "fit"—their atomic weights seemed wrong. But instead of discarding his model, he chose to ignore the anomalous weights, concluding instead that perhaps they had been measured incorrectly to begin with. And sure enough, it was later discovered that the accepted atomic weights were wrong because the presence of certain isotopes distorted the measurements. There is much truth to Sir Arthur Eddington's famously paradoxical remark "Don't believe the results of experiments until they're confirmed by theory."

But we must not ignore every anomaly, since some of them have the potential for driving paradigm shifts. Our wisdom lies in being able to tell which anomaly is trivial and which one is a potential gold mine. Unfortunately, there's no simple formula for distinguishing trivia from gold, but as a rule of thumb, if an odd, inconsistent observation has been lying around for ages and has not been *empirically* confirmed despite repeated honest attempts, then it is probably a trivial one. (I regard telepathy and repeated Elvis sightings as belonging to this category.) On the other hand, if the observation in question has resisted several attempts at disproof and is regarded as an oddity *solely* because it resists explanation in terms of our current conceptual scheme, then you are probably looking at a genuine anomaly.

One famous example is continental drift. Around the turn of this century (1912), the German meteorologist Alfred Wegener noticed that the east coast of South America and the west coast of Africa "fit" neatly together like the pieces of a giant jigsaw puzzle. He also noticed that fossils of a small freshwater reptile "mesosaurus" were found in only two parts of the earth—in Brazil and in West Africa. How could a freshwater lizard swim across the Atlantic, he wondered? Is it conceivable that in the distant past these two continents were in fact parts of a single large landmass that had subsequently split and drifted apart? Obsessed with this idea, he sought additional evidence and found it in the form of dinosaur fossils scattered in identical rock strata, again in the west coast of Africa and the east coast of Brazil. This was compelling evidence indeed, but surprisingly it was rejected by the entire geological establishment, who argued that the dinosaurs must have walked across an ancient and now submerged land bridge connecting the two continents. As recently as 1974, at St. John's College in Cambridge, England, a professor of geology shook his head when I mentioned Wegener. "A lot of rot," he said with exasperation in his voice.

Yet we now know that Wegener was right. His idea was rejected simply because there was no mechanism that people could conceive of that would cause whole continents to drift. If there's one thing we all regard as axiomatic, it is the stability of terra firma. But once plate tectonics—the study of rigid plates moving about on a hot gooey mantle below—was discovered, Wegener's idea became credible and won universal acceptance.

The moral of this tale is that you should not reject an idea as outlandish simply because you can't think of a mechanism that explains it. And this argument is valid whether you are talking about continents, heredity, warts or pseudocyesis. After all, Darwin's theory of evolution was proposed and widely accepted long before the mechanisms of heredity were clearly understood.

A second example of a genuine anomaly is multiple personality disorder or MPD, which in my view may turn out to be just as important for medicine as continental drift was for geology. To this day MPD continues to be ignored by the medical community even though it provides a valuable testing ground for the claims of mind-body medicine. In this syndrome—immortalized by Robert Louis Stevenson in *Dr. Jekyll and Mr. Hyde*—a person can assume two or more distinct personalities, each of which is completely unaware, or only dimly aware, of the others. Again, there have been occasional reports in the clinical literature that one personality can be diabetic while the other is not, or that various vital signs and hormone profiles can be different in the two personalities. There is even a claim that one personality can be allergic to a substance while the other is not and that one might be myopic—or nearsighted—whereas the other has 20/20 vision.[9]

MPD defies common sense. How can two personalities dwell in one body? In Chapter 7, we learned that the mind is constantly struggling to create a coherent belief system from a multiplicity of life experiences. When there are minor discrepancies, you usually readjust your beliefs or engage in the kinds of denials and rationalizations that Sigmund Freud talked about. But consider what might happen if you held two sets of beliefs—each internally consistent and rational—but these two sets were completely in conflict with one another? The best solution might be to balkanize the beliefs, to wall them off from each other by creating two personalities.

There is of course an element of this "syndrome" in all of us. We talk about whore/madonna fantasies and say things like "I was of two minds," "I'm not feeling myself today" or "He's a different person when you're around." But in some rare instances, it's possible that this schism becomes literal so that you end up with two "separate minds." Assume that one set of beliefs says, "I am Sue, the sexy woman who lives on 123 Elm Street in Boston, goes to bars at night to pick up studs, drinks straight shots of Wild Turkey and has never bothered to get an AIDS test." Another says, "I am Peggy, the bored housewife who lives on 123 Elm Street in Boston, watches TV at night, drinks nothing stronger than herbal tea and goes to the doctor for every minor ailment." These two stories are so different that they obviously refer to two different people. But Peggy Sue has a problem: She is both of these people. She occupies one body, indeed one brain! Perhaps the only way for her to avoid internal civil war is to "split" her beliefs into two clusters, like soap bubbles, resulting in the strange phenomenon of multiple personalities.

According to many psychiatrists, some cases of MPD are a consequence of childhood sexual or physical abuse. The child, growing up, finds the abuse so emotionally intolerable that she gradually walls it off into Sue's world, not Peggy's. What is truly remarkable, though, is that to keep the illusion going, she actually invests each personality with different voices, intonations, motivations, mannerisms and even different immune systems—almost two bodies, one is tempted to say. Perhaps she needs such elaborate devices to keep these minds separate and avoid the ever-present danger of having them coalesce and create unbearable internal strife.

I would like to carry out experiments on people like Peggy Sue but have thus far been thwarted by the lack of what I would call a clear-cut case of MPD. When I telephone friends in psychiatry, asking for names of patients, they tell me that they have seen such patients but most of them have several personalities rather than just two. One apparently had nineteen "alters" inside him. Claims of this sort have made me deeply suspicious of the whole phenomenon. Given limited time and resources, a scientist always has to strike a balance between wasting time on tenuous and unrepeatable "effects" (such as cold fusion, poly-water or Kirlian photography) and being open-minded (keeping in mind the lessons from continental drift or asteroid impacts). Perhaps the best strategy is to focus only on claims that are relatively easy to prove or disprove.

If I ever locate an MPD patient with just two personalities, I intend to eliminate doubt by sending the person two bills. If he pays both, I'll know he's for real. If he doesn't, I'll know he's a fake. In either case I can't lose.

On a more serious note, it would be interesting to carry out systematic studies on immune function when the patient is in the two different states by measuring specific aspects of the immune response (such as cytokine production by lymphocytes and monocytes and interleukin production by T cells provoked by mitogens—factors that stimulate cell division). Such experiments may seem tedious and esoteric, but only by doing them can we achieve the right blend of East and West and create a new revolution in medicine. Most of my professors scoffed at ancient "touchy-feely" Hindu practices such as Ayurvedic medicine, Tantra and meditation. Yet ironically, some of the most potent drugs we now use can trace their ancestry to ancient folk remedies such as willow bark (aspirin), digitalis and reserpine. Indeed, it has been estimated that over 30 percent of drugs used in Western medicine are derived from plant products. (If you think of molds—antibiotics—as "herbs," the percentage is even higher. In ancient Chinese medicine, mold was often rubbed into wounds.)

The moral of all this is not that we should have blind faith in the "wisdom of the East" but that there are sure to be many nuggets of insight in these ancient practices. However, unless we conduct systematic "Western-style" experiments, we'll never know which ones really work (hypnosis and meditation) and which ones don't (crystal healing). Several laboratories throughout the world are poised to launch such experiments, and the first half of the next century will, in my view, be remembered as a golden age of neurology and mind-body medicine. It will be a time of great euphoria and celebration for novice researchers entering the field.

CHAPTER 12

Do Martians See Red?

All of modern philosophy consists of unlocking, exhuming and recanting what has been said before.

—V.S. RAMACHANDRAN

Why is thought, being a secretion of the brain, more wonderful than gravity, a property of matter?

—CHARLES DARWIN

In the first half of the next century, science will confront its greatest challenge in trying to answer a question that has been steeped in mysticism and metaphysics for millennia: What is the nature of the self? As someone who was born in India and raised in the Hindu tradition, I was taught that the concept of the self—the "I" within me that is aloof from the universe and engages in a lofty inspection of the world around me—is an illusion, a veil called *maya*. The search for enlightenment, I was told, consists of lifting this veil and realizing that you are really "One with the cosmos." Ironically, after extensive training in Western medicine and more than fifteen years of research on neurological patients and visual illusions, I have come to realize that there is much truth to this view—that the notion of a single unified self "inhabiting" the brain may indeed be an illusion. Everything I have learned from the intensive study of both normal people and patients who have sustained damage to various parts of their brains points to an unsettling notion: that you create your own "reality" from mere fragments of information, that what you "see" is a reliable—but not always accurate—representation of what exists in the world, that you are completely unaware of the vast majority of events going on in your brain. Indeed, most of your actions are carried out by a host of unconscious zombies who exist in peaceful harmony along with you (the "person") inside your body! I hope that the stories you have heard so far have helped convince you that the problem of self—far from being a metaphysical riddle—is now ripe for scientific inquiry.

Nevertheless, many people find it disturbing that all the richness of our mental life—all our thoughts, feelings, emotions, even what we regard as our intimate selves—arises entirely from the activity of little wisps of protoplasm in the brain. How is this possible? How could something as deeply mysterious as consciousness emerge from a chunk of meat inside the skull? The problem of mind and matter, substance and spirit, illusion and reality, has been a major preoccupation of both Eastern and Western philosophy for millennia, but very little of lasting value has emerged. As the British psychologist Stuart Sutherland has said, "Consciousness is a fascinating but elusive phenomenon: it is impossible to specify what it is, what it does, or why it evolved. Nothing worth reading has been written on it."

I won't pretend to have solved these mysteries,[1] but I do think there's a new way to study consciousness by treating it not as a philosophical, logical or conceptual issue, but rather as an empirical problem.

Except for a few eccentrics (called panpsychists) who believe everything in the universe is conscious, including things like anthills, thermostats, and Formica tabletops, most people now agree that consciousness arises in brains and not in spleens, livers, pancreases or any other organ. This is already a good start. But I will narrow the scope of inquiry even further and suggest that consciousness arises not from the whole brain but rather from certain specialized brain circuits that carry out a particular style of computation. To illustrate the nature of these circuits and the special computations they perform, I'll draw from the many examples in perceptual psychology and neurology that we have already considered in this book. These examples will show that the circuitry that embodies the vivid subjective quality of consciousness resides mainly in parts of the temporal lobes (such as the amygdala, septum, hypothalamus and insular cortex) and a single projection zone in the frontal lobes—the cingulate gyrus. And the activity of these structures must fulfill three important criteria, which I call (with apologies to Isaac Newton, who described the three basic laws of physics) the "three laws of qualia" ("qualia" simply means the raw feel of sensations such as the subjective quality of "pain" or "red" or "gnocchi with truffles"). My goal in identifying these three laws and the specialized structures embodying them is to stimulate further inquiry into the biological origin of consciousness.

The central mystery of the cosmos, as far as I'm concerned, is the following: Why are there always two parallel descriptions of the universe—the first-person account ("I see red") and the third-person account ("He says that he sees red when certain pathways in his brain encounter a wavelength of six hundred nanometers")? How can these two accounts be so utterly different yet complementary? Why isn't there only a third-person account, for according to the objective worldview of the physicist and neuroscientist, that's the only one that really exists? (Scientists who hold this view are called behaviorists.) Indeed, in their scheme of "objective science," the need for a first-person account doesn't even arise—implying that consciousness simply doesn't exist. But we all know perfectly well that can't be right. I'm reminded of the old quip about the behaviorist who, just having made passionate love, looks at his lover and says, "Obviously that was good for you, dear, but was it good for me?" This need to reconcile the first-person and third-person accounts of the universe (the "I" view versus the "he" or "it" view) is the single most important unsolved problem in science. Dissolve this barrier, say the Indian mystics and sages, and you will see that the separation between self and nonself is an illusion—that you are really One with the cosmos.

Philosophers call this conundrum the riddle of *qualia* or subjective sensation. How can the flux of ions and electrical currents in little specks of jelly—the neurons in my brain—generate the whole subjective world of sensations like red, warmth, cold or pain? By what magic is matter transmuted into the invisible fabric of feelings and sensations? This problem is so puzzling that not everyone agrees it is even a problem. I will illustrate this so-called qualia riddle with two simple thought experiments of the kind that philosophers love to make up. Such whimsical pretend experiments are virtually impossible to carry out in real life. My colleague Dr. Francis Crick is deeply suspicious of thought experiments, and I agree with him that they can be very misleading because they often contain hidden question-begging assumptions. But they can be used to clarify logical points, and I will use them here to introduce the problem of qualia in a colorful way.

First, imagine that you are a future superscientist with a complete knowledge of the workings of the human brain. Unfortunately you are also completely color-blind. You don't have any cone receptors (the structures in your retina that allow your eyes to discriminate the different colors), but you do have rods (for seeing black and white), and you also have the correct machinery for processing colors higher up inside your brain. If your eyes could distinguish colors, so could your brain.

Now suppose that you, the superscientist, study my brain. I am a normal color perceiver—I can see that the sky is blue, the grass is green and a banana is yellow—and you want to know what I mean by these color terms. When I look at objects and describe them as turquoise, chartreuse or vermilion, you don't have any idea what I'm talking about. To you, they all look like shades of gray.

But you are intensely curious about the phenomenon, so you point a spectrometer at the surface of a ripe red apple. It indicates that light with a wavelength of six hundred nanometers is emanating from the fruit. But you still have no idea what *color* this might correspond to because you can't experience it. Intrigued, you study the light-sensitive pigments of my eye and the color pathways in my brain until you eventually come up with a complete description of the laws of wavelength processing. Your theory allows you to trace the entire sequence of color perception, starting from the receptors in my eye and passing all the way into my brain, where you monitor the neural activity that generates the word "red." In short, you completely understand the laws of color vision (or more strictly, the laws of wavelength processing), and you can tell me in advance which word I will use to describe the color of an apple, orange or lemon. As a superscientist, *you have no reason to doubt the completeness of your account.*

Satisfied, you approach me with your flow diagram and say, "Ramachandran, this is what's going on in your brain!"

But I must protest. "Sure, that's what's going on. But I also *see* red. Where is the red in this diagram?"

"What is that?" you ask.

"That's part of the actual, ineffable experience of the color, which I can never seem to convey to you because you're totally color-blind."

This example leads to a definition of "qualia": they are aspects of my brain state that seem to make the scientific description incomplete—from my point of view.

As a second example, imagine a species of Amazonian electric fish that is very intelligent, in fact, as intelligent and sophisticated as you or I. But it has something we lack—namely, the ability to sense electrical fields using special organs in its skin. Like the superscientist in the previous example, you can study the neurophysiology of this fish and figure out how the electrical organs on the sides of its body transduce electrical current, how this information is conveyed to the brain, what part of the brain analyzes this information and how the fish uses this information to dodge predators, find prey and so on. If the fish could talk, however, it would say, "Fine, but you'll never know what it *feels* like to sense electricity."

These examples clearly state the problem of why qualia are thought to be essentially private. They also illustrate why the problem of qualia is not necessarily a scientific problem. Recall that your *scientific* description is complete. It's just that the your account is incomplete epistemologically because the actual experience of electric fields or redness is something you never will know. For you, it will forever remain a "third-person" account.

For centuries philosophers have assumed that this gap between brain and mind poses a deep epistemological problem—a barrier that simply cannot be crossed. But is this really true? I agree that the barrier hasn't yet been crossed, but does it follow that it can *never* be crossed? I'd like to argue that there is in fact no such barrier, no great vertical divide in nature between mind and matter, substance and spirit. Indeed, I believe that this barrier is only apparent and that it arises as a result of language. This sort of obstacle emerges when there is ***any translation*** from one language to another.[2]

How does this idea apply to the brain and the study of consciousness? I submit that we are dealing here with two mutually unintelligible languages. One is the language of nerve impulses—the spatial and temporal patterns of neuronal activity that allow us to see red, for example. The second language, the one that allows us to communicate what we are seeing to others, is a natural spoken tongue like English or German or Japanese—rarefied, compressed waves of air traveling between you and the listener. Both are languages in the strict technical sense, that is, they are information-rich messages that are intended to convey meaning, across synapses between different brain parts in one case and across the air between two people in the other.

The problem is that I can tell you, the color-blind superscientist, about my qualia (my experience of seeing red) only by using a spoken language. But the ineffable "experience" itself is lost in the translation. The actual "redness" of red will remain forever unavailable to you.

But what if I were to skip spoken language as a medium of communication and instead hook a cable of neural pathways (taken from tissue culture or from another person) from the color-processing areas in my brain directly into the color-processing regions of your brain (remember that your brain has the machinery to see color even though your eyes cannot discriminate wavelengths because they have no color receptors)? The cable allows the color information to go straight from my brain to neurons in your brain without intermediate translation. This is a far-fetched scenario, but there is nothing logically impossible about it.

Earlier when I said "red," it didn't make any sense to you because the mere use of the word "red" already involves a translation. But if you skip the translation and use a cable, so that the nerve impulses themselves go directly to the color area, then perhaps you'll say, "Oh, my God, I see exactly what you mean. I'm having this wonderful new experience."[3]

This scenario demolishes the philosophers' argument that there is an insurmountable logical barrier to understanding qualia. In principle, you *can* experience another creature's qualia, even the electric fish's. If you could find out what the electroceptive part of the fish brain is doing and if you could somehow graft it onto the relevant parts of your brain with all the proper associated connections, then you would start experiencing the fish's electrical qualia. Now, we could get into a philosophical debate over whether you need to be a *fish* to experience it or whether as a human being you could experience it, but the debate is not relevant to my argument. The logical point I am making here pertains only to the electrical qualia—not to the whole experience of being a fish.

The key idea here is that the qualia problem is not unique to the mind-body problem. It is no different in kind from problems that arise from *any* translation, and thus there is no need to invoke a great division in nature between the world of qualia and the material world. There is only one world with lots of translation barriers. If you can overcome them, the problems vanish.

This may sound like an esoteric, theoretical debate, but let me give you a more realistic example—an experiment we are actually planning to do. In the seventeenth century the English astronomer William Molyneux posed a challenge (another thought experiment). What would happen, he asked, if a child were raised in complete darkness from birth to age twenty-one and were then suddenly allowed to see a cube? Would he recognize the cube? Indeed, what would happen if the child were suddenly allowed to see ordinary daylight? Would he experience the light, saying, "Aha! I now see what people mean by light!" or would he act utterly bewildered and continue to be blind? (For the sake of argument, the philosopher assumes that the child's visual pathways have not degenerated from the deprivation and that he has an intellectual concept of seeing, just as our superscientist had an intellectual concept of color before we used the cable.)

This turns out to be a thought experiment that can actually be answered empirically. Some unfortunate individuals are born with such serious damage to their eyes that they have never seen the world and are curious about what "seeing" really is: To them it's as puzzling as the fish's electroception is to you. It's now possible to stimulate small parts of their brains directly with a device called a transcranial magnetic stimulator—an extremely powerful, fluctuating magnet that activates neural tissue with some degree of precision. What if one were to stimulate the visual cortex of such a person with magnetic pulses, thereby bypassing the nonfunctional optics of the eye? I can imagine two possible outcomes. He might say, "Hey, I feel something funny zapping the back of my head," but nothing else. Or he might say, "Oh, my God, this is extraordinary! I now understand what all of you folks are talking about. I am finally experiencing this abstract thing called vision. So this is light, this is color, this is seeing!"

This experiment is logically equivalent to the neuron cable experiment we did on the superscientist because we are bypassing spoken language and directly hitting the blind person's brain. Now you may ask, If he does experience totally novel sensations (what you and I call seeing), how can we be sure that it is in fact true vision? One way would be to look for evidence of topography in his brain. I could stimulate different parts of his visual cortex and ask him to point to various regions of the outside world where he experiences these strange new sensations. This is akin to the way you might see stars "out there" in the world when I hit you on the head with a hammer; you don't experience the stars as being inside your skull. This exercise would provide convincing evidence that he was indeed experiencing for the first time something very close to our experience of seeing, although it might not be as discriminating or sophisticated as normal seeing.[4]

•

Why did qualia—subjective sensation—emerge in evolution? Why did some brain events come to have qualia? Is there a particular *style* of information processing that produces qualia, or are there some *types* of neurons exclusively associated with qualia? (The Spanish neurologist Ramón y Cajal calls these neurons the "psychic neurons.") Just as we know that only a tiny part of the cell, namely, the deoxyribonucleic acid (DNA) molecule, is directly involved in heredity and other parts such as proteins are not, could it be that only some neural circuits are involved in qualia and others aren't? Francis Crick and Christof Koch have made the ingenious suggestion that qualia arise from a set of neurons in the lower layers of the primary sensory areas, because these are the ones that project to the frontal lobes where many so-called higher functions are carried out. Their theory has galvanized the entire scientific community and served as a catalyst for those seeking biological explanations for qualia. Others have suggested that the actual patterns of nerve impulses (spikes) from widely separated brain regions become "synchronized" when you pay attention to something and become aware of it.[5] In other words, it is the synchronization itself that leads to conscious awareness. There's no direct evidence for this yet, but it's encouraging to see that people are at least trying to explore the question experimentally.

These approaches are attractive for one main reason, namely, the fact that reductionism has been the single most successful strategy in science. As the English biologist Peter Medawar defines it, "Reductionism is the belief that a whole may be represented as a function (in the mathematical sense) of its constituent parts, the functions having to do with the spatial and temporal ordering of the parts and with the precise way in which they interact." Unfortunately, as I stated at the beginning of this book, it's not always easy to know a priori what the appropriate level of reductionism is for any given scientific problem. For understanding consciousness and qualia there wouldn't be much point in looking at ion channels that conduct nerve impulses, at the brain stem reflex that mediates sneezing or at the spinal cord reflex arc that controls the bladder, even though these are interesting problems in themselves (at least to some people). They would be no more useful in understanding higher brain functions like qualia than looking at silicon chips in a microscope in an attempt to understand the logic of a computer program. And yet this is precisely the strategy most neuroscientists use in trying to understand the higher functions of the brain. They argue either that the problem doesn't exist or that it will be solved some fine day as we plod along looking at the activity of individual neurons.[6]

Philosophers offer another solution to this dilemma when they say that consciousness and qualia are "epiphenomena." According to this view, consciousness is like the whistling sound that a train makes or the shadow of a horse as it runs: It plays no causal role in the real work done by the brain. After all, you can imagine a "zombie" unconsciously doing everything in exactly the same manner that a conscious being does. A sharp tap on the tendon near your knee joint sets in motion a cascade of neural and chemical events that causes a reflex knee jerk (stretch receptors in the knee connect to nerves in the spinal cord, which in turn send messages to the muscles). Consciousness doesn't enter into this picture; a paraplegic has an excellent knee jerk even though he can't feel the tap. Now imagine a much more complex cascade of events starting with long-wavelength light striking your retina and various relays, leading to your saying "red." Since you can imagine this more complex cascade happening without conscious awareness, doesn't it follow that consciousness is irrelevant to the whole scheme? After all, God (or natural selection) could have created an unconscious being that does and says all the things you do, even though "it" is not conscious.

This argument sounds reasonable but in fact it is based on the fallacy that because you can imagine something to be logically possible, therefore it is actually possible. But consider the same argument applied to a problem in physics. We can all imagine something traveling faster than the speed of light. But as Einstein tells us, this "commonsense" view is wrong. Simply being able to imagine that something is logically possible does not guarantee its possibility in the real world, even in principle. Likewise, even though you can imagine an unconscious zombie doing everything you can do, there may be some deep natural cause that prevents the existence of such a being! Notice that this argument does not prove that consciousness must have a causal role; it simply proves that you cannot use statements that begin, "After all, I can imagine" to draw conclusions about any natural phenomenon.

I would like to try a somewhat different approach to understanding qualia, which I will introduce by asking you to play some games with your eyes. First, recall the discussion in Chapter 5 concerning the so-called blind spot—the place where your optic nerve exits the back of your eyeball. Again, if you close your right eye, fix your gaze on the black spot in Figure 5.2 and slowly move the page toward or away from your eye, you will see that the hatched disk disappears. It has fallen into your natural blind spot. Now close your right eye again, hold up the index finger of your right hand and aim your left eye's blind spot at the middle of your ex-

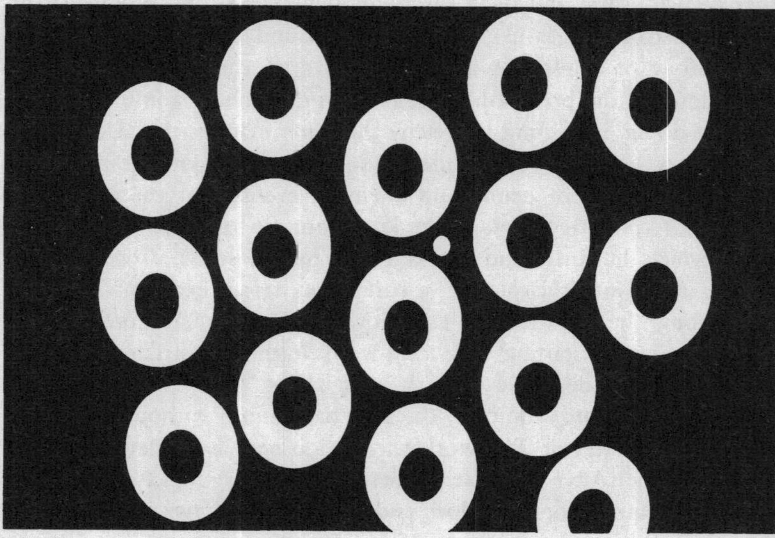

Figure 12.1 *A field of yellow doughnuts (shown in white here). Shut your right eye and look at the small white dot near the middle of the illustration with your left eye. When the page is about six to nine inches from your face, one of the doughnuts will fall exactly around your left eye's blind spot. Since the black hole in the center of the doughnut is slightly smaller than your blind spot, it should disappear and the blind spot then is "filled in" with yellow (white) qualia from the ring so that you see a yellow disk rather than a ring. Notice that the disk "pops out" conspicuously against the background of rings. Paradoxically, you have made a target more conspicuous by virtue of your blind spot. If the illusion doesn't work, try using an enlarged photocopy and shifting the white dot horizontally.*

tended finger. The middle of the finger *should* disappear, just as the hatched disk does, and yet it doesn't; it looks continuous. In other words, the qualia are such that you do not merely *deduce* intellectually that the finger is continuous—"After all, my blind spot is there"—you literally *see* the "missing piece" of your finger. Psychologists call this phenomenon "filling in," a useful if somewhat misleading phrase that simply means that you see something in a region of space where nothing exists.

This phenomenon can be demonstrated even more dramatically if you look at Figure 12.1. Again, with your right eye shut look at the small white dot on the right with your left eye and gradually move the book toward you until one of the "doughnuts" falls on your blind spot. Since the inner diameter of the doughnut—the small black disk—is slightly smaller than your blind spot, it should disappear and the white ring should encompass the blind spot. Say the doughnut (the ring) is yellow. What you will see if your vision is normal is a complete yellow homogeneous disk, which will indicate that your brain "filled in" your blind spot with yellow qualia (or white in Figure 12.1). I emphasize this because some people have argued that we all simply ignore the blind spot and don't notice what's going on, meaning that there really is no filling in. But this can't be right. If you show someone several rings, one of which is concentric with the blind spot, that concentric one will look like a homogeneous disk and will actually "pop out" perceptually against a background of rings. How can something you are ignoring pop out at you? This means that the blind spot does have qualia associated with it and, moreover, that the qualia can provide actual "sensory support." In other words, you don't merely deduce that the center of the doughnut is yellow; you literally *see* it as yellow.[7]

Now consider a related example. Suppose I put one finger crosswise in front of another finger (as in a plus sign) and look at the two fingers. Of course, I see the finger in the back as being continuous. I know it's continuous. I sort of see it as continuous. But if you asked me whether I *literally see* the missing piece of finger, I would say no—for all I know, someone could have actually sliced two pieces of finger and put them on either side of the finger in front to fool me. I cannot be certain that I really see that missing part.

Compare these two cases, which are similar in that the brain supplies the missing information both times. What's the difference? What does it matter to you, the conscious person, that the yellow doughnut now has qualia in the middle and that the occluded part of your finger does not? The difference is that *you cannot change your mind* about the yellow in the middle of the doughnut. You can't think, "Maybe it's yellow, but maybe it's pink, or maybe it's blue." No, it's shouting at you, "I am yellow," with an explicit representation of yellowness in its center. In other words, the filled-in yellow is not revocable, not changeable by you.

In the case of the occluded finger, however, you can think, "There's a high probability that there is a finger there, but some malicious scientist could have pasted two half fingers on either side of it." This scenario is highly improbable, but not inconceivable.

In other words, I can choose to assume that there might be something else behind the occluding finger, but I cannot do so with the filled-in yellow of the blind spot. Thus the crucial difference between a qualia-laden perception and one that doesn't have qualia is that the qualia-laden perception is irrevocable by higher brain centers and is therefore "tamper-resistant," whereas the one that lacks qualia is flexible; you can choose any one of a number of different "pretend" inputs using your imagination. Once a qualia-laden perception has been created, you're stuck with it. (A good example of this is the dalmatian dog in Figure 12.2. Initially, as you look, it's all fragments. Then suddenly everything clicks and you see the dog. Loosely speaking, you've now got the dog qualia. The next time you see it, there's no way you can avoid seeing the dog. Indeed, we have recently shown that neurons in the brain have permanently altered their connections once you have seen the dog.)[8]

These examples demonstrate an important feature of qualia—it must be irrevocable. But although this feature is necessary, it's not sufficient to explain the presence of qualia. Why? Well, imagine that you are in a coma and I shine a light into your eye. If the coma is not too deep, your pupil will constrict, even though you will have no subjective awareness of any qualia caused by the light. The entire reflex arc is irrevocable, and yet there are no qualia associated with it. You can't change your mind about it. You can't do anything about it, just as you couldn't do anything about the yellow filling in your blind spot in the doughnut example. So why does only the latter have qualia? The key difference is that in the case of the pupil's constriction, there is only one output—one final outcome—available and hence no qualia. In the case of the yellow disk, even though the representation that was created is irrevocable, you have the luxury of a choice; what you can do with the representation is open-ended. For instance, when you experienced yellow qualia, you could say yellow, or you could think of yellow bananas, yellow teeth, the yellow skin of jaundice and so on. And when you finally saw the dalmatian, your mind would be poised to conjure up any one of an infinite set of dog-related associations—the word "dog," the dog's bark, dog food or even fire engines. And there is apparently no limit to what you can choose. This is the second important feature of qualia: Sensations that are qualia-laden afford the luxury of choice. So now we have identified *two* functional features of qualia: irrevocability on the input side and flexibility on the output side.

There is a third important feature of qualia. In order to make decisions on the basis of a qualia-laden representation, the representation needs to exist long enough for you to work with it. Your brain needs to hold the representation in an intermediate buffer or in so-called immediate memory. (For example, you hold the phone number you get from the information operator just long enough to dial it with your fingers.) Again this

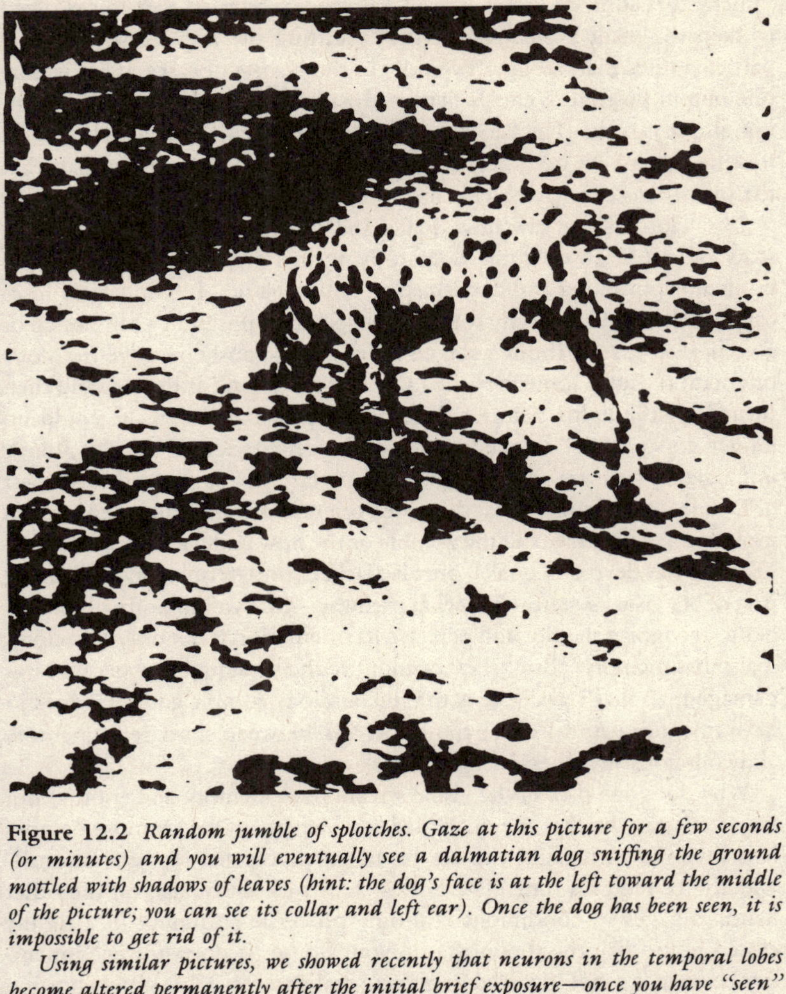

Figure 12.2 *Random jumble of splotches. Gaze at this picture for a few seconds (or minutes) and you will eventually see a dalmatian dog sniffing the ground mottled with shadows of leaves (hint: the dog's face is at the left toward the middle of the picture; you can see its collar and left ear). Once the dog has been seen, it is impossible to get rid of it.*

Using similar pictures, we showed recently that neurons in the temporal lobes become altered permanently after the initial brief exposure—once you have "seen" the dog (*Tovee, Rolls and Ramachandran, 1996*). Dalmatian dog photographed by Ron James.

condition is not enough in itself to generate qualia. A biological system can have other reasons, besides making a choice, for holding information in a buffer. For example, Venus's-flytrap snaps shut only if its trigger hairs inside the trap are stimulated twice in succession, apparently retaining a memory of the first stimulus and comparing it with the second to "infer" that something has moved. (Darwin suggested that this evolved to help the plant avoid inadvertently shutting the trap if hit by a dust particle rather than a bug.) Typically in these sorts of cases, there is only one output possible: Venus's-flytrap ***invariably*** closes shut. There's nothing else it can do. The second important feature of qualia—choice—is missing. I think we can safely conclude, contrary to the panpsychists, that the plant does not have qualia linked to bug detection.

In Chapter 4, we saw how qualia and memory are connected in the story of Denise, the young woman living in Italy who suffered carbon monoxide poisoning and developed an unusual kind of "blindsight." Recall that she could correctly rotate an envelope to post it in a horizontal or a vertical slot, even though she could not consciously perceive the slot's orientation. But if someone asked Denise first to look at the slot and then turned off the lights before asking her to post the letter, she could no longer do so. "She" seemed to forget the orientation of the slot almost immediately and was unable to insert the letter. This suggests that the part of Denise's visual system that discerned orientation and controlled her arm movements—what we call the zombie or the how pathway in Chapter 4—not only was devoid of qualia, but also lacked short-term memory. But the part of her visual system—the what pathway—that would normally enable her to recognize the slot and perceive its orientation is not only conscious, it also has memory. (But "she" cannot use the what pathway because it is damaged; all that's available is the unconscious zombie and "it" doesn't have memory.) And I don't think this link between short-term memory and conscious awareness is coincidental.

Why does one part of the visual stream have memory and another not have it? It may be that the qualia-laden what system has memory because it is involved in making choices based on perceptual representations—and choice requires time. The how system without qualia, on the other hand, engages in continuous real-time processing running in a tightly closed loop—like the thermostat in your house. It does not need memory because it is not involved in making real choices. Thus simply posting the letter does not require memory, but choosing which letter to post and deciding where to mail it do require memory.

This idea can be tested in a patient like Denise. If you set up a situation in which she was forced to make a *choice*, the zombie system (still intact in her) should go haywire. For example, if you asked Denise to mail a letter and you showed her two slots (one vertical, one horizontal) simultaneously, she should fail, for how could the zombie system choose between the two? Indeed, the very idea of an unconscious zombie making choices seems oxymoronic—for doesn't the very existence of free will imply consciousness?

To summarize thus far—for qualia to exist, you need potentially infinite implications (bananas, jaundice, teeth) but a stable, finite, irrevocable representation in your short-term memory as a starting point (yellow). But if the starting point is revocable, then the representation will not have strong, vivid qualia. Good examples of the latter are a cat that you "infer" under the sofa when you only see its tail sticking out, or your ability to imagine that there is a monkey sitting on that chair. These do not have strong qualia, for good reason, because if they did you would confuse them with real objects and wouldn't be able to survive long, given the way your cognitive system is structured. I repeat what Shakespeare said: "You cannot cloy the hungry edge of appetite by bare imagination of a feast." Very fortunate, for otherwise you wouldn't eat; you would just generate the qualia associated with satiety in your head. In a similar vein, any creature that simply imagines having orgasms is unlikely to pass on its genes to the next generation.

Why don't these faint, internally generated images (the cat under the couch, the monkey in the chair) or beliefs, for that matter, have strong qualia? Imagine how confusing the world would be if they did. Actual perceptions need to have vivid, subjective qualia because they are driving decisions and you cannot afford to hesitate. Beliefs and internal images, on the other hand, should not be qualia-laden because they need to be tentative and revocable. So you believe—and you can imagine—that under the table there is a cat because you see a tail sticking out. But there *could* be a pig under the table with a transplanted cat's tail. You must be willing to entertain that hypothesis, however implausible, because every now and then you might be surprised.

What is the functional or computational advantage to making qualia irrevocable? One answer is stability. If you constantly changed your mind about qualia, the number of potential outcomes (or "outputs") would be infinite; nothing would constrain your behavior. At some point you need to say "this is it" and plant a flag on it, and it's the planting of the flag that we call qualia. The perceptual system follows a rationale something like this: Given the available information, it is 90 percent certain that what you are seeing is yellow (or dog or pain or whatever). Therefore, for the sake of argument, I'll assume that it *is* yellow and act accordingly, because if I keep saying, "Maybe it's not yellow," I won't be able to take the next step of choosing an appropriate course of action or thought. In other words, if I treated perceptions as beliefs, I would be blind (as well as being paralyzed with indecision). Qualia are irrevocable ***in order to eliminate hesitation and to confer certainty*** to decisions.[9] And this, in turn, may depend on which particular neurons are firing, how strongly they're firing and what structures they project to.

•

When I see the cat's tail sticking out from under the table, I "guess" or "know" there is a cat under the table, presumably attached to the tail. But I don't literally see the cat, even though I literally see the tail. And this raises another fascinating question: Are seeing and knowing—the qualitative distinction between perception and conception—completely different, mediated by different types of brain circuitry perhaps, or is there a gray area in between? Let's go back to the region corresponding to the blind spot in my eye, where I can't see anything. As we saw in the Chapter 5 discussion on Charles Bonnet syndrome, there is another kind of blind spot—the enormous region behind my head—where I also can't see anything (although people don't generally use the term "blind spot" for this region). Of course, ordinarily you don't walk around experiencing a huge gap behind your head, and therefore you might be tempted to jump to the conclusion that you are in some sense filling in the gap in the same way that you fill in the blind spot. But you don't. You can't. There is no visual neural representation in the brain corresponding to this area behind your head. You fill it in only in the trivial sense that if you are standing in a bathroom with wallpaper in front of you, you assume that the wallpaper continues behind your head. But even though you assume that there is wallpaper behind your head, you don't literally see it. In other words, this sort of "filling in" is purely metaphorical and does not fulfill our criterion of being irrevocable. In the case of the "real" blind spot, as we saw earlier, you can't change your mind about the area that has been filled in. But regarding the region behind your head, you are free to think, "In all likelihood there is wallpaper there, but who knows, maybe there is an elephant there."

Filling in of the blind spot is therefore fundamentally different from your failure to notice the gap behind your head. But the question remains, Is the distinction between what is going on behind your head and the blind spot qualitative or quantitative? Is the dividing line between "filling in" (of the kind seen in the blind spot) and mere guesswork (for things that might be behind your head) completely arbitrary? To answer this, consider another thought experiment. Imagine we continue evolving in such a way that our eyes migrate toward the sides of our heads, while preserving the binocular visual field. The fields of view of the two eyes encroach farther and farther behind our heads until they are almost touching. At that point let's assume you have a blind spot behind your head (between your eyes) that is identical in size to the blind spot that is in front of you. The question then arises, Would the completion of objects across the blind spot behind your head be true filling in of qualia, as with the real blind spot, or would it still be conceptual, revocable imagery or guesswork of the kind that you and I experience behind our heads? I think that there will be a definite point when the images become irrevocable, and when robust perceptual representations are created, perhaps even re-created and fed back to the early visual areas. At that point the blind region behind your head becomes functionally equivalent to the normal blind spot in front of you. The brain will then suddenly switch to a completely novel mode of representing the information; it will use neurons in the sensory areas to signal the events behind your head irrevocably (instead of neurons in the thinking areas to make educated but tentative guesses as to what might be lurking there).

Thus even though blind-spot completion and completion behind your head can be logically regarded as two ends of a continuum, evolution has seen fit to separate them. In the case of your eye's blind spot, the chance that something significant is lurking there is small enough that it pays simply to treat the chance as zero. In the case of the blind area behind your head, however, the odds of something important being there (like a burglar holding a gun) are high enough that it would be dangerous to fill in this area irrevocably with wallpaper or whatever pattern is in front of your eyes.

•

So far we have talked about three laws of qualia—three logical criteria for determining whether a system is conscious or not—and we have considered examples from the blind spot and from neurological patients. But you may ask, How general is this principle? Can we apply it to other specific instances when there is a debate or doubt about whether consciousness is involved? Here are some examples:

It's known that bees engage in very elaborate forms of communication including the so-called bee waggle dance. A scout bee, having located a source of pollen, will travel back to the hive and perform an elaborate dance to designate the location of the pollen to the rest of the hive. The question arises, Is the bee conscious when it's doing this?[10] Since the bee's behavior, once set in motion, is irrevocable and since the bee is obviously acting on some short-term memory representation of the pollen's location, at least two of the three criteria for consciousness are met. You might then jump to the conclusion that the bee is conscious when it engages in this elaborate communication ritual. But since the bee lacks the third criterion—flexible output—I would argue that it is a zombie. In other words, even though the information is very elaborate, is irrevocable and held in short-term memory, the bee can only do one thing with that information; only one output is possible—the waggle dance. This argument is important, for it implies that mere complexity or elaborateness of information processing is no guarantee that there is consciousness involved.

One advantage my scheme has over other theories of consciousness is that it allows us unambiguously to answer such questions as, Is a bee conscious when it performs a waggle dance? Is a sleepwalker conscious? Is the spinal cord of a paraplegic conscious—does it have its own sexual qualia—when he (it) has an erection? Is an ant conscious when it detects pheromones? In each of these cases, instead of the vague assertion that one is dealing with various degrees of consciousness—which is the standard answer—one should simply apply the three criteria specified. For example, can a sleepwalker (while he's sleepwalking) take the "Pepsi test"—that is, choose between a Pepsi Cola and a Coca Cola? Does he have short-term memory? If you showed him the Pepsi, put it in a box, switched off the room lights for thirty seconds and then switched them on again, would he reach for the Pepsi (or utterly fail like the zombie in Denise)? Does a partially comatose patient with akinetic mutism (seemingly awake and able to follow you with his eyes but unable to move or talk) have short-term memory? We can now answer these questions and avoid endless semantic quibbles over the exact meaning of the word "consciousness."

•

Now you might ask, "Does any of this yield clues as to where in the brain qualia might be?" It is surprising that many people think that the seat of consciousness is the frontal lobes, because nothing dramatic happens to qualia and consciousness per se if you damage the frontal lobes—even though the patient's personality can be profoundly altered (and he may have difficulty switching attention). I would suggest instead that most of the action is in the temporal lobes because lesions and hyperactivity in these structures are what most often produce striking disturbances in consciousness. For instance, you need the amygdala and other parts of the temporal lobes for seeing the significance of things, and surely this is a vital part of conscious experience. Without this structure you are a zombie (like the fellow in the famous Chinese room thought experiment proposed by the philosopher John Searle[11]) capable only of giving a single correct output in response to a demand, but with no ability to sense the meaning of what you are doing or saying.

Everyone would agree that qualia and consciousness are not associated with the early stages of perceptual processing as at the level of the retina. Nor are they associated with the final stages of planning motor acts when behavior is actually carried out. They are associated, instead, with the intermediate stages of processing[12]—a stage where stable perceptual representations are created (yellow, dog, monkey) and that have meaning (the infinite implications and possibilities for action from which you can choose the best one). This happens mainly in the temporal lobe and associated limbic structures, and, in this sense, the temporal lobes are the interface between perception and action.

The evidence for this comes from neurology; brain lesions that produce the most profound disturbances in consciousness are those that generate temporal lobe seizures, whereas lesions in other parts of the brain only produce minor disturbances in consciousness. When surgeons electrically stimulate the temporal lobes of epileptics, the patients have vivid conscious experiences. Stimulating the amygdala is the surest way to "replay" a full experience, such as an autobiographical memory or a vivid hallucination. Temporal lobe seizures are often associated not only with alterations in consciousness in the sense of personal identity, personal destiny and personality, but also with vivid qualia—hallucinations such as smells and sounds. If these are mere memories, as some claim, why would the person say, "I literally feel like I'm reliving it"? These seizures are characterized by the vividness of the qualia they produce. The smells, pains, tastes and emotional feelings—all generated in the temporal lobes—suggest that this brain region is intimately involved in qualia and conscious awareness.

Another reason for choosing the temporal lobes—especially the left one—is that this is where much of language is represented. If I see an apple, temporal lobe activity allows me to apprehend all its implications almost simultaneously. Recognition of it as a fruit of a certain type occurs in the inferotemporal cortex, the amygdala gauges the apple's significance for my well-being and Wernicke's and other areas alert me to all the nuances of meaning that the mental image—including the word "apple"—evokes; I can eat the apple, I can smell it; I can bake a pie, remove its pith, plant its seeds; use it to "keep the doctor away," tempt Eve and on and on. If one enumerates all of the attributes that we usually associate with the words "consciousness" and "awareness," each of them, you will notice, has a correlate in temporal lobe seizures, including vivid visual and auditory hallucinations, "out of body" experiences and an absolute sense of omnipotence or omniscience.[13] Any one of this long list of disturbances in conscious experience can occur individually when other parts of the brain are damaged (for instance, disturbances of body image and attention in parietal lobe syndrome), but it's only when the temporal lobes are involved that they occur simultaneously or in different combinations; that again suggests that these structures play a central role in human consciousness.

•

Until now we have discussed what philosophers call the "qualia" problem—the essential privacy and noncommunicability of mental states—and I've tried to transform it from a philosophical problem into a scientific one. But in addition to qualia (the "raw feel" of sensations), we also have to consider the self—the "I" inside you who actually experiences these qualia. Qualia and self are really two sides of the same coin; obviously there is no such thing as free-floating qualia not experienced by anyone and it's hard to imagine a self devoid of all qualia.

But what exactly is the self? Unfortunately, the word "self" is like the word "happiness" or "love"; we all know what it is and know that it's real, but it's very hard to define it or even to pinpoint its characteristics. As with quicksilver, the more you try to grasp it the more it tends to slip away. When you think of the word "self," what pops into your mind? When I think about "myself," it seems to be something that unites all my diverse sensory impressions and memories (unity), claims to be "in charge" of my life, makes choices (has free will) and seems to endure as a single entity in space and time. It also sees itself as embedded in a social context, balancing its checkbook and maybe even planning its own funeral. Actually we can make a list of all the characteristics of the "self"—just as we can for happiness—and then look for brain structures that are involved in each of these aspects. Doing this will someday enable us to develop a clearer understanding of self and consciousness—although I doubt that there will be a single, grand, climactic "solution" to the problem of the self in the way that DNA is the solution to the riddle of heredity.

What are these characteristics that define the self? William Hirstein, a postdoctoral fellow in my lab, and I came up with the following list:

The embodied self: My Self is anchored within a single body. If I close my eyes, I have a vivid sense of different body parts occupying space (some parts more felt than others)—the so-called body image. If you pinch my toe, it is "I" who experiences the pain, not "it." And yet the body image, as we have seen, is extremely malleable, despite all its appearance of stability. With a few seconds of the right type of sensory stimulation, you can make your nose three feet long or project your hand onto a table (Chapter 3)! And we know that circuits in the parietal lobes, and the regions of the frontal lobes to which they project, are very much involved in constructing this image. Partial damage to these structures can cause gross distortions in body image; the patient may say that her left arm belongs to her mother or (as in the case of the patient I saw with Dr. Riita Hari in Helsinki) claim that the left half of her body is still sitting in the chair when she gets up and walks! If these examples don't convince you that your "ownership" of your body is an illusion, then nothing will.

The passionate self: It is difficult to imagine the self without emotions—or what such a state could even mean. If you don't see the meaning or significance of something—if you cannot apprehend all its implications—in what sense are you really aware of it consciously? Thus your emotions—mediated by the limbic system and amygdala—are an essential aspect of self, not just a "bonus." (It is a moot point whether a purebred Vulcan, like Spock's father in the original *Star Trek*, is really conscious or whether he is just a zombie—unless he is also tainted by a few human genes as Spock is.) Recall that the "zombie" in the "how" pathway is unconscious, whereas the "what" pathway is conscious, and I suggest that the difference arises because only the latter is linked to the amygdala and other limbic structures (Chapter 5).

The amygdala and the rest of the limbic system (in the temporal lobes) ensures that the cortex—indeed, the entire brain—serves the organism's basic evolutionary goals. The amygdala monitors the highest level of perceptual representations and "has its fingers on the keyboard of the autonomic nervous system"; it determines whether or not to respond emotionally to something and what kinds of emotions are appropriate (fear in response to a snake or rage to your boss and affection to your child). It also receives information from the insular cortex, which in turn is driven partially by sensory input not only from the skin but also from the viscera—heart, lung, liver, stomach—so that one can also speak of a "visceral, vegetative self" or of a "gut reaction" to something. (It is this "gut reaction," of course, that one monitors with the GSR machine, as we showed in Chapter 9, so that you could argue that the visceral self isn't, strictly speaking, part of the conscious self at all. But it can nevertheless profoundly intrude on your conscious self; just think of the last time you felt nauseous and threw up.)

Pathologies of the emotional self include temporal lobe epilepsy, Capgras' syndrome and Klüver-Bucy syndrome. In the first, there may be a heightened sense of self that may arise partly through a process that Paul Fedio and D. Bear call "hyperconnectivity"—a strengthening of connections between the sensory areas of the temporal cortex and the amygdala. Such hyperconnectivity may result from repeated seizures that cause a permanent enhancement (kindling) of these pathways, leading the patient to ascribe deep significance to everything around him (including himself!). Conversely, people with Capgras' syndrome have reduced emotional response to certain categories of objects (faces) and people with Klüver-Bucy or Cotard's syndrome have more pervasive problems with emotions (Chapter 8). A Cotard's patient feels so emotionally remote from the world and from himself that he will actually make the absurd claim that he is dead or that he can smell his flesh rotting.

Interestingly, what we call "personality"—a vital aspect of your self that endures for life and is notoriously impervious to "correction" by other people or even by common sense—probably also involves the very same limbic structures and their connections with the ventromedial frontal lobes. Damage to the frontal lobes produces no obvious, immediate disturbance in consciousness, but it can profoundly alter your personality. When a crowbar pierced the frontal lobes of a railway worker named Phineas Gage, his close friends and relatives remarked, "Gage wasn't Gage anymore." In this famous example of frontal lobe damage, Gage was transformed from a stable, polite, hardworking young man into a lying, cheating vagabond who could not hold down a job.[14]

Temporal lobe epilepsy patients like Paul in Chapter 9 also show striking personality changes, so much so that some neurologists speak of a "temporal lobe epilepsy personality." Some of them (the patients, not the neurologists) tend to be pedantic, argumentative, egocentric and garrulous. They also tend to be obsessed with "abstract thoughts." If these traits are a result of hyperfunctioning of certain parts of the temporal lobe, what exactly is the normal function of these areas? If the limbic system is concerned mainly with emotions, why would seizures in these areas cause a tendency to generate abstract thought? Are there areas in our brains whose role is to produce and manipulate abstract thoughts? This is one of the many unsolved problems of temporal lobe epilepsy.[15]

The executive self: Classical physics and modern neuroscience tell us that you (including your mind and brain) inhabit a deterministic billiard ball universe. But you don't ordinarily experience yourself as a puppet on a string; you feel that you are in charge. Yet paradoxically, it is always obvious to you that there are some things you can do and others you cannot given the constraints of your body and of the external world. (You know you can't lift a truck; you know you can't give your boss a black eye, even if you'd like to.) Somewhere in your brain there are *representations* of all these possibilities, and the systems that plan commands (the cingulate and supplementary motor areas in the frontal lobes) need to be aware of this distinction between things they can and cannot command you to do. Indeed, a "self" that sees itself as completely passive, as a helpless spectator, is no self at all, and a self that is hopelessly driven to action by its impulses and urgings is equally effete. A self needs free will—what Deepak Chopra calls "the universal field of infinite possibilities"—even to exist. More technically, conscious awareness has been described as a "conditional readiness to act."

To achieve all this, I need to have in my brain not only a representation of the world and various objects in it but also a representation of myself, including my own body within that representation—and it is this peculiar recursive aspect of the self that makes it so puzzling. In addition, the representation of the external object has to interact with my self-representation (including the motor command systems) in order to allow me to make a choice. (He's your boss; don't sock him. It's a cookie; it's within your reach to grab it.) Derangements in this mechanism can lead to syndromes like anosognosia or somatoparaphrenia (Chapter 7) in which a patient will with a perfectly straight face claim that her left arm belongs to her brother or to the physician.

What neural structure is involved in representing these "embodied" and "executive" aspects of the self? Damage to the anterior cingulate gyrus results in a bizarre condition called "akinetic mutism"—the patient simply lies in bed unwilling to do or incapable of doing anything even though he appears to be fully aware of his surroundings. If there's such a thing as absence of free will, this is it.

Sometimes when there is partial damage to the anterior cingulate, the very opposite happens: The patient's hand is uncoupled from her conscious thoughts and intentions and attempts to grab things or even perform relatively complex actions without her permission. For example, Dr. Peter Halligan and I saw a patient at Rivermead Hospital in Oxford whose left hand would seize the banister as she walked down the steps and she would have to use her other hand forcibly to unclench the fingers one by one, so she could continue walking. Is the alien left hand controlled by an unconscious zombie, or is it controlled by parts of her brain that have qualia and consciousness? We can now answer this by applying our three criteria. Does the system in her brain that moves her arm create an irrevocable representation? Does it have short-term memory? Can it make a choice?

Both the executive self and the embodied self are deployed while you are playing chess and assume you're the queen as you plan "her" next move. When you do this, you can almost feel momentarily that you are inhabiting the queen. Now one could argue that you're just using a figure of speech here, that you're not literally assimilating the chess piece into your body image. But can you really be all that sure that the loyalty of your mind to your ***own*** body is not equally a "figure of speech"? What would happen to your GSR if I suddenly punched the queen? Would it shoot up as though I were punching your own body? If so, what is the justification for a hard-and-fast distinction between her body and yours? Could it be that your tendency normally to identify with your "own" body rather than with the chess piece is also a matter of convention, albeit an enduring one? Might such a mechanism also underlie the empathy and love you feel for a close friend, a spouse or a child who is literally made from your own body?

The mnemonic self: Your sense of personal identity—as a single person who endures through space and time—depends on a long string of highly personal recollections: your autobiography. Organizing these memories into a coherent story is obviously vital to the construction of self.

We know that the hippocampus is required for acquiring and consolidating new memory traces. If you lost your hippocampi ten years ago, then you will not have any memories of events that occurred after that date. You are still fully conscious, of course, because you have all the memories prior to that loss, but in a very real sense your existence was frozen at that time.

Profound derangement to the mnemonic self can lead to multiple personality disorder or MPD. This disorder is best regarded as a malfunction of the same coherencing principle I alluded to in the discussion of denial in Chapter 7. As we saw, if you have two sets of mutually incompatible beliefs and memories about yourself, the only way to prevent anarchy and endless strife may be to create two personalities within one body—the so-called multiple personality disorder. Given the obvious relevance of this syndrome to understanding the nature of self, it is astonishing how little attention it has received from mainstream neurology.

Even the mysterious trait called hypergraphia—the tendency of temporal lobe epilepsy patients to maintain elaborate diaries—may be an exaggeration of the same general tendency: the need to create and sustain a coherent worldview or autobiography. Perhaps kindling in the amygdala causes every external event and internal belief to acquire deep significance for the patient, so there is an enormous proliferation of spuriously self-relevant beliefs and memories in his brain. Add to this the compelling need we all have from time to time to take stock of our lives, see where we stand; to review the significant episodes of our lives periodically—and you have hypergraphia, an exaggeration of this natural tendency. We all have random thoughts during our day-to-day musings, but if these were sometimes accompanied by miniseizures—producing euphoria—then the musings themselves might evolve into obsessions and entrenched beliefs that the patient would keep returning to whether in his speech or in his writing. Could similar phenomena provide a neural basis for zealotry and fanatacism?

The unified self—imposing coherence on consciousness, filling in and confabulation: Another important attribute of self is its unity—the internal coherence of its different attributes. One way to approach the question of how our account of qualia relates to the question of the self is to ask why something like filling in of the blind spot with qualia occurs. The original motive many philosophers had for arguing that the blind spot is ***not*** filled in was that there is no person in the brain to fill it in for—that no little homunculus is watching.

Since there's no little man, they argued, the antecedent is also false: Qualia are not filled in, and thinking so is a logical fallacy. Since I argue that qualia are in fact filled in, does this mean that I believe they are filled in for a homunculus? Of course not. The philosopher's argument is really a straw man. The line of reasoning should run, If qualia are filled in, they are filled in for ***something*** and what is that "something"? There exists in certain branches of psychology the notion of an executive, or a control process, which is generally thought to be located in the prefrontal and frontal parts of the brain. I would like to suggest that the "something" that qualia are filled in for is not a "thing" but simply another brain process, namely, executive processes associated with the limbic system including parts of the anterior cingulate gyrus. This process connects your perceptual qualia with specific emotions and goals, enabling you to make choices—very much the sort of thing that the self was traditionally supposed to do. (For example, after having lots of tea, I have the sensation or urge—the qualia—to urinate but I'm giving a lecture so I choose to delay action until the talk is finished but also choose to excuse myself at the end instead of taking questions.) An executive process is not something that has all the properties of a full human being, of course. It is not a homunculus. Rather, it is a process whereby some brain areas such as those concerned with perception and motivation influence the activities of other brain areas such as ones dealing with the planning of motor output.

Seen this way, filling in is a kind of treating and "preparing" of qualia to enable them to interact properly with limbic executive structures. Qualia may need to be filled in because gaps interfere with the proper working of these executive structures, reducing their efficiency and their ability to select an appropriate response. Like our general who ignores gaps in data given to him by scouts to avoid making a wrong decision, the control structure also finds a way to avoid gaps—by filling them in.[15]

Where in the limbic system are these control processes? It might be a system involving the amygdala and the anterior cingulate gyrus, given the amygdala's central role in emotion and the anterior cingulate's apparent executive role. We know that when these structures are disconnected, disorders of "free will" occur, such as akinetic mutism[16] and alien hand syndrome. It is not difficult to see how such processes could give rise to the mythology of a self as an active presence in the brain—a "ghost in the machine."

The vigilant self: A vital clue to the neural circuitry underlying qualia and consciousness comes from two other neurological disorders—penduncular hallucinosis and "vigilant coma" or akinetic mutism.

The anterior cingulate and other limbic structures also receive projections from the intralaminar thalamic nuclei (cells in the thalamus), which in turn are driven by clusters of cells in the brain stem (including the cholinergic lateral tegmental cells and the penduncolopontine cells). Hyperactivity of these cells can lead to visual hallucinations (penduncular hallucinosis), and we also know that schizophrenics have a doubling of cell number in these very same brain stem nuclei—which may contribute to their hallucinations.

Conversely, damage to the intralaminar nucleus or to the anterior cingulate results in coma vigilance or akinetic mutism. Patients with this curious disorder are immobile and mute and react sluggishly, if at all, to painful stimuli. Yet they are apparently awake and alert, moving their eyes around and tracking objects. When the patient comes out of this state, he may say, "No words or thoughts would come to my mind. I just didn't want to do or think or say anything." (This raises a fascinating question: Can a brain stripped of all motivation record any memories at all? If so, how much detail does the patient remember? Does he recall the neurologist's pinprick? Or the cassette tape that his girlfriend played for him?) Clearly these brain stem and thalamic circuits play an important role in consciousness and qualia. But it remains to be seen whether they merely play a "supportive" role for qualia (as indeed the liver and heart do!) or whether they are an integral part of the circuitry that embodies qualia and consciousness. Are they analogous to the power supply of a VCR or TV set or to the actual magnetic recording head and the electron gun in the cathode-ray tube?

The conceptual self and the social self: In a sense, our concept of self is not fundamentally different from any other abstract concept we have—such as "happiness" or "love." Therefore, a careful examination of the different ways in which we use the word "I" in ordinary social discourse can provide some clues as to what the self is and what its function might be.

For instance, it is clear that the abstract self-concept also needs to have access to the "lower" parts of the system, so that the person can acknowledge or claim responsibility for different self-related facts: states of the body, body movements and so on (just as you claim to "control" your thumb when hitching a ride but not your knee when I tap the tendon with my rubber hammer). Information in autobiographical memory and information about one's body image need to be accessible to the self-concept, so that thought and talk about self are possible. In the normal brain there are specialized pathways that allow such access to occur, but when one or more of these pathways is damaged, the system tries to do it anyway, and confabulation results. For instance, in the denial syndrome discussed in Chapter 7, there is no access channel between information about the left side of the body and the patient's self-concept. But the self-concept is set up to try automatically to include that information. The net result of this is anosognosia or denial syndrome; the self "assumes" that the arm is okay and "fills in" the movements of that arm.

One of the attributes of the self-representation system is that the person will confabulate to try to cover up deficits in it. The main purposes of doing this, as we saw in Chapter 7, are to prevent constant indecisiveness and to confer stability on behavior. But another important function may be to support the sort of created or narrative self that the philosopher Dan Dennett talks about—that we present ourselves as unified in order to achieve social goals and to be understandable to others. We also present ourselves as acknowledging our past and future identity, enabling us to be seen as part of society. Acknowledging and taking credit or blame for things we did in the past help society (usually kin who share our genes) incorporate us effectively in its plans, thereby enhancing the survival and perpetuation of our genes.[17]

If you doubt the reality of the social self, ask yourself the following question: Imagine that there is some act you've committed about which you are extremely embarrassed (love letters and Polaroid photographs from an illicit affair). Assume further that you now have a fatal illness and will be dead in two months. If you know that people rummaging through your belongings will discover your secrets, will you do your utmost to cover your tracks? If the answer is yes, the question arises, Why bother? After all, you know you won't be around, so what does it matter what people think of you after you're gone? This simple thought experiment suggests that the idea of the social self and its reputation is not just an abstract yarn. On the contrary, it is so deeply ingrained in us that we want to protect it even after death. Many a scientist has spent his entire life yearning obsessively for posthumous fame—sacrificing everything else just to leave a tiny scratchmark on the edifice.

So here is the greatest irony of all: that the self that almost by definition is entirely private is to a significant extent a social construct—a story you make up for others. In our discussion on denial, I suggested that confabulation and self-deception evolved mainly as by-products of the need to impose stability, internal consistency and coherence on behavior. But an added important function might stem from the need to conceal the truth from other people.

The evolutionary biologist Robert Trivers[18] has proposed the ingenious argument that self-deception evolved mainly to allow you to lie with complete conviction, as a car salesman can. After all, in many social situations it might be useful to lie—in a job interview or during courtship ("I'm not married"). But the problem is that your limbic system often gives the game away and your facial muscles leak traces of guilt. One way to prevent this, Trivers suggests, may be to deceive yourself first. If you actually believe your lies, there's no danger your face will give you away. And this need to lie efficiently provided the selection pressure for the emergence of self-deception.

I don't find Trivers's idea convincing as a *general* theory of self-deception, but there is one particular class of lies for which the argument carries special force: lying about your abilities or boasting. Through boasting about your assets you may enhance the likelihood of getting more dates, thereby disseminating your genes more effectively. The penalty you pay for self-deception, of course, is that you may become delusional. For example, telling your girlfriend that you're a millionaire is one thing; actually believing it is a different thing altogether, for you may start spending money you don't have! On the other hand, the advantages of boasting successfully (reciprocation of courtship gestures) may outweigh the disadvantage of delusion—at least up to a point. Evolutionary strategies are always a matter of compromsie.

So can we do experiments to prove that self-deception evolved in a social context? Unfortunately, these are not easy ideas to test (as with all evolutionary arguments), but again our patients with denial syndrome whose defenses are grossly amplified may come to our rescue. When questioned by the physician, the patient denies that he is paralyzed, but would he deny his paralysis to *himself* as well? Would he do it when nobody was watching? My experiments suggest that he probably would, but I wonder whether the delusion is amplified when others are present. Would his skin register a galvanic response as he confidently asserted that he could arm wrestle? What if we showed him the word "paralysis"? Even though he denies the paralysis, would he be disturbed by the word and register a strong GSR? Would a normal child show a skin change when confabulating (children are notoriously prone to such behavior)? What if a neurologist were to develop anosognosia (the denial syndrome) as the result of a stroke? Would he continue to lecture on this topic to his students—blissfully unaware that he himself was suffering from denial? Indeed, how do I know that I am not such a person? It's only through raising questions such as these that we can begin to approach the greatest scientific and philosophical riddle of all—the nature of the self.

Our revels now are ended. These our actors,
As I foretold you, were all spirits and
Are melted into air, into thin air. . . .
We are such stuff
As dreams are made on,
And our little life
Is rounded with a sleep.

—WILLIAM SHAKESPEARE

During the last three decades, neuroscientists throughout the world have probed the nervous system in fascinating detail and have learned a great deal about the laws of mental life and about how these laws emerge from the brain. The pace of progress has been exhiliarating, but—at the same time—the findings make many people uncomfortable. It seems somehow disconcerting to be told that your life, all your hopes, triumphs and aspirations simply arise from the activity of neurons in your brain. But far from being humiliating, this idea is ennobling, I think. Science—cosmology, evolution and especially the brain sciences—is telling us that we have no privileged position in the universe and that our sense of having a private nonmaterial soul "watching the world" is really an illusion (as has long been emphasized by Eastern mystical traditions like Hinduism and Zen Buddhism). Once you realize that far from being a spectator, you are in fact part of the eternal ebb and flow of events in the cosmos, this realization is very liberating. Ultimately this idea also allows you to cultivate a certain humility—the essence of all authentic religious experience. It is not an idea that's easy to translate into words but comes very close to that of the cosmologist Paul Davies, who said:

> Through science, we human beings are able to grasp at least some of nature's secrets. We have cracked part of the cosmic code. Why this should be, just why *Homo sapiens* should carry the spark of rationality that provides the key to the universe, is a deep enigma. We, who are children of the universe—animated stardust—can nevertheless reflect on the nature of that same universe, even to the extent of glimpsing the rules on which it runs. How we have become linked into this cosmic dimension is a mystery. Yet the linkage cannot be denied.
>
> What does it mean? What is Man that we might be party to such privilege? I cannot believe that our existence in this universe is a mere quirk of fate, an accident of history, an incidental blip in the great cosmic drama. Our involvement is too intimate. The physical species *Homo* may count for nothing, but the existence of mind in some organism on some planet in the universe is surely a fact of fundamental significance. Through conscious beings the

> universe has generated self-awareness. This can be no trivial detail, no minor by-product of mindless, purposeless forces. We are truly meant to be here.

Are we? I don't think brain science alone, despite all its triumphs, will ever answer that question. But that we can ask the question at all is, to me, the most puzzling aspect of our existence.

Acknowledgments

My sojourns into neurology during the last ten years have been fascinating, full of all sorts of unexpected twists and turns as each plot unfolded. My companions during this journey have been my numerous students and colleagues, the many books from which I have drawn inspiration and the images of my old teachers from Cambridge and India still fresh in my mind. In particular I would like to thank the following individuals:

First and foremost, my parents—Vilayanur Subramanian and Vilayanur Meenakshi—who strongly encouraged my early interest in science. (My dad bought me a Zeiss research microscope when I was ten years old, and my mother whetted my appetite for chemistry by giving me Partington's textbook of inorganic chemistry and helping me set up a small lab under our staircase.) My brother, Vilayanur Ravi, got me interested in poetry and literature, which have more in common with science than many people realize. My wife, Diane, has been my collaborator in exploring the brain and helped me think through many of the chapters. Two of my uncles, Parameswara Hariharan and Alladi Ramakrishnan, fueled my latent interest in vision and brain science (when I was still in my teens, Dr. Ramakrishman urged me to submit to *Nature* a paper that was accepted and published). I also owe an enormous debt to former teachers John Pettigrew, Oliver Braddick, Colin Blakemore, David Whitteridge, Horace Barlow, Fergus Campbell, Richard Gregory, Donald MacKay, K.V. Thiruvengadam and P.K. Krishnan Kutty, and to various colleagues, friends and students, Reid Abraham, Tom Albright, Krishnaswami Alladi, John Allman, Stuart Anstis, Carrie Armel, Richard Attiyeh, Elizabeth Bates, Floyd Bloom, Mark Bode, Patrick Cavanagh, Steve Cobb, Diana Deutsch, Paul Drake, Sally Duensing, Rosetta Ellis, Martha Farah, David Galin, Sir Alan Gilchrist, Chris Gillin, Rick Grush, Ishwar Hariharan, Laxmi Hariharan, Steve Hillyer, David Hubel, Mumtaz Jahan, Jonathan Khazi, Julie Kindy, Ranjit Kumar, Margaret Livingstone, Donald MacLeod, M.K. Mani, Rama Mani, Jonathan Miller, Ken Nakayama, Kumpati Narenda, David Pearlmutter, Dan Plummer, Mike Posner, Alladi Prabhakar, David Presti, Mark Raichle, Chandramani Ramachandran, William Rosar, Vivian Roum, Krish Sathian, Nick Schiff, Terry Sejnowski, Margaret Sereno, Marty Sereno, Alan Snyder, Subramanian Sriram, Arnie Starr, L. Stone, Gene Stoner, R. Sudarshan,

Christopher Tyler, Claude Valenti, T.R. Vidyasagar, Ben Williams and Tony Yang. And special thanks to Miriam Alaboudi, Eric Altschuler, Gerald Arcilla, Roger Bingham, Joe Bogen, Pat Churchland, Paul Churchland, Francis Crick, Odile Crick, Hanna Damasio, Tony Damasio, Art Flippin, Harold Forney, William Hirstein, Bela Julesz, Leah Levi, Charlie Robbins, Irvin Rock, Oliver Sacks, Elsie Schwartz, Nithya Shiva, John Smythies and Christopher Wills.

I also thank the University of California, San Diego, and the Center for Brain and Cognition (Center for Human Information Processing: CHIP) for providing a superb academic environment; in a recent survey by the National Research Council, the UCSD campus was ranked number one in the country in neuroscience. The university is also fortunate in having a symbiotic relationship with many neighbors, including the Salk Institute, the Scripps Clinic and the Neuroscience Institute, making La Jolla a mecca for neuroscientists from all over the world.

Many of the investigations I describe in this book were carried out in La Jolla, but I also conduct studies on patients in India during my annual visits there. I thank the Institute of Neurology, Madras General Hospital, and the Tata Institute of Fundamental Research in Bangalore for their hospitality.

Some of the ideas discussed in the book emerged from discussions I had with students and colleagues—Eric Altschuler (experiments on placebos and somatoparaphrenia), Roger Bingham (evolutionary psychology), Francis Crick (consciousness and qualia; the term "zombie" for the how pathway in the parietal lobe), Anthony Deutsch (analogy with talking pig), Ilya Farber (arm movement sensations in a denial patient), Stephen Jay Gould (alerting me to Freud's idea on scientific revolutions), Richard Gregory (qualia, filling in and mirrors), Laxmi Hariharan (pediatric diagnosis), Mark Hauser (consciousness of bees), William Hirstein (with whom an early draft of Chapter 12 was written), Ardon Lyon (blind spots), John Pettigrew (talent as a marker of brain size), Bob Rafael (somatoparaphrenia), Diane Rogers-Ramachandran (the mock injection experiment), Alan Snyder (similarities between Nadia's horses and those of da Vinci in the section on savant syndrome) and Christopher Wills (who helped with an early draft of Chapter 5).

I am also grateful to my agent, John Brockman, president of the EDGE Foundation, not only for urging me to write this book but also for doing everything he has to help bridge the "two cultures." Like the Earl of Bridgewater, who commissioned many popular science books in Victorian England, Brockman has been a potent force in the dissemination of science in the latter part of this century. Thanks also to Sandra Blakeslee and Toni Sciarra, who kept goading me to finish this project and helped make the book accessible to a wider readership.

Finally, I owe a very important debt to my patients, who often sat through long hours of tedious testing, many of them as intensely curious about their predicament as I was. I have sometimes learned more from chatting with them or reading their letters than I have from my medical colleagues at conferences.

Notes

Chapter 1: The Phantom Within

1. I am of course talking about style here, not content. Modesty aside, I doubt whether any observation in this book is as important as one of Faraday's discoveries, but I do think that all experimental scientists should strive to emulate his style.
2. Of course, one doesn't want to make a fetish out of low-tech science. My point is simply that poverty and crude equipment can sometimes, paradoxically, actually serve as a catalyst rather than a handicap, for they force you to be inventive.

   There is no denying, though, that innovative technology drives science just as surely as ideas do. The advent of new imaging techniques like PET, fMRI and MEG is likely to revolutionize brain science in the next millennium by allowing us to watch living brains in action, as people engage in various mental tasks. (See Posner and Raichle, 1997, and Phelps and Mazziotta, 1981.)

   Unfortunately, there is currently a lot of gee whiz going on (almost a repeat of nineteenth-century phrenology). But if used intelligently, these toys can be immensely helpful. The best experiments are ones in which imaging is combined with clear, testable hypotheses of how the mind actually works. There are many instances where tracing the flow of events is vital for understanding what is happening in the brain and we will encounter some examples in this book.
3. This question can be answered more easily using insects, which have specific stages, each with a fixed life span. (For instance, the cicada species ***Magicicada septendecim*** spends seventeen years as an immature nymph and just a few weeks as an adult!) Using the metamorphosis hormone ecdysone or an antibody to it or mutant insects, which lack the gene for the hormone, one could theoretically manipulate the duration of each stage separately to see how it contributes to the total life span. For example, would blocking ecdysone allow the caterpillar to enjoy an indefinitely long life, and conversely would changing it into a butterfly allow it to enjoy a longer life as a butterfly?
4. Long before the role of deoxyribonucleic acid (DNA) in heredity was explained by James Watson and Francis Crick, Fred Griffiths proved in 1928 that when a chemical substance obtained from a heat-killed bacterium of one species—called strain S pneumococcus—was injected simultaneously into mice along with another strain (strain R), the latter actually became "transformed" into strain S! It was clear that something was present in S bacteria that was causing the R form to become S. Then, in the 1940s, Oswald Avery, Colin Macleod and Maclyn McCarty showed that this reaction is caused by a chemical substance, DNA. The implication—that DNA contains the genetic code—should have sent shock waves through the world of biology but caused only a small stir.
5. Historically there have been many different ways of studying the brain. One method, popular with psychologists, is the so-called black box approach: You systematically vary the input to the system to see how the output changes and

construct models of what is going on in between. If you think this sounds boring, it is. Nevertheless, the approach has had some spectacular successes, such as the discovery of trichromacy as the mechanism of color vision. Researchers found that all the colors that you can see could be made by simply combining different proportions of three primary ones—red, green and blue. From this they deduced that we have only three receptors in the eye, each of which responds maximally to one wavelength but also reacts to a lesser extent to other wavelengths.

One problem with the black box approach is that, sooner or later, one ends up with multiple competing models and the only way to discover which one is correct is to open up the black box—that is, do physiological experiments on humans and animals. For example, I doubt very much whether anyone could have figured out how the digestive system works by simply looking at its output. Using this strategy alone, no one could have deduced the existence of mastication, peristalsis, saliva, gastric juices, pancreatic enzymes or bile nor realized that the liver alone has over a dozen functions to help assist the digestive process. Yet a vast majority of psychologists—called functionalists—cling to the view that we can understand mental processes from a strictly computational, behaviorist or "reverse engineering perspective"—without bothering with the messy stuff in the head.

When dealing with biological systems, understanding structure is crucial to understanding function—a view that is completely antithetical to the functionalist or black box approach to brain function. For example, consider how our understanding of the anatomy of the DNA molecule—its double-helical structure—completely transformed our understanding of heredity and genetics, which until then had remained a black box subject. Indeed, once the double helix was discovered, it became obvious that the structural logic of this DNA molecule *dictates* the functional logic of heredity.

6. For over half a century, modern neuroscience has been on a reductionist path, breaking things down into ever smaller parts with the hope that understanding all the little pieces will eventually explain the whole. Unfortunately, many people think that because reductionism is so often useful in solving problems, it is therefore also *sufficient* for solving them, and generations of neuroscientists have been raised on this dogma. This misapplication of reductionism leads to the perverse and tenacious belief that somehow reductionism itself will tell us how the brain works, when what is really needed are attempts to bridge different levels of discourse. The Cambridge physiologist Horace Barlow recently pointed out at a scientific meeting that we have spent five decades studying the cerebral cortex in excruciating detail, but we still don't have the foggiest idea of how it works or what it does. He shocked the audience by suggesting that we are all like asexual Martians visiting earth who spend fifty years examining the detailed cellular mechanisms and biochemistry of the testicles without knowing anything at all about sex.

7. The doctine of modularity was carried to its most ludicrous extremes by Franz Gall, an eighteenth-century psychologist who founded the fashionable pseudoscience of phrenology. One day while giving a lecture, Gall noted that one particular student, who was very bright, had prominent eyeballs. Gall started thinking, Why does he have prominent eyeballs? Maybe the frontal lobes have something to do with intelligence. Maybe they are especially large in this boy,

pushing his eyeballs forward. On the basis of this tenuous reasoning, Gall embarked on a series of experiments that involved measuring the bumps and depressions on people's skulls. Finding differences, Gall began to correlate the shapes with various mental functions. Phrenologists soon "discovered" bumps for such esoteric traits as veneration, cautiousness, sublimity, acquisitiveness and secretiveness. In an antique shop in Boston, a colleague of mine recently saw a phrenology bust that depicted a bump for the "Republican spirit"! Phrenology was still popular in the late nineteenth and early twentieth centuries.

Phrenologists were also interested in how brain size is related to mental capacity, asserting that heavier brains are more intelligent than lighter ones. They claimed that, on average, the brains of black people are smaller than white people's and that women's brains are smaller than men's and argued that the difference "explained" differences in average intelligence between these groups. The crowning irony is that when Gall died, people actually weighed *his* brain and found that it was a few grams lighter than the average female brain. (For an eloquent description of the pitfalls of phrenology, see Stephen Jay Gould's *The Mismeasure of Man.*)

8. These two examples were great favorites of the Harvard neurologist Norman Geschwind when he gave lectures to lay audiences.

9. Hints about the role of medial temporal lobe structures, including the hippocampus, in memory formation go all the way back to the Russian psychiatrist Sergei Korsakov. Patient H.M. and other amnesics like him have been studied elegantly by Brenda Milner, Larry Weiskrantz, Elizabeth Warrington and Larry Squire.

   The actual cellular changes that strengthen connections between neurons have been explored by several researchers, most notably Eric Kandel, Dan Alkon, Gary Lynch and Terry Sejnowski.

10. Our ability to engage in numerical computations (add, subtract, multiply and divide) seems so effortless that it's easy to jump to the conclusion that it is "hardwired." But, in fact, it *became* effortless only after the introduction of two basic concepts—place value and zero—in India during the third century A.D. These two notions and the idea of negative numbers and of decimals (also introduced in India) laid the foundation of modern mathematics.

    It has even been claimed that the brain contains a "number line," a sort of graphical, scalar representation of numbers with each point in the graph being a cluster of neurons signaling a particular numerical value. The abstract mathematical concept of a number line goes all the way back to the Persian poet and mathematician Omar Khayyám, in the ninth century, but is there any evidence that such a line exists in the brain? When normal people are asked which of two numbers is larger, it takes them longer to make the decision if the numbers are closer together than if they are wider apart. In Bill, the number line seems unaffected because he is okay at making crude quantitative estimates—which number is bigger or smaller or why it seems inappropriate to say the dinosaur bones are sixty million and three years old. But there is a separate mechanism for numerical computation, for juggling numbers about in your head, and for this you need the angular gyrus in the left hemisphere. For a very readable account of dyscalculias, see Dehaene, 1997.

My colleague here at UCSD Dr. Tim Rickard has shown by using functional magnetic resonance imaging (fMRI) that the "numerical calculation area" actually lies not entirely in the classical left angular gyrus itself but slightly in front of it, but this doesn't affect my main argument and it's only a matter of time before someone also demonstrates the "number line" using modern imaging techniques.

Chapter 2: "Knowing Where to Scratch"

1. Throughout this book I use fictitious names for patients. The place, time and circumstances have also been altered substantially, but the clinical details are presented as accurately as possible. For more detailed clinical information, the reader should consult the original scientific articles.

   In one or two instances when I describe a classic syndrome (such as the neglect syndrome in Chapter 6) I use several patients to create composites of the kind used in neurology textbooks in order to emphasize salient aspects of the disorder, even though no single patient may display all the symptoms and signs described.
2. Silas Weir Mitchell, 1872; Sunderland, 1972.
3. Aristotle was an astute observer of natural phenomena, but it never occurred to him that you could do experiments; that you could generate conjectures and proceed to test them systematically. For instance, he believed that women had fewer teeth than men; all he needed to do to verify or refute the theory was to ask a number of men and women to open their mouths so he could count their teeth. Modern experimental science really began with Galileo. It astonishes me when I sometimes hear developmental psychologists assert that babies are "born scientists," because it is perfectly clear to me that even *adults* are not. If the experimental method is completely natural to the human mind—as they assert—why did we have to wait so many thousands of years for Galileo and the birth of the experimental method? Everyone believed that big, heavy objects fall much faster than light ones, and all it took was a five-minute experiment to disprove it. (In fact, the experimental method is so alien to the human mind that many of Galileo's colleagues dismissed his experiments on falling bodies even after seeing them with their own eyes!) And even to this day, three hundred years after the scientific revolution began, people have great difficulty in understanding the need for a "control experiment" or "double-blind" studies. (A common fallacy is, I got better after I took pill A, therefore I got better because I took pill A.)
4. Penfield and Rasmussen, 1950.

   The reason for this peculiar arrangement is unclear and probably lost in our phylogenetic past. Martha Farah of the University of Pennsylvania has proposed a hypothesis that is consistent with my view (and Merzenich's) that brain maps are highly malleable. She points out that in the curled-up fetus, the arms are usually bent at the elbow with the hands touching the cheek and the legs are bent with the feet touching the genitals. The repeated coactivation of these body parts and the synchronous firing of corresponding neurons in the fetus may have resulted in their being laid down close to each other in the brain. Her idea is ingenious, but it doesn't explain why in other brain areas (S2 in the cortex) the foot (not just the hand) lies next to the face as well. My own bias is to think that even though the maps are modifiable by experience, the basic blueprint for them is genetic.

5. The first clear experimental demonstration of "plasticity" in the central nervous system was provided by Patrick Wall of the University College, London, 1977, and by Mike Merzenich, a distinguished neuroscientist at the University of California in San Francisco, 1984.

   The demonstration that sensory input from the hand can activate the "face area" of the cortex in adult monkeys comes from Tim Pons and his colleagues, 1991.

6. When people are pitched from a motorcycle at high speed, one arm is often partially wrenched from the shoulder, producing a kind of naturally occurring rhizotomy. As the arm is pulled, both the sensory (dorsal) and motor (ventral) nerve roots going from the arm into the spine are yanked off the spinal cord so that the arm becomes completely paralyzed and devoid of sensation even though it remains attached to the body. The question is, How much function—if any—can people recover in the arm during rehabilitation? To explore this, physiologists cut the sensory nerves going from the arm into the spinal cord in a group of monkeys. Their goal was to try to reeducate the monkeys to use the arm, and a great deal of valuable information was obtained from studying these animals (Taub et al., 1993). Eleven years after this study was done these monkeys became a cause célèbre when animal rights activists complained that the experiment was needlessly cruel. The so-called Silver Spring monkeys were soon sent to the equivalent of an old age home for primates and, because they were said to be suffering, scheduled to be killed.

   Dr. Pons and his collaborators agreed to the euthanasia but decided first to record from their brains to see whether anything had changed. The monkeys were anesthetized before the recordings were made, so that they would not feel any pain during the procedure.

7. Ramachandran et al., 1992a, b; 1993; 1994; 1996.

   Ramachandran, Hirstein and Rogers-Ramachandran, 1998.

8. It had been noticed by many previous researchers (Weir Mitchell, 1871) that stimulating certain trigger points on the stump often elicits sensations from missing fingers. William James (1887) once wrote, "A breeze on the stump is felt as a breeze on the phantom" (see also an important monograph by Cronholm, 1951). Unfortunately, neither Penfield's map nor the results of Pons and his collaborators were available at the time, and these early observations were therefore open to several interpretations. For example, the severed nerves in the stump would be expected to reinnervate the stump; if they did, that might explain why sensations from this region are referred to the fingers. Even when points remote from the stump elicited referred sensations, the effect was often attributed to diffuse connections in a "neuromatrix" (Melzack, 1990). What was novel about our observations is that we discovered an actual topographically organized map on the face and also found that relatively complex sensations such as "trickling," "metal" and "rubbing" (as well as warmth, cold and vibration) were referred from the face to the phantom hand in a modality-specific manner. Obviously, this cannot be attributed to accidental stimulation of nerve

endings on the stump or to "diffuse" connections. Our observations imply instead that highly precise and organized new connections can be formed in the adult brain with extreme rapidity, at least in some patients.

Furthermore, we have tried to relate our findings in a systematic way to physiological results, especially the "remapping" experiments of Pons et al., 1991. We have suggested, for example, that the reason we often see two clusters of points—one on the lower face region and a second set near or around the amputation line—is that the map of the hand on the sensory homunculus in the cortex and the thalamus is flanked on one side by the face and the other side by the upper arm, shoulder and axilla. If the sensory input from the face and from the upper arm above the stump were to "invade" the cortical territory of the hand, one would expect precisely this sort of clustering of points. This principle allows one to dissociate proximity of points on the body surface from proximity of points in brain maps, an idea that we refer to as the remapping hypothesis of referred sensations. If the hypothesis is correct, then one would also expect to see referral from the genitals to the foot after leg amputation, since these two body parts are adjacent on the Penfield map. (See Ramachandran, 1993b; Aglioti et al., 1994) But one would never see referral from the face to a phantom foot or from the genitals to a phantom arm. Also see note 10.

9. Recently David Borsook, Hans Breiter and their colleagues at the Massachusetts General Hospital (MGH) have shown that in some patients sensations such as touch, paintbrush, rubbing and pinpricks are referred (in a modality-specific manner) from the face to the phantom just a few hours after amputation (Borsook et al., 1998). This makes it clear that disinhibition or "masking" of preexisting connections must at least contribute to the effect, although some sprouting of new connections probably occurs as well.

10. If the remapping hypothesis is correct, then cutting the trigeminal nerve (supplying half the face) should result in the exact opposite of what we noticed in Tom. In such a patient, touching the hand should cause sensations to emerge in the face (Ramachandran, 1994). Stephanie Clark and her colleagues recently tested this prediction in an elegant and meticulous series of experiments. Their patient had the trigeminal nerve ganglion cut because a tumor had to be removed in its vicinity, and two weeks later they found that when the hand was touched, the patient felt the sensations emerging from the face—even though the nerves from the face were cut. In her brain, the sensory input from the skin of the hand had invaded territory vacated by the sensory input from her face.

Intriguingly, in this patient the sensations were felt only on the face—not on the hand—when the hand was touched. One possibility is that during the initial remapping there is a sort of "overshoot"—the new sensory input from hand skin to the face area of the cortex is actually stronger than the original connections and as a result the sensations are felt predominantly on the face, masking the weaker hand sensations.

11. Caccace et al., 1994.

12. Referred sensations provide an opportunity for studying changing cortical maps in the adult human brain, but the question remains, What is the ***function*** of remapping? Is it an epiphenomenon—residual plasticity left over from infancy—or does it continue to have a function in the adult brain? For example, would

the larger cortical area devoted to the face after arm amputation lead to improved sensory discrimination—measured by two-point discrimination—or tactile hyperacuity on the face? Would such improvement, if it occurred at all, be seen only after the abnormal referred sensations have disappeared, or would it be seen immediately? Such experiments would settle, once and for all, the question of whether or not remapping is actually useful for the organism.

Chapter 3: Chasing the Phantom

1. Mary Ann Simmel (1962) originally claimed that very young children do not experience phantoms after amputation and that children born with limbs missing also do not experience phantoms, but this idea has been challenged by others. (A lovely series of studies was conducted recently by Ron Melzack and his colleagues at McGill University; Melzack et al., 1997.)
2. The importance of frontal brain structures in planning and executing movements has been discussed in fascinating detail by Fuster, 1980; G. Goldberg, 1987; Pribram et al., 1967; Shallice, 1988; E. Goldberg et al., 1987; Benson, 1997; and Goldman-Rakic, 1987.
3. Next I asked Philip to move his index finger and thumb of both hands and simultaneously look in the mirror but this time the phantom thumb and finger remained paralyzed; they were not revived. This is an important observation, for it rules out the possibility that the previous result was simply a confabulation in response to the peculiar circumstances surrounding our experiment. If it was confabulatory, why is it he was able to move his whole hand and elbow but not individual fingers?

   Our experiments of the use of mirrors to revive movements in phantom limbs were originally reported in *Nature* and *Proceedings of the Royal Society of London B* (Ramachandran, Rogers-Ramachandran and Cobb, 1995; Ramachandran and Rogers-Ramachandran, 1996a and b).
4. The notion of learned paralysis is provocative and may have implications beyond treating paralyzed phantom limbs.

   As an example, take writer's cramp (focal dystonia). The patient can wiggle his fingers, scratch his nose or tie his necktie with no problem, but all of a sudden his hand is incapable of writing. Theories about what causes the condition range all the way from muscle cramps to a form of "hysterical paralysis." But could it be another example of learned paralysis? If so, would as simple a trick as using a mirror help these patients as well?

   The same argument might also apply to other syndromes that straddle the boundary between overt paralysis and a reluctance to move a limb—a sort of mental block. Ideomotor apraxia—the inability to perform skilled movements on command (the patient can write a letter independently but not pretend to wave good-bye or to stir a cup of tea when asked to do so)—is certainly not "learned" in the sense that a paralyzed phantom might be learned. But could it also be based on some sort of temporary neural inhibition or block? And if so, can visual feedback help overcome the block?

   Finally, there is Parkinson's disease, which causes rigidity, tremor and poverty of movements (akinesia) involving the entire body including the face (a masklike expression). Early in this disease, the rigidity and tremor affect only one hand, so, in principle, one could try the mirror technique, using the reflection of the good hand for feedback. Since it is known that visual feedback can indeed influence Parkinson's disease (for example, the patient ordinarily can't walk, but if the floor has alternate black and white tiles, he can), perhaps the mirror technique will help them as well.

5. Another fascinating observation on Mary deserves comment. In the previous ten years she had never felt a phantom elbow or wrist; her phantom fingers were dangling from the stump above the elbow, but upon looking into the mirror, she gasped, exclaiming that she could now actually feel—not merely see—her long-lost elbow and wrist. This raises the fascinating possibility that even for an arm lost a long time ago, a dormant ghost still survives somewhere in the brain and can be resurrected instantly by the visual input. If so, this technique may have application for amputees contemplating the use of a prosthetic arm or leg, since they often feel the need to animate the prosthesis with a phantom and complain that the prosthesis feels "unnatural" once the phantom is gone.

   Perhaps transsexual women contemplating becoming men can try out a dress rehearsal and revive a dormant brain image of a penis (assuming something like this even exists in a female brain) using a trick similar to the mirror device used on Mary.

6. Forked phantoms were described by Kallio, 1950. Multiple phantoms in a child were described by La Croix et al., 1992.

7. These are highly speculative explanations, although at least some of them can be tested with the help of imaging procedures such as MEG and functional magnetic resonance imaging (fMRI). These devices allow us to see different parts of the living brain light up as a patient performs different tasks. (In the child with three separate phantom feet, would there be three separate representations in her brain that could be visualized using these techniques?)

8. Our phantom nose effect (Ramachandran and Hirstein, 1997) is quite similar to one reported by Lackner (1988) except that the underlying principle is different. In Lackner's experiment, the subject sits blindfolded at a table, with his arm flexed at the elbow, holding the tip of his own nose. If the experimenter now applies a vibrator to the tendon of the biceps, the subject feels not only that his arm is extended—because of spurious signals from muscle stretch receptors—but also that his nose has actually lengthened. Lackner invokes Helmholtzian "unconscious inference" as an explanation for this effect (I am holding my nose; my arm is extended; therefore, my nose must be long). The illusion we have described, on the other hand, does not require a vibrator and seems to depend entirely on a Bayesian principle—the sheer statistical improbability of two tactile sequences being identical. (Indeed, our illusion cannot be produced if the subject simply holds the accomplice's nose.) Not all subjects experience this effect, but that it happens at all—that a lifetime's evidence concerning your nose can be negated by just a few seconds of intermittent tactile input—is astonishing.

   Our GSR experiments are mentioned in Ramachandran and Hirstein, 1997, and Ramachandran, Hirstein and Rogers-Ramachandran, 1998.

9. Botvinik and Cohen, 1998.

Chapter 4: The Zombie in the Brain

1. Milner and Goodale, 1995.
2. For lively introductions to the study of vision, see Gregory, 1966; Hochberg, 1964; Crick, 1993; Marr, 1981; and Rock, 1985.
3. Another line of evidence is the exact converse: Your perception can remain constant even though the image changes. For example, every time you swivel your eyeballs while observing everyday scenes, the image on each retina races across your photoreceptors at tremendous speed—much like the blur you see when you pan your video camera across the room. But when you move your eyes around, you don't see objects darting all over the place or the world zooming past you at warp speed. The world seems perfectly stable—it doesn't seem to move around even though the image is moving on your retina. The reason is that your brain's visual centers have been "tipped off" in advance by motor centers controlling your eye movements. Each time a motor area sends a command to your eyeball muscles, causing them to move, it also sends a command to visual centers saying, "Ignore this motion; it's not real." Of course, all this takes place without conscious thought. The computation is built into the visual modules of your brain to prevent you from being distracted by spurious motion signals each time you glance around the room.
4. Ramachandran, 1988a and b, 1989a and b; Kleffner and Ramachandran, 1992. Ask a friend to hold the page (with the pictures of shaded disks) upright while you bend down and look at the page with your head hanging upside down between your legs. The page will then be upside down with respect to your retina. You will find once again that the eggs and cavities have switched places (Ramachandran, 1988a). This is quite astonishing because it implies that in judging shape from shading, the brain now assumes that the sun is shining from below: That is, your brain is making the assumption that the sun is stuck to your head when you rotate your head! Even though the world still looks upright because of correction from the balance organ in the ear, your visual system is unable to use this knowledge to interpret shape from shading (Ramachandran, 1988b).

   Why does the visual system incorporate such a foolish assumption? Why not correct for head tilt when interpreting the shaded images? The answer is that as we walk around the world, most of the time we keep our heads upright, not tilted or upside down. So the visual system can take advantage of this to avoid the additional computational burden of sending the vestibular information all the way back to the shape from shading module. You can get away with this "shortcut" because, statistically speaking, your head is usually upright. Evolution doesn't strive for perfection; your genes will get passed down on to your offspring so long as you survive long enough to leave babies.
5. The architecture of this brain region has been studied in fascinating detail by David Hubel and Torsten Weisel at Harvard University; their research culminated in a Nobel Prize. During the two decades 1960–1980 more was learned about the visual pathways as a result of their work than during the preceding two hundred years, and they are rightly regarded as the founding fathers of modern visual science.

6. The evidence that these extrastriate cortical areas are exquisitely specialized for different functions comes mainly from six physiologists—Semir Zeki, John Allman, John Kaas and David Van Essen, Margaret Livingstone and David Hubel. These researchers first mapped out these cortical areas systematically in monkeys and recorded from individual nerve cells; it quickly became clear that the cells had very different properties. For example, any given cell in the area called MT, the middle temporal area, will respond best to targets in the visual field moving in one particular direction but not other directions, but the cell isn't particularly fussy about what color or shape the target is. Conversely, cells in an area called V4 (in the temporal lobes) are very sensitive to color but don't care much about direction of motion. These physiological experiments strongly hint that these two areas are specialized for extracting different aspects of visual information—motion and color. But overall, the physiological evidence is still a bit messy, and the most compelling evidence for this division of labor comes, once again, from patients in whom one of these two areas has been selectively damaged.

   A description of the celebrated case of the motion blind patient can be found in Zihl, von Cramon and Mai, 1983.
7. For a description of the original blindsight syndrome, see Weiskrantz, 1986. For an up-to-date discussion of the controversies surrounding blindsight see Weiskrantz, 1997.
8. For a very stimulating account of many aspects of cognitive science, see Dennett, 1991. The book also has a brief account of "filling in."
9. See especially the elegant work of William Newsome, Nikos Logotethis, John Maunsell, Ted DeYoe, and Margaret Livingstone and David Hubel.
10. Aglioti, DeSouza and Goodale, 1995.
11. Here and elsewhere, when I say that the self is an "illusion," I simply mean that there is probably no *single* entity corresponding to it in the brain. But in truth we know so little about the brain that it is best to keep an open mind. I see at least two possibilities (see Chapter 12). First, when we achieve a more mature understanding of the different aspects of our mental life and the neural processes that mediate them, the word "self" may disappear from our vocabulary. (For instance, now that we understand DNA, the Krebs cycle and other biochemical mechanisms that characterize living things, people no longer worry about the question "What is life?") Second, the self may indeed be a useful biological construct based on specific brain mechanisms—a sort of organizing principle that allows us to function more effectively by imposing coherence, continuity and stability on the personality. Indeed many authors, including Oliver Sacks, have spoken eloquently of the remarkable endurance of self—whether in health or disease—amid the vicissitudes of life.

Chapter 5: The Secret Life of James Thurber

1. For an excellent biography of Thurber, see Kinney, 1995. This book also has a bibliography of Thurber's works.
2. Bonnet, 1760.

3. My blind-spot experiments were originally described in *Scientific American* (1992). For the claim that genuine completion does not occur in scotomas, see Sergent, 1988. For the demonstration that it does occur, see Ramachandran, 1993b, and Ramachandran and Gregory, 1991.

4. The famous Victorian physicist Sir David Brewster was so impressed by this filling-in phenomenon that he concluded, as Lord Nelson did for phantom limbs, that it was proof for the existence of God. In 1832 he wrote, "We should expect, whether we use one eye or both eyes, to see a black or dark spot on every landscape within fifteen degrees of the point which most particularly attracts our notice. The Divine Artificer, however, has not left his work thus imperfect . . . the spot, in place of being black, has always the same color as the ground." Curiously, Sir David was apparently not troubled by the question of why the Divine Artificer would have created an imperfect eye to begin with.

5. In modern terminology, "filling in" is a convenient phrase that some scientists use when referring to this completion phenomenon—the tendency to see the same color in the blind region as in the surround or background. But we must be careful not to fall into the trap of assuming that the brain recreates a pixel-by-pixel rendering of the visual image in this region, for that would defeat the whole purpose of vision. There is, after all, no homunculus—that little man inside the brain—watching an internal mental screen who would benefit from such filling in. (For instance, you don't say the brain "fills in" the tiny spaces between retinal receptors.) I like to use the term simply as a shorthand to indicate that the person quite literally sees something in a region of visual space from which no light or other information is reaching the eye. The advantage of this "theory-neutral" definition is that it keeps open a door to doing experiments, allowing us to search for neural mechanisms of vision and perception.

6. Jerome Lettvin of Rutgers University (1976) performed this clever experiment. The explanation of this effect—as having something to do with stereoscopic vision—is my own (see note 7).

   I have also seen the same effect in patients with scotomas of cortical origin: the lining up of horizontally misaligned vertical bars (Ramachandran, 1993b).

7. Since you look at the world from two slightly different vantage points corresponding to the two eyes, there are differences between the retinal images of the two eyes that are proportional to the relative distances of objects in the world. The brain therefore compares the two images, measures the horizontal separations and "fuses" the images so that you see a single unified picture of the world—not two. In other words, you already have in place in your visual pathway a neural mechanism for "lining up" horizontally separated vertical edges. But since your eyes are separated horizontally and not vertically, you have no such mechanism for lining up horizontal edges that are vertically misaligned. In my view you are tapping the very same mechanism when you are trying to deal with edges that are "misaligned" across a blind spot. This would explain why the vertical lines get "fused" into a continuous line, whereas your visual system fails to cope with the horizontal lines. The fact that you are using only one eye in the blind spot experiment doesn't negate this argument because you may very well be unconsciously deploying the same neural circuits even when you close the other eye.

8. These exercises are amusing for those of us with normal vision and natural blind spots, but what would life be like with a damaged retina, so that you developed an artificial blind spot? Would the brain compensate by "filling in" the blind regions of the visual field? Or might there be remapping; do adjacent parts of the visual field now map onto the region that's no longer getting any input?

   What would be the consequence of the remapping? Would the patient experience double vision? Imagine I hold up a pencil next to his scotoma. He's looking straight ahead and obviously sees the original pencil, but since it now also stimulates the patch of cortex corresponding to the scotoma, he should see a second, "ghost" image of the pencil in his scotoma. He should therefore see two pencils instead of one, just as Tom felt sensations on both his face and hand.

   To explore this possibility, we tested several patients who had a hole in one retina, but not one person saw double. My immediate conclusion was, Oh, well, who knows, maybe vision is different. And then suddenly I realized that although one eye has a scotoma, the patient has *two* eyes, and the corresponding patch in the other eye is still sending information to the primary visual cortex. The cells are stimulated by the good eye, so perhaps remapping does not occur. To get the double vision effect, you'd have to remove the good eye.

   A few months later I saw a patient who had a scotoma in the lower left quadrant of her left eye and had completely lost her right eye. When I presented spots of light in the normal visual field, she did not see a doubling, but to my amazement if I *flickered* the spot at about ten hertz (ten cycles per second), she saw two spots— one where it actually was and a ghostlike double inside her scotoma.

   I can't yet explain why Joan only sees double when the stimulus is flickering. She often has the experience while driving, amid sunlight, foliage and constant movement. It may be that a flickering stimulus preferentially activates the magnocellular pathway—a visual system involved in motion perception—and that this pathway is more prone to remapping than others.

9. Ramachandran, 1992.

10. Sergent, 1988.

11. I subsequently verified that this happened every time I tested Josh and also observed the same phenomenon in one of Dr. Hanna Damasio's patients (Ramachandran, 1993b).

12. An early draft of this chapter, based on my clinical notes, was written in collaboration with Christopher Wills, but the text has been completely rewritten for this work. I have, however, retained one or two of his more colorful metaphors, including this one about the fun house.

13. Kosslyn, 1996; Farah, 1991.

14. Evidence for this comes from the fact that even though most Charles Bonnet patients don't remember having seen the same images before (perhaps they are from the distant past), in some patients the images are either objects that they saw just a few seconds or minutes ago or things that might be logically associated with objects near the scotoma. For example, Larry often saw multiple copies of his own shoe (one that he had seen a few seconds earlier) and had difficulty reaching out for the "real" one. Others have told me that when they're driving a car, a vivid scene that they had passed several minutes ago suddenly reemerges in the scotoma.

   Thus the Charles Bonnet syndrome blends into another well-known visual syndrome, called palinopsia (which neurologists often encounter after a patient's head injury or brain disease that has damaged the visual pathways), in which patients report that when an object moves, it leaves behind multiple copies of itself. Although ordinarily conceived of as a motion detection problem, palinopsia may have more in common with Charles Bonnet syndrome than ophthalmologists realize. The deeper implication of both syndromes is that we may all be subconsciously rehearsing recently encountered visual images for minutes or even hours (after they have been seen) and this rerunning emerges to the surface, becoming more obviously manifest, when there is no real input coming from the retina (as can happen after injury to the visual pathway).

Humphrey (1992) has also suggested the idea that the deafferentation is somehow critical for visual hallucinations and that such hallucinations may be based on back-projections. Any claim to novelty by me derives from the observation that in both my patients the hallucination was confined entirely to the inside of the scotoma, never spilling across the margins. This observation gave me the clue that this phenomenon can only be explained by back-projections (since back-projections are topographically organized) and that no other hypothesis is viable.

15. If this theory is correct, why don't we all hallucinate when we close our eyes or walk into a darkroom? After all, there's no visual input coming in. For one thing, when people are completely deprived of sensory input (as when they float in a sensory isolation tank), they do indeed hallucinate. The more important reason, however, is that even when you close your eyes, the neurons in your retina and the early stages of your visual pathways are continuously sending baseline activity (we call it spontaneous activity) to higher centers, and this might suffice to veto the top-down induced activity. But when the pathways (retina, primary visual cortex and optic nerve) are damaged or lost, producing a scotoma, even this little spontaneous activity is gone, thereby permitting the internal images—the hallucinations—to emerge. Indeed, one could argue that spontaneous activity in the early visual pathways, which has always been a puzzle, evolved mainly to provide such a "null" signal. The strongest evidence for this comes from our two patients in whom the hallucinations were sharply confined within the margins of their scotoma.

16. This somewhat radical view of perception, I suggest, holds mainly for recognizing specific objects in the ventral stream—a shoe, a kettle a friend's face—where it makes good computational sense to use your high-level semantic knowledge base to help resolve ambiguity. Indeed, it could hardly be otherwise, given how underconstrained this aspect of perception—object perception—really is.

For the other more "primitive" or "early" visual processes—such as motion, stereopsis and color—such interactions may occur on a more limited scale since you can get away with just using *generic* knowledge of surfaces, contours, textures, and so on, which can be incorporated into the neural architecture of early vision (as emphasized by David Marr, although Marr did not make the particular distinction that I am making here). Yet even with these low-level visual modules, the evidence suggests that the interactions across modules and with "high-level" knowledge are much greater than generally assumed (see Churchland, Ramachandran and Sejnowski, 1994).

The general rule seems to be that interactions occur whenever it would be useful for them to occur and do not (and cannot) occur when it isn't. Discovering which interactions are weak and which are strong is one of the goals of visual psychophysics and neuroscience.

Chapter 6: Through the Looking Glass

1. For descriptions of neglect, see Critchley, 1966; Brain, 1941; Halligan and Marshall, 1994.
2. No one has described the selective function of consciousness more eloquently than the eminent psychologist William James (1890) in his famous essay "The Stream of Thought." He wrote, "We see that the mind is at every stage a theatre of simultaneous possibilities. Consciousness consists in the comparison of these with each other, the selection of some, and the suppression of the rest by the reinforcing and inhibiting agency of attention. The highest and most elaborated mental products are filtered from the data chosen by the faculty next beneath, out of the mass offered by the faculty below that, which mass in turn was sifted from a still larger amount of yet simpler material, and so on. The mind, in short, works on the data it receives very much as a sculptor works on his block of stone. In a sense the statue stood there from eternity. But there were a thousand different ones beside it, and the sculptor alone is to thank for having extricated this one from the rest. We may, if we like, by our reasonings unwind things back to that black and jointless continuity of space and moving clouds of swarming atoms which science calls the only real world. But all the while the world we feel and live in will be that which our ancestors and we, by slowly cumulative strokes of choice, have extricated out of this, like sculptors, by simply rejecting certain portions of the given stuff. Other sculptors, other statues, from the same stone! Other minds, other worlds from the same monotonous and inexpressive chaos! My world is but one in a million alike embedded, alike real to those who may abstract them. How different must be the world in the consciousness of ant, cuttlefish or crab!"
3. This positive feedback loop involved in orienting has been described by Heilman, 1991.
4. Marshall and Halligan, 1988.
5. Sacks, 1985.
6. Gregory, 1997.
7. What would happen if I were to throw a brick at you from the backseat so that you saw the brick coming at you in the mirror? Would you duck forward (as you should), or would you be fooled by the expanding image in the mirror and duck backward? Perhaps the intellectual correction for the mirror reflection, deducing accurately where the real object is located, is performed by the conscious what pathway (object pathway) in the temporal lobes, whereas ducking to avoid a missile is done by the how pathway (spatial stream) in the parietal lobe. If so, you might get confused and duck incorrectly—it's your zombie that's ducking!
8. Edoardo Bisiach added a brilliant twist to this line-bisection test that suggests that this interpretation can't be the whole story, although it's a reasonable first-pass explanation. Instead of having the patient bisect a predrawn horizontal line, he simply gave him a sheet of paper with a tiny vertical line in the middle and said, "Pretend that this vertical mark is the bisector of a horizontal line and draw

the horizontal line." The patient confidently drew the line, but once again the portion of the line on the right side was about half the size of the portion on the left. This suggests that more than simple inattention is going on. Bisiach argues that the whole representation of space is squished to enlarge the healthy right visual field and shrink the left. So the patient has to make the left side of the line longer than the right to make them appear equal to his own eyes.

9. The good news is that many patients with neglect syndrome—caused by damage to the right parietal lobe—recover spontaneously in a few weeks. This is important, for it implies that many of the neurological syndromes that we've come to regard as permanent—involving destroyed neural tissue—may in fact be "functional deficits," involving a temporary imbalance of transmitters. The popular analogy between brains and digital computers is highly misleading, but in this particular instance I am tempted to use it. A functional deficit is akin to a software malfunction, a bug in a program rather than a problem with the hardware. If so, there may be hope yet for the millions of people who suffer from disorders that have traditionally been deemed "incurable" because up to now we have not known how to debug their brain's software.

   To illustrate this more directly, let me mention another patient, who, as a result of damage to parts of his left hemisphere, had a striking problem called dyscalculia. Like many patients with this syndrome, he was intelligent, articulate and lucid in most respects but when it came to arithmetic he was hopelessly inept. He could discuss the weather, what happened in the hospital that day and who had visited him. And yet if you asked him to subtract 7 from 100, he was stymied. But surprisingly, he didn't merely fail to solve the arithmetic problem. My student Eric Altschuler and I noticed that every time he even attempted to do so, he confidently produced incomprehensible gibberish—what Lewis Carroll would call jabberwocky—and he seemed unaware that it was gibberish. The "words" were fully formed but devoid of any meaning—the sort of thing you see in language disorders such as Wernicke's aphasia (indeed even the words were largely neologisms). It was as if the mere confrontation with a math problem caused him to insert a "language floppy disk" with a bug in it.

   Why does he produce gibberish instead of remaining silent? We are so used to thinking about autonomous brain modules—one for math, one for language, one for faces—that we forget the complexity and magnitude of the interactions among the modules. His condition, in particular, makes sense only if you assume that the very deployment of a module depends on the current demands placed on the organism. The ability to sequence bits of information rapidly is a vital part of mathematical operations as well as the generation of language. Perhaps his brain has a "sequencing bug." There may be a requirement of a certain special type of sequencing that is common to both math and language that is deranged. He can carry on ordinary conversation because he has so many more clues—so many backup options—to go by that he doesn't need the sequencing mechanism in full gear. But when presented with a math problem, he is forced to rely on it to a much larger extent and is therefore thrown off completely. Needless to say, all this is pure speculation, but it provides food for thought.

10. Some sort of conversation between the what system in the temporal lobe and the how pathway in the parietal lobe must obviously occur in normal people,

and this communication is perhaps compromised in patients with the looking glass syndrome. Released from the influence of the what pathway, the zombie reaches straight into the mirror.

11. Some patients with right parietal disease actually deny that their left arm belongs to them—a disorder called somatoparaphrenia; we consider such patients in Chapter 7. If you grab the patient's lifeless left arm, raise it and move it into the patient's right visual field, he will insist that the arm belongs to you, the physician, or to his mother, brother or spouse. The first time I saw a patient with this disorder, I remember saying to myself, "This must be the strangest phenomenon in all of neurology—if not in all of science!" How could a perfectly sane, intelligent person assert that his arm belongs to his mother?

    Robert Rafael, Eric Altschuler and I recently tested two patients with this disorder and found that when they looked at their left arm in a mirror (placed on the right to elicit the looking glass syndrome), they suddenly started agreeing that it was indeed their arm! Could a mirror "cure" this disorder?

Chapter 7: The Sound of One Hand Clapping

1. This may seem harsh, but it's frustrating for the physical therapist to begin rehabilitating patients when they're in denial, so overcoming the delusion is of great practical importance in the clinic.
2. For descriptions of anosognosia see Critchley, 1966; Cutting, 1978; Damasio, 1994; Edelman, 1989; Galin, 1992; Levine, 1990; McGlynn and Schacter, 1989; Feinberg and Farah, 1997.
3. The distinguished evolutionary psychologist Robert Trivers at the University of California in Santa Cruz has proposed a clever explanation for the evolution of self-deception (Trivers, 1985). According to Trivers, there are many occasions in daily life when we need to lie—say, during a tax audit or an adulterous affair or in an effort to protect someone's feelings. Other research has shown that liars, unless they are very practiced, almost always give the game away by producing an unnatural smile, a slightly flawed expression or a false tone of voice that others can detect (Ekman, 1992). The reason is that the limbic system (involuntary, prone to truth telling) controls spontaneous expressions, whereas the cortex (responsible for voluntary control, also the location where the lies are concocted) controls the facial expressions displayed when we are fibbing. Consequently, when we lie with a smile, it's a fake smile, and even if we try to keep a straight face, the limbic system invariably leaks traces of deceit.

    There is a solution to this problem, argues Trivers. To lie effectively to another person, all you have to do is first lie to yourself. If you believe it's true, your expressions will be genuine, without a trace of guile. So by adopting this strategy, you can come up with some very convincing lies—and sell a lot of snake oil.

    But it seems to me there is an internal contradiction in this scenario. Suppose you're a chimp who has hidden some bananas under a tree branch. Along comes the alpha male chimp, who knows you have bananas and demands you give them to him. What do you do? You lie to your superior and say that the bananas are across the river, but you also run the risk of his detecting your lie by the expression on your face. So then what do you do? According to Trivers, you adopt the simple device of first convincing yourself that the bananas really are on the other side of the river, and you say that to the alpha male, who is fooled, and you are off the hook. But there's a problem. What if you later got hungry and went looking for the bananas? Since you now believe that the food is across the river, that's where you'd go look for it. In other words, the strategy proposed by Trivers defeats the whole purpose of lying, for the very definition of a lie is that you must continue to have access to the truth—otherwise there'd be no point to the evolutionary strategy.

One escape from this dilemma would be to suggest that a "belief" is not necessarily a unitary thing. Perhaps self-deception is mainly a function of the left hemisphere—as it tries to communicate its knowledge to others—whereas the right hemisphere continues to "know" the truth. One way to approach this experimentally would be to obtain galvanic skin responses in anosognosics and, indeed, in normal people (for example, children) when they are confabulating. When a normal person generates a false memory—or when a child confabulates—would he/she nevertheless register a strong galvanic skin response (as he would if he were lying)?

Finally, there is another type of lie for which Trivers's argument may indeed be valid, and that concerns lying about one's own abilities—boasting. Of course, a false belief about your abilities can also get you into trouble ("I am a big strong fellow, not puny and weak") if it leads you to strive for unrealistic goals. But this disadvantage may be outweighed in many instances by the fact that a convincing boaster may get the best dates on Saturday night and may therefore disseminate his genes more widely and more frequently so that the "successful boasting through self-deception" genes quickly become part of the gene pool. One prediction for this would be that men should be more prone to both boasting and self-deception than women. To my knowledge this prediction has never been tested in a systematic way, although various colleagues assure me that it is true. Women, on the other hand, should be better at detecting lies since they have a great deal more at stake—an arduous nine-month pregnancy, a risky labor and a long period of caring for a child whose "maternity" is in no doubt.

4. Kinsbourne, 1989; Bogen, 1975; and Galin, 1976, have all warned us repeatedly of the dangers of "dichotomania," of ascribing cognitive functions entirely to one hemisphere versus the other. We must bear in mind that the specialization in most instances is likely to be *relative* rather than absolute and that the brain has a front and a back and a top and a bottom, and not just left and right. To make matters worse, an elaborate pop culture and countless self-help manuals are based on the notion of hemispheric specialization. As Robert Ornstein (1997) has noted, "It's a cliché in general advice to managers, bankers and artists, it's in cartoons. It's an advertisement. United Airlines offers reasons to fly both sides of you coast to coast. The music for one side and the good value for the other. The Saab automobile company offered their Turbo charged sedan as 'a car for both sides of your brain.' A friend of mine, unable to remember a name, excused this by describing herself as a 'right atmosphere sort of person.' " But the existence of such a pop culture shouldn't cloud the main issue—the notion that two hemispheres may indeed be specialized for different functions. The tendency to ascribe mysterious powers to the right hemisphere isn't new—it goes all the way back to the nineteenth-century French neurologist Charles Brown-Sequard, who started a fashionable right hemisphere aerobics movement.

For an up-to-date review of ideas on hemispheric specialization, see Springer and Deutsch, 1998.

5. Much of our knowledge of hemispheric specialization comes from the groundbreaking work of Gazzaniga, Bogen and Sperry, 1962, whose research on split brain patients is well known. When the corpus callosum bridging the two hemispheres is cut, the cognitive capacities of each hemisphere can be studied separately in the laboratory.

   What I'm calling "the general" is not unlike what Gazzaniga, 1992, calls "the interpreter" in the left hemisphere. However, Gazzaniga does not consider the evolutionary origin or biological rationale for having an interpreter (as I attempt to do here), nor does he postulate an antagonistic mechanism in the right hemisphere.

   Ideas on hemispheric specialization similar to mine have also been proposed by Kinsbourne, 1989, not to explain anosognosia, but to explain laterality effects seen in depression following stroke. Although he does not discuss Freudian defenses or "paradigm shifts," he has made the ingenious proposal that the left hemisphere may be needed for maintaining ongoing behavior, whereas right hemisphere activation may be required for interrupting behavior and producing an orienting response.

6. I would like to emphasize that the specific theory of hemispheric specialization that I am proposing certainly doesn't explain *all* forms of anosognosia. For example, the anosognosia of Wernicke's aphasics probably arises because the very part of the brain that would ordinarily represent beliefs about language is itself damaged. Anton's syndrome (denial of cortical blindness), on the other hand, may require the simultaneous presence of a right hemisphere lesion. (I have seen a single "two-lesion" case like this, with Dr. Leah Levi, but additional research is needed to settle the matter.) Would a Wernicke's aphasic become more aware of his deficit if his ear were irrigated with cold water?

7. Ramachandran, 1994, 1995a, 1996.

8. We are still a long way from understanding the neural basis of such delusions, but the important recent work of Graziano, Yap and Gross, 1994, may be relevant. They found single neurons in the monkey supplementary motor area that had visual receptive fields "superimposed" on somatosensory fields of the monkey's hand. Curiously, when the monkey moved its hand, the visual receptive field moved with the hand, but eye movements had no effect on the receptive field. These hand-centered visual receptive fields ("monkey see, monkey do cells") may provide a neural substrate for the kinds of delusions I see in my patients.

9. The notion that there is a mechanism in the right hemisphere not only for detecting and orienting to discrepancies of body image (as suggested by our virtual reality box and by Ray Dolan and Chris Frith's experiment) but also for other kinds of anomalies receives support from three other studies that have been reported in the literature. First, it has been known for some time that patients with left hemisphere damage tend to be more depressed and pessimistic than those with right hemisphere strokes (Gainotti, 1972; Robinson et al., 1983), a difference that is usually attributed to the fact that the right hemisphere is more "emotional." I would argue instead that because of damage to the left hemisphere, the patient does not have even the minimal "defense mechanisms" that

you and I would use for coping with the minor discrepancies of day-to-day life, so that every trifling anomaly becomes potentially destabilizing.

Indeed, I have argued (Ramachandran, 1996) that even idiopathic depression seen in a psychiatric setting may arise from a failure by the left hemisphere to deploy Freudian defense mechanisms—perhaps as a result of transmitter imbalances or clinically undetectable damage to the left frontal region of the brain. The old experimental observation that depressed people are actually more sensitive to subtle inconsistencies (such as a briefly presented red ace of spades) than normal people is consistent with this line of speculation. I am currently administering similar tests to patients with anosognosia.

A second set of experiments supporting this idea comes from the important observation (Gardner, 1993) that after damage to the right (but not left) hemisphere patients have trouble recognizing the absurdity of "garden path sentences" in which there is an unexpected twist at the ending that contradicts the beginning. I interpret this finding as a failure of the anomaly detector.

10. Bill's denials would seem comical if they were not tragic. But his behavior "makes sense" in that he is doing his utmost to protect his "ego" or self. When one is faced with a death sentence, what's wrong with denial? But even though Bill's denial may be a healthy response to a hopeless situation, its magnitude is surprising and it raises another interesting question. Do patients like him who have been delusional as a result of ventromedial frontal lobe involvement confabulate mainly to protect the integrity of "self," or can they be provoked to confabulate about other abstract matters as well? If you were to ask such a patient, "How many hairs does Clinton have on his head?" would he confabulate or would he admit ignorance?

In other words, would the very act of questioning by an authority figure be sufficient to make him confabulate? There have been no systematic studies to address these issues, but unless a patient has dementia (loosely speaking, mental retardation due to diffuse cortical damage) he is usually quite "honest" in admitting ignorance of matters that don't pose any immediate threat to his well-being.

11. Clearly denial runs very deep. But even though it's fascinating to watch, it's also a source of great frustration and practical concern for the patient's relatives (although by definition not for the patient!). For instance, given that patients tend to deny the immediate consequences of the paralysis (having no inkling that the cocktail tray will surely topple or that they can't tie laces), do they also deny its remote consequences—what's going to happen next week, next month, next year? Or are they dimly aware in the back of their minds that something is amiss, that they are disabled? Would the denial stop them from writing a will?

I have not explored this question on a systematic basis, but on the few occasions when I raised this question, patients responded as if they were completely unaware of how deeply the paralysis would affect their future lives. For example, the patient may confidently assert that he intends to drive back home from the hospital or that he would like to resume golf or tennis. So it is clear that he is not merely suffering from a mere sensory/motor distortion—a failure to update his current body image (although that is certainly a major component of this illness). Rather, his whole range of beliefs about himself and his means of survival have been radically altered to accommodate his present denial. Mercifully such delusions can often be a considerable solace and comfort to these patients, even though their attitude comes into direct conflict with one of the goals of rehabilitation—restoring the patient's insight into his predicament.

Another way to approach the domain specificity and depth of denial would be to flash the word "paralysis" on the screen and obtain a galvanic skin response. Would the patient find the word threatening—and register a big GSR—even though she is unaware of her paralysis? How would she rate the word for unpleasantness on a scale of 1 to 10, if asked to do so? Would her rating be higher (or indeed lower) than that of a normal person?

12. There are even patients with right frontal lobe stroke who manifest symptoms that are halfway between anosognosia and multiple personality disorder syndrome. Dr. Riita Hari and I saw one such patient recently in Helsinki. As a result of two lesions—one in the right frontal region and one in the cingulate—the patient's brain was apparently unable to "update" her body image in the way that normal brains do. When she sat on a chair for a minute and then got up to start walking, she would experience her body as splitting into two halves—the left half still sitting in the chair and the right half walking. And she would look back in horror to ensure that she hadn't abandoned the left half of her body.

13. Recall that when we are awake, the left hemisphere processes incoming sensory data, imposing consistency, coherence and temporal ordering on our everyday experiences. In doing so it rationalizes, denies, represses and otherwise censors much of this incoming information.

Now consider what happens during dreams and REM sleep. There are at least two possibilities that are not mutually exclusive. First, REM may have an important "vegetative" function related to wet-ware (for example, maintenance and "uploading" of neurotransmitter supplies), and dreams may just be epiphenomenal—irrelevant by-products. Second, dreams themselves may have an important cognitive/emotional function, and REM may simply be a vehicle for bringing this about. For example, they may enable you to try out various hypothetical scenarios that would be potentially destabilizing if rehearsed during wakefulness. In other words, dreams may allow a sort of "virtual reality" stimulation using various forbidden thoughts that are ordinarily eclipsed by the conscious mind; such thoughts might be brought out tentatively to see whether they can be assimilated into the story line. If they can't be, then they are repressed and once again forgotten.

Why we cannot carry out these rehearsals in our imagination, while fully awake, is not obvious, but two ideas come to mind. First, for the rehearsals to be effective, they must look and feel like the real thing, and this may not be possible when we are awake, since we know that the images are internally generated. As we noted earlier, Shakespeare said, "You cannot cloy the hungry edge of appetite with bare imagination of a feast." It makes good evolutionary sense that imagery cannot substitute for the real thing.

Second, unmasking disturbing memories when awake would defeat the very purpose of repressing them and could have a profound destabilizing effect on the brain. But unmasking such memories during dreams may permit a realistic and emotionally charged simulation to take place while preventing the penalties that would result if you were to do this when awake.

There are many opinions on the functions of dreams. For stimulating reviews on the subject see Hobson, 1988, and Winson, 1986.

14. This isn't true for all people. One patient, George, vividly remembered that he had denied his paralysis. "I could see that it wasn't moving," he said, "but my mind didn't want to accept it. It was the strangest thing. I guess I was in denial." Why one person remembers and the other forgets is not clear, but it could have something to do with residual damage to the right hemisphere. Perhaps George had recovered more fully than Mumtaz or Jean and was therefore able to confront reality squarely. It is clear from my experiments, though, that at least some patients who recover from denial will "deny their denials" even though they are mentally lucid and have no other memory problems.

    Our memory experiments also raise another interesting question: What if a person were to have an automobile accident that caused peripheral nerve damage and rendered her left arm paralyzed? Then suppose she suffered a stroke some months later, the kind that leads to left body paralysis and denial syndrome. Would she then suddenly say, "Oh, my God, doctor, my arm that has been paralyzed all along is suddenly moving again." Going back to my theory that the patient tends to cling to a preexisting worldview, would she cling to her updated worldview and therefore say that the left arm was paralyzed—or would she go back to her earlier body image and assert that her arm was in fact moving again?

15. I emphasize that this is a single case study and we need to repeat the experiment more carefully on additional patients. Indeed, not every patient was as cooperative as Nancy. I vividly recall one patient, Susan, who vigorously denied her left arm paralysis and who agreed to be part of our experiments. When I told her that I was going to inject her left arm with a local anesthetic, she stiffened in her wheelchair, leaned forward to look me straight in the eye and without batting an eyelid, said, "But doctor, is that fair?" It was as though Susan was playing some sort of game with me and I had suddenly changed the rules and this was forbidden. I didn't continue the experiment.

    I wonder, though, whether mock injections may pave the way for an entirely new form of psychotherapy.

16. Another fundamental problem arises when the left hemisphere tries to read and interpret messages from the right hemisphere. You will recall from Chapter 4 that the visual centers of the brain are segregated into two streams, called the how and what pathways (parietal and temporal lobes). Crudely speaking, the right hemisphere tends to use an analogue—rather than digital—medium of representation, emphasizing body image, spatial vision and other functions of the how pathway. The left hemisphere, on the other hand, prefers a more logical style related to language, recognizing and categorizing objects, tagging objects with verbal labels and representing them in logical sequences (done mainly by the what pathway). This creates a profound *translation barrier*. Every time the left hemisphere tries to interpret information coming from the right—such as trying to put into words the ineffable qualities of music or art—at least some forms of confabulation may arise because the left hemisphere starts spinning a yarn when it doesn't get the expected information from the right (because the latter is either damaged or disconnected from the left). Can such a failure of translation explain at least some of the more florid

confabulations that we see in patients with anosognosia? (See Ramachandran and Hirstein, 1997.)

Chapter 8: "The Unbearable Likeness of Being"

1. J. Capgras and J. Reboul-Lachaux, 1923; H.D. Ellis and A.W. Young, 1990; Hirstein and Ramachandran, 1997.
2. This disorder is called prosopagnosia. See Farah, 1990; Damasio, Damasio and Van Hoesen, 1982.

   Cells in the visual cortex (area 17) respond to simple features like bars of light, but in the temporal lobes they often respond to complex features such as faces. These cells may be part of a complex network specialized for recognizing faces. See Gross, 1992; Rolls, 1995; Tovee, Rolls and Ramachandran, 1996.

   The functions of the amygdala which figures prominently in this chapter, have been discussed in detail by LeDoux, 1996, and Damasio, 1994.
3. The clever idea that Capgras' delusion may be a mirror image of prosopagnosia was first proposed by Young and Ellis (1990), but they postulate a disconnection between dorsal stream and limbic structures rather than the IT amygdala disconnection that we suggest in this chapter. Also see Hirstein and Ramachandran, 1997.
4. Another question: Why does the mere absence of this emotional arousal lead to such an extraordinarily far-fetched delusion? Why doesn't the patient just think, I know that this is my father but for some reason I no longer feel the warmth? One answer is that some additional lesion, perhaps in the right frontal cortex, may be required to generate such extreme delusions. Recall the denial patients in the last chapter whose left hemispheres sought to preserve global consistency by explaining away discrepancies and whose right hemispheres kept things in balance by monitoring and responding to inconsistency. To develop full-blown Capgras' syndrome, one might need a conjunction of two lesions—one that affects the brain's ability to attach emotional significance to a familiar face and one that disturbs the global "consistency-checking" mechanism in the right hemisphere. Additional brain imaging studies are needed to resolve this.
5. Baron-Cohen, 1995.

Chapter 9: God and the Limbic System

1. At present the device is effective mainly for stimulating parts of the brain near the surface but we may eventually be able to stimulate deeper structures.
2. See Papez, 1937, for the original description and Maclean, 1973, for a comprehensive review full of fascinating speculations.

   It's no coincidence that the rabies virus "chooses" to lodge itself mainly in the limbic structures. When dog A bites dog B, the virus travels from the peripheral nerves near the bite into the spinal cord and then eventually up to the victim's limbic system, turning Benji into Damien. Snarling and foaming at the mouth, the once-placid pooch bites another victim and the virus is thus passed on, infecting those very brain structures that drive aggressive biting behavior. And as part of this diabolical strategy, the virus initially leaves other brain structures completely unaffected so that the dog can remain alive just long enough to transmit the virus. But how the devil does a virus travel all the way from peripheral nerves near the bite to cells deep inside the brain while sparing all other brain structures along the way? When I was a student I often wondered whether it might be possible to stain the virus with a fluorescent dye in order to "light up" these brain areas—thereby allowing us to discover pathways specifically concerned with biting and aggression, in much the same way one uses PET scans these days. In any event, it is clear that as far as the rabies virus is concerned, a dog is just another way of making a virus—a temporary vehicle for passing on its genome.

3. Useful descriptions of temporal lobe epilepsy can be found in Trimble, 1992, and Bear and Fedio, 1977. Waxman and Geschwind, 1975, have championed the view that there is a constellation of personality traits more frequently found in temporal lobe epilepsy patients than in age-matched controls. Although this notion is not without its critics, several studies have confirmed such an association: Gibbs, 1951; Gastaut, 1956; Bear and Fedio, 1977; Nielsen and Kristensen, 1981; Rodin and Schmaltz, 1984: Adamec, 1989; Wieser, 1983.

   The presumed link between "psychiatric disturbances" and epilepsy, of course, goes back to antiquity, and, in the past, there has been an unfortunate stigma attached to the disorder. But as I have stressed repeatedly in this chapter, there is no basis for concluding that any of these traits is "undesirable" or that the patient is worse off because of them. The best way to eliminate the stigma, of course, is to explore the syndrome in greater depth.

   Slater and Beard (1963) noted "mystical experiences" in 38 percent of their series of cases, and Bruens (1971) made a similar observation. Frequent religious conversions are also seen in some patients (Dewhurst and Beard, 1970).

   It is important to recognize that only a minority of patients display esoteric traits, like religiosity or hypergraphia, but that does not make the association any less real. By way of analogy, consider the fact that kidney or eye changes (complications of diabetes) occur only in a minority of diabetics, but no one would deny that the association exists. As Trimble (1992) has noted, "It is most likely that personality traits such as religiosity and hypergraphia seen in patients with epilepsy represent an all-or-none phenomenon and are seen in a minority of patients. It is not a graded characteristic, for example like obsessionality, and therefore does not emerge as a prominent factor in questionnaire studies unless a sufficiently large number of patients are evaluated."

4. To complicate matters, it is entirely possible that some clinically undetectable damage in the temporal lobes also underlies schizophrenia and manic-depressive disorders, so the fact that psychiatric patients sometimes experience religious feelings doesn't negate my argument.

5. Similiar views have been put forward by Crick, 1993; Ridley, 1997; and Wright, 1994, although they do not invoke specialized structures in the temporal lobe.

   This argument smacks of group selection—a taboo phrase in evolutionary psychology—but it doesn't have to. After all, most religions, even though they pay lip service to the "brotherhood" of mankind, tend mainly to emphasize loyalty to one's own clan or tribe (hence those who probably share many of the same genes).

6. Bear and Fedio (1977) offered the ingenious suggestion that there has been hyperconnectivity in the limbic system that makes the patients see cosmic sig-

nificance in everything. Their idea predicts a heightened GSR to everything the patient looks at, a prediction that held up in some preliminary studies. But other studies showed either no change or a reduction in GSR to most categories. The picture is complicated also by the extent to which the patient is on medication while the GSR is measured.

Our own preliminary studies, on the other hand, suggest that there can be a *selective* enhancement of GSR responses to some categories and not others—thereby altering the patients' emotional landscape permanently (Ramachandran, Hirstein, Armel, Tecoma and Iragui, 1997). But this finding, too, should be taken with a generous scoop of salt until it is confirmed on a large number of patients.

7. Moreover, even if the changes in the patient's brain were originally mediated by the temporal lobes—the actual repository of the changes—"a religious outlook" probably involves many different brain areas.
8. For lucid and lively expositions of Darwin's ideas, see Dawkins, 1976; Maynard Smith, 1978; Dennett, 1995.

   There is an acrimonious debate going on at the high table of evolution over whether every trait (or almost every trait) is a direct result of natural selection or whether there are other laws or principles governing evolution. We will take up this debate in Chapter 10, where I discuss the evolution of humor and laughter.
9. Much of this discussion appears in a book by Loren Eisley (1958).
10. This idea is clearly described in a delightful book by Christopher Wills (1993). See also Leakey, 1993, and Johanson and Edward, 1996.
11. The savant who could produce the cube-root is described by Hill, 1978. The idea that savants have learned some simple shortcuts or tricks for discovering primes or for factoring has been around for some time. But it doesn't work. When a professional mathematician learned the appropriate algorithm, he still took almost a minute to generate all primes between 10,037 and 10,133—whereas a nonverbal autistic man, naive to this task, took only ten seconds (Hermelin and O'Connor, 1990).

    There are algorithms for generating primes at a high frequency—with occasional rare errors. It would be interesting to see whether prime number savants make exactly the same rare errors that these algorithms do; that would tell us whether the savants were tacitly using the same algorithm.
12. Another possible explanation of the savant syndrome is based on the notion that the absence of certain abilities may actually make it easier to take advantage of what's left over and to focus attention on more esoteric skills. For instance, as you encounter events in the external world, you obviously do not record every trivial detail in your mind; that would be maladaptive. Our brains first gauge the significance of events and engage in an elaborate censoring and editing of the information—before storing it. But what if this mechanism goes awry? Then you might start recording at least some events in needless detail like the words in a book that you read ten years ago. This, to you or me, might seem to be an astounding talent. But in truth, it emerges from a damaged brain that cannot censor daily experience. Similarly, an autistic child is locked in a world where others are not welcome, save one or two channels of interest to the outside. The child's ability to focus all her attention on a single subject to the exclusion of all else can lead to apparently exotic abilities—but, again, her brain is not normal and she remains profoundly retarded.

A related but more ingenious argument is proposed by Snyder and Thomas (1997), who suggest that savants are for some reason less concept-driven because of their retardation and this in turn allows them access to earlier levels of the processing hierarchy, which is not available to most of us (hence the obsessively detailed drawings of Stephen Wiltshire, which contrast sharply with the tadpole figures or the conceptual cartoonlike drawings of normal children).

This idea is not inconsistent with mine. One could argue that the shift in emphasis from concept-driven perception (or conception) to allow access to early processes may depend on the hypertrophy of the "early" modules in precisely the manner I have suggested. Snyder's idea could therefore be seen as being halfway between the traditional attention theory and my theory proposed in this chapter.

One problem is that although drawings of some savants seem excessively detailed (for example, Stephen Wiltshire's, described by Sacks), there are others whose drawings seem genuinely beautiful (for example, the da Vinci–like drawings of horses produced by Nadia). Her sense of perspective, shading and so on seem hypernormal in a manner predicted by my argument.

What all these ideas have in common is that they imply a *shift in emphasis* from one set of modules to the other. Whether this results simply from the lack of function of one set (with more attention paid to others) or from actual hypertrophy of what's left remains to be seen.

The attention shift idea also doesn't appeal to me for two other reasons. First, saying that you automatically become skilled at something by deploying attention doesn't really tell us very much unless you know what attention is, and we don't. Second, if this argument is correct, then why don't *adult* patients with damaged large portions of their brains suddenly become very skilled at other things—by shifting attention? I have yet to come across a dyscalculic who suddenly became a musical savant or a neglect patient who became a calculating prodigy. In other words, the argument doesn't explain why savants are born, not made.

The hypertrophy theory can, of course, be readily tested by using magnetic resonance imaging (MRI) on different types of savants.

13. Patients like Nadia also bring us face-to-face with an even deeper question: What is art? Why are some things pretty, while others are not? Is there a universal grammar underlying all visual aesthetics?

An artist is skilled at grasping the essential features (what Hindus call *rasa*) of an image he is trying to portray and eliminating superfluous detail, and in doing so he is essentially imitating what the brain itself has evolved for. But the real question is: Why should this be aesthetically pleasing?

In my view, all art is "caricature" and hyperbole, so if you understand why caricatures are effective you understand art. If you teach a rat to discriminate a square from, say, a rectangle and reward it for the latter, then it will soon start recognizing the rectangle and show a preference for it. But paradoxically, it will respond even more vigorously to a skinnier "caricature" rectangle (e.g., with an aspect ratio of 3:1 instead of 2:1) than to the original prototype! The paradox is resolved when you realize that what the rat learns is a *rule*—"rectangularity"—rather than a particular exemplar of that rule. And the way the visual form area in the brain is structured, amplifying the rule (a skinnier rectangle) is especially reinforcing (pleasing) to the rat, providing an incentive for the rat's visual system to "discover" the rule. In a similar vein, if you subtract a generic average face from Nixon's face and then amplify the differences, you end up with a caricature that is more Nixon-like than the original. In fact, the visual system is constantly struggling to "discover the rule." My hunch is that very early in evolution, many of the extrastriate visual areas that are specialized for extracting correlations and rules and binding features along different dimensions (form, motion, shading, color, etc.) are directly linked to limbic structures to produce a pleasant sensation, since this would enhance the animal's survival. Consequently, amplifying a specific rule and eliminating irrelevant detail makes the picture look even more attractive. I would suggest also that these mechanisms and associated limbic connections are more prominent in the right hemisphere. There are many cases in the literature of patients with left-hemisphere stroke whose drawings actually ***improved*** after the stroke—perhaps because the right hemisphere is then free to amplify the rule. A great painting is more evocative than a photograph because the photograph's details may actually ***mask*** the underlying rule—a masking that is eliminated by the artist's touch (or by a left-hemisphere stroke!).

This is not a complete explanation of art, but it's a good start. We still need to explain why artists often use incongruous juxtapositions deliberately (as in humor) and why a nude seen behind a shower curtain or a diaphanous veil is more attractive than a nude photograph. It's as though the rule discovered after a struggle is even more reinforcing than one that is instantly obvious, a point that has also been made by the art historian Ernest Gombrich. Perhaps natural selection has wired up the visual areas in such a way that the reinforcement is actually stronger if it obtained after "work"—in order to ensure that the effort itself is pleasant rather than unpleasant. Hence the eternal appeal of puzzle-pictures such as the dalmatian dog on page 239 or "abstract" pictures of faces with strong shadows. A pleasant feeling occurs when the picture finally clicks and the splotches are correctly linked together to form a figure.

Chapter 10: The Woman Who Died Laughing

1. Ruth and Willy (pseudonyms) are reconstructions of patients originally described in an article by Ironside (1955). The clinical details and autopsy reports, however, have not been altered.
2. Fried, Wilson, MacDonald and Behnke, 1998.
3. The discipline of evolutionary psychology was foreshadowed by the early writings of Hamilton (1964), Wilson (1978) and Williams (1966). The modern manifesto of this discipline is by Barkow, Cosmides and Tooby (1992), who are regarded as founders of the field. (Also see Daly and Wilson, 1983, and Symons, 1979.)

   The clearest exposition of these ideas can be found in Pinker's book *How the Mind Works*, which contains many stimulating ideas. My disagreement with him on specific details of evolutionary theory doesn't detract from the value of his contributions.
4. This idea is intriguing, but as with all problems in evolutionary psychology it is difficult to test. To emphasize this further, I'll mention another equally untestable idea. Consider Margie Profet's clever suggestion that women get morning sickness in the first three months of pregnancy to curtail appetite, thus avoiding the natural poisons in many foods that might lead to abortion (Profet, 1997). My colleague

Dr. Anthony Deutsch has proposed an even more ingenious argument. He suggests, tongue-in-cheek, that the odor of vomitus prevents the male from wanting to have sex with a pregnant woman, thereby reducing the likelihood of intercourse, which in turn is known to increase the risk of abortion. It's instantly obvious this is a silly argument, but why is the argument about toxins any less silly?

5. V.S. Ramachandran, 1997. Here is what they fell for:

Now ask yourself, "Why do gentlemen prefer blondes?" In Western cultures, it is widely believed that men have a distinct sexual and aesthetic preference for blondes over brunettes (Alley and Hildebrandt, 1988). A similar preference for women of lighter than average skin color is also seen in many non-Western cultures. (This has been formally confirmed by "scientific" surveys; Van der Berghe and Frost, 1986.) Indeed, in many countries, there is an almost obsessive preoccupation with "improving one's complexion"—a mania that the cosmetic industry has been quick to pander to with innumerable useless skin products. (Interestingly, there appears to be no such preference for men of lighter skin, hence the phrase "tall, dark and handsome.")

The well-known American psychologist Havelock Ellis suggested fifty years ago that men prefer rotund features (which indicate fecundity) in women and that blonde hair emphasizes the roundness by blending in better with the body outline. Another view is that infants' skin and hair color tend to be lighter than adults' and the preference for blonde women may simply reflect the fact that in humans, neotenous babylike features in females may be secondary sexual characteristics.

I'd like to propose a third theory, which is not incompatible with these two but has the added advantage of being consistent with more general biological theories of mate selection. But to understand my theory, you have to consider why sex evolved in the first place. Why not reproduce asexually since you could then pass on *all* your genes to your offspring rather than just half of them? The surprising answer is that sex evolved mainly to avoid parasites (Hamilton and Zuk, 1982)! Parasitic infestation is extremely common in nature and parasites are always trying to fool the host immune system into thinking that they are part of the host body. Sex evolved to help the host species shuffle its genes so that it always stays one step ahead of the parasites. (This is called the Red Queen strategy, a term inspired by the queen in *Alice in Wonderland*, who had to keep running just to stay in one place.) Similarly, we can ask why secondary sexual characteristics such as the peacock's tail or the rooster's wattles evolved. The answer again is parasites. These displays—a shimmering large tail or blood red wattles—may serve the purpose of "informing" the female that the suitor is healthy and free of skin parasites.

Might being blonde or light skinned serve a similar purpose? Every medical student knows that anemia, usually caused by either intestinal or blood parasites; cyanosis (a sign of heart disease); jaundice (a sick liver) and skin infection are much easier to detect in fair-skinned people than in brunettes. This is true for both skin and eyes. Infestation with intestinal parasites must have been very common in early agricultural settlements, and such infestation can cause severe anemia in the host. There must have been considerable selection pressures for the early detection of anemia in nubile young women since anemia can interfere with fertility, pregnancy and the birth of a healthy child. So the blonde is in effect telling your eyes, "I am pink, healthy and free of parasites. Don't trust that brunette. She could be concealing her ill health and parasitic infestation."

A second, related reason for the preference might be that the absence of protection from ultraviolet radiation by melanin causes the skin of blondes to "age" faster than that of brunettes and the dermal signs of aging—age spots and wrinkles—are usually easier to detect. Since fertility in women declines rapidly with age, perhaps aging men prefer very young women as sexual partners (Stuart Anstis, personal communication). So blondes might be preferred not only because the signs of aging occur earlier but also because the signs are easier to detect in them.

Third, certain external signs of sexual interest like social embarrassment and blushing, as well as sexual arousal (the "flush" of orgasm), might be more difficult to detect in dark-skinned women. Thus the likelihood that one's courtship gestures will be reciprocated and consummated can be predicted with greater confidence when courting blondes.

The reason that the preference is not so marked for light-skinned ***men*** might be that anemia and parasites are mainly a risk during pregnancy and men don't get pregnant. Furthermore, a blonde woman would have greater difficulty than a brunette in lying about an affair she just had since the blush of embarrassment and guilt would give her away. For a man, detecting such a blush in a woman would be especially important because he is terrified of being cuckolded, whereas a woman need not worry about this—her main goals are to find and keep a good provider. (This paranoia in the man is not unreasonable; recent surveys show that as many as 5 to 10 percent of fathers are not genetic fathers. There are probably many more milkman genes in the population than anyone realizes.)

One last reason for preferring blondes concerns the pupils. Pupil dilation—another obvious sign of sexual interest—would be more evident when seen against the blue iris of a blonde than against the dark iris of a brunette. This may also explain why brunettes are often considered "sultry" and mysterious (or why women use belladonna to dilate pupils and why men try to seduce women by candlelight; the drug and dim light dilate the pupils, enhancing the sexual interest display).

Of course, all these arguments would apply equally well to any woman of lighter skin. Why does the blond ***hair*** make any difference, if indeed it does? The preference for lighter skin has been established by conducting surveys, but the question of blond hair has not been studied. (The existence of bleached blondes doesn't negate our argument since evolution couldn't have anticipated the invention of hydrogen peroxide. Indeed, the fact that there is no such thing as a "fake brunette" but only a "fake blonde" suggests that such a preference does exist; after all, most blondes don't dye their hair black.) I suggest that the blond hair serves as a "flag" so that even from a great distance it's obvious to a male that a light-skinned woman is in the neighborhood.

The take-home message: Gentlemen prefer blondes so they can easily detect the early signs of parasitic infection and aging, both of which reduce fertility and offspring viability and can also detect blushing and pupil size, which are indices of sexual interest and fidelity. (That fair skin may itself be an indicator of youth and hormonal status was proposed in 1995 by Don Symons, a distinguished evolutionary psychologist from UCSB, but he did not put forward specific arguments concerning the easier detection of parasites, anemia, blushing or pupils in blondes being advocated here.)

As I said earlier, I concocted this whole ridiculous story as a satire on ad hoc sociobiological theories of human mate selection—the mainstay of evolutionary psychology. I give it less than a 10 percent chance of being true, but even so it's at least as viable as many other theories of human courtship currently in vogue. If you think my theory is silly, then you should read some of the others.

6. Ramachandran, 1998.
7. The important link between humor and creativity has also been emphasized by the English physician, playwright and polymath Jonathan Miller.
8. The notion that a smile is related to a threat grimace goes all the way back to Darwin and often resurfaces in the literature. But to my knowledge, no one has pointed out that it has the same ***logical form*** as laughter: an aborted response to a potential threat when an approaching stranger turns out to be a friend.
9. Any theory that purports to explain humor and laughter has to account for ***all*** of the following features—not just one or two: first, the logical structure of jokes and events that elicit laughter—that is, the input; second, the evolutionary reason why the input has to take the particular form that it does, a buildup of a model followed by a sudden paradigm shift that is of trivial consequence; third, the loud explosive sound; fourth, the relation of humor to tickling and why tickling might have evolved (I suggest it has the same logical form as humor but may represent "play" rehearsal for adult humor); fifth, the neurological structures involved and how the functional logic of humor maps onto the "structural logic" of these parts of the brain; sixth, whether humor has any other functions than the one it originally evolved for (for example, we suggest that adult cognitive humor may provide rehearsal for creativity and may also serve internally to "deflate" potentially disturbing thoughts that you can't do anything about); seventh, why a smile is a "half laugh" and often precedes laughter (the reason I suggest is that it has the same logical form—deflation of potential threat—that humor and laughter have because it evolved in response to approaching strangers).

   Laughter may also facilitate a kind of social bonding or "grooming," especially since it frequently occurs in response to a spurious violation of social contracts or taboos (e.g., when someone is lecturing on the podium with his fly open). Telling jokes or laughing at someone may allow an individual to recalibrate frequently the social mores of the group to which he belongs and help consolidate a shared sense of values. (Hence the popularity of ethnic jokes.)

   The psychologist Wallace Chafe (1987) has proposed an ingenious theory of laughter that is in some ways the converse of mine—although he doesn't consider the neurobiology. The main function of laughter, he says, is to serve as a "disabling" device—the physical act is so exhausting that it literally immobilizes you momentarily and allows you to relax when you realize that the threat isn't genuine. I find this idea attractive for two reasons. First, when you stimulate the left supplementary motor cortex, not only do you get fits of laughter but the patient is effectively immobilized; he can't do anything else (Fried et al., 1998). Second, in a strange disorder called catalepsy, listening to a joke causes the patient to become paralyzed and collapse to the ground while remaining fully conscious. It seems plausible that this might be a pathological expression of the "immobilization reflex" that Chafe is alluding to. However, Chafe's theory doesn't explain how a laugh is related to a smile or how it is related to tickling; nor why a laugh should take the particular form that it does—the rhythmic, loud explosive sounds.

Why not just stop dead in your tracks like an opossum? This, of course, is a general problem in evolutionary psychology; you can come up with several reasonable-sounding scenarios of how something might have evolved, but it is often difficult to retrace the particular route taken by the trait to get where it is now.

Finally, even if I am correct in asserting that laughter evolved as an "it's OK" or "all is well" signal for communication, we have to explain the rhythmic head and body movements (in addition to the sounds) that accompany laughter. Can it be a coincidence that so many other pleasurable activities such as dancing, sex and music also involve rhythmic movements? Could it be that they all tap partially into the same circuits? Jacobs (1994) has proposed that both autistic children and normal people may enjoy rhythmic movements because such movements activate the serotinergic raphe system, releasing the "reward transmitter" serotonin. One wonders whether laughter activates the same mechanism. I knew of at least one autistic child who frequently engaged in uncontrollable, socially inappropriate laughter for relief.

10. In saying this, I have no intention of providing ammunition for creationists. These "other factors" should be seen as mechanisms that complement rather than contradict the principle of natural selection. Here are some examples:

a. Contingency—plain old luck—must have played an enormous role in evolution. Imagine two different species that are slightly different genetically—let's call them hippo A and hippo B—on two different islands, island A and island B. Now if a huge asteroid hits both islands, perhaps hippo B is better adapted to asteroid impacts, survives and passes on its gene via natural selection. But it's equally possible that the asteroid may not have hit island B and its hippos. Say it hit only island A and wiped out all hippo A's. Hippo B's therefore survived and passed on their genes not because they had "asteroid-resistance genes" but simply because they were *lucky* and the asteroid never hit them.

This idea is so obvious that I find it astonishing that people argue about it. In my view, it encapsulates the whole debate over the Burgess shale creatures. Whether Gould is right or wrong about the particular creatures unearthed there, his general argument about the role of contingency is surely correct. The only sensible counterargument would be the many instances of convergent evolution. My favorite example is the evolution of intelligence and complex types of learning—such as imitation learning—independently in octopuses and higher vertebrates. How does one explain the independent emergence of such complex traits in both vertebrates and invertebrates, if contingency rather than natural selection was playing the major role? Doesn't it imply that if the tape of evolution were played again, intelligence would evolve yet again? If it evolved twice, why not three times?

Yet such instances of astonishing convergence are not fatal to the notion of contingency; after all, they occur very rarely. Intelligence evolved twice, not dozens of times. Even the apparent convergent evolution of eyes in vertebrates and invertebrates—such as squids—is probably not a true case of convergence, since it has recently been shown that the same genes are involved.

b. When certain neural systems reach a critical level of complexity, they may suddenly acquire unforeseen properties, which again are not a direct result of selection. There is nothing mystical about these properties; one can show mathematically that even completely random interactions can lead to these little eddies of order from complexity. Stuart Kauffman, a theoretical biologist at the Santa Fe

Institute, has argued that this might explain the punctuated nature of organic evolution—that is, the sudden emergence of new species in novel phylogenetic lines.

c. The evolution of morphological traits may be driven, to a significant extent, by perceptual mechanisms. If you teach a rat to discriminate a square (1:1 aspect ratio) from a rectangle (of 1:2 aspect ratio) and reward it for the rectangle alone, then the rat is found to respond even more vigorously to a skinnier (1:4 ratio) rectangle than to the original prototype rectangle, which it was trained on. This paradoxical result—called the "peak shift effect"—suggests that the animal is learning a rule—rectangularity—rather than a response to a single stimulus. I suggest that this basic propensity—wired into the visual pathways of all animals—can help explain the emergence of new species and of new phylogenetic trends. Consider the classic problem of how the giraffe got its long neck. Assume first that an ancestral group of giraffes evolved a slightly longer neck as a result of competition for food, that is, through conventional Darwinian selection. Once such a trend had been set up, however, it would be important for long-necked giraffes to mate only with other long-necked giraffes to ensure viability and fertility of the offspring. Once the longer neck became a distinguishing trait for the new species, then this trait must become "wired" into the visual centers of the giraffe's brain to help locate potential mates. Once this "giraffe = long neck" rule has been wired into a freely interbreeding group of giraffes, given the peak shift principle, any giraffe would tend to prefer mating with the most "giraffe-like" individual that it could spot—that is, the most long-necked individual in the herd. The net result would be a progressive increase in "long neck" alleles in the population *even in the absence of a specific selection pressure from the environment*. The final outcome would be a race of giraffes with almost comically exaggerated necks of the kind we see today.

This process will lead to a positive feedback "gain amplification" of any preexisting evolutionary trends; it will exaggerate morphological and behavioral differences between a given species and its immediate ancestor. This amplification will occur as a direct consequence of a psychological law rather than a result of environmental selection pressures. The theory makes the interesting prediction that there should be many instances in evolution of progressive caricaturization of species. Such trends do occur and can be seen clearly in the evolution of elephants, horses and rhinoceroses. As we trace their evolution, they appear to become more and more "mammothlike" or "horselike" or "rhinolike" with the passage of time.

This idea is quite similar to Darwin's own explanation for the origin of secondary sexual characteristics—his so-called theory of sexual selection. The progressive enlargement of the male peacock tail, for example, is thought to arise from a female's preference for mates with larger tails. The key difference between our idea and Darwinian sexual selection is that the latter idea was put forth specifically to explain differences between the sexes, whereas our idea accounts for morphological differences between species as well. Mate selection involves choosing partners that have more salient "sexual markers" (secondary sexual characteristics) and have species "markers" (labels that serve to differentiate one species from another). Consequently, our idea might help explain the evolution of *external morphological traits in general* and the progressive caricaturization of species, and not just the emergence of flamboyant sexual display signals and ethological "releasers."

One wonders whether the explosive enlargement of brain (and head) size in hominid evolution is a consequence of the same principle. Perhaps we find infantile, neotenous features, such as a disproportionately large head, appealing because such features are usually diagnostic of a helpless infant, and genes that promote the care of infants would quickly multiply in a population. But once this perceptual mechanism is in place, infants' heads would become larger and larger (since large-head genes would produce neotenous features and elicit greater care) and a large brain might simply be a bonus!

To this long list we can add others—Lynn Margulis's idea that symbiotic organisms can "fuse" to evolve into new phylogenetic lines (for example, mitochondria have their own DNA and may have started out as intracellular parasites). A detailed description of her ideas is outside the scope of this book, which, after all, is about the brain, not evolution.

Chapter 11: "You Forgot to Deliver the Twin"

1. This story is a reconstruction based on a case originally described by Silas Weir Mitchell. See Bivin and Klinger, 1937.
2. Christopher Wills told me the story of an eminent professor of obstetrics who was fooled by a patient sufficiently that he actually presented her as a case of normal pregnancy to his residents and medical students during Grand Rounds. The students promptly elicited all the classic symptoms and signs of pregnancy in the unfortunate lady. They even claimed to hear the fetal heartbeat with their gleaming new stethoscopes—until one student remembered the "protruding umbilicus" sign and risked embarrassing her professor by revealing the correct diagnosis.
3. Pseudocyesis is a fossil disease, so rare that one hardly sees it anymore. The condition was first described by Hippocrates in 300 B.C. It afflicted Mary Tudor, queen of England, who was falsely pregnant twice, with one episode lasting thirteen months. Anna O., one of Freud's most famous patients, suffered through a false pregnancy. And the more recent medical literature even describes two transsexuals who experienced it! For recent work on pseudocyesis, see Brown and Barglow, 1971, and Starkman et al., 1985.
4. Follicle-stimulating hormone (FSH), luteinizing hormone (LH) and prolactin are produced by the anterior pituitary; they regulate the menstrual cycle and ovulation. FSH causes the initial ripening of the ovarian follicle and LH causes ovulation. The combined action of FSH and LH augments the release of estrogen by the ovaries and later of both estrogen and progesterone by the corpus luteum (what remains of the follicle after release of the egg). Last, prolactin also acts on the corpus luteum, causing it to secrete estrogen and progesterone and preventing it from becoming involuted (and therefore preventing subsequent menstruation if the ovum is fertilized).
5. For the effects of suggestion on warts, see Spanos, Stenstrom and Johnston, 1988. For a report on unilateral wart remission, see Sinclair-Gieben and Chalmers, 1959.
6. See Ader, 1981, and Friedman, Klein and Friedman, 1996.
7. Hypnosis is a good example. Its a topic that's sometimes taught even in the most conservative medical establishments, and yet every time the word is mentioned at scientific meetings, there is an uncomfortable shuffling of feet. Even

though hypnosis has a venerable tradition going all the way back to one of the founding fathers of modern neurology, Jean Martin Charcot, it seems to enjoy a curious dual reputation, being accepted as real on the one hand and yet also regarded as the orphan child of "fringe medicine." Charcot claimed that if the right side of a normal person's body is temporarily paralyzed as the result of a hypnotic suggestion, then that person also has problems with language, suggesting that the trance is actually inhibiting brain mechanisms in the left hemisphere (recall that language is in the left). A similar trance-induced paralysis of the left side of the body does not produce language problems. We have tried replicating this result in our lab, without success.

The key question about hypnosis is whether it is simply an elaborate form of "role playing" (in which you temporarily suspend disbelief as you do while watching a horror movie) or whether it is a fundamentally different mental state.

Richard Brown, Eric Altschuler, Chris Foster and I have begun to try to answer this question using a technique called Stroop interference. The words "red" and "green" are printed either in the correct color (red ink for the word "red," green for "green") or with the colors reversed (the word "green" in red ink). If a normal subject is asked just to name the color of the ink and ignore the word, he is slowed down considerably if the word and color don't match. He's apparently unable voluntarily to ignore the word, and so the word interferes with color naming (Stroop interference). Now the question arises, What would happen if you implanted the hypnotic suggestion in the subject's mind that he's a native Chinese who can't read the English alphabet but can still name colors? Would this suddenly eliminate Stroop interference? This test would prove once and for all that hypnosis is real—not playacting—for there is no way a subject can voluntarily ignore the word. (As a "control" one could simply offer him a large cash reward for voluntarily overcoming the interference.)

8. The placebo response is a much maligned but poorly understood phenomenon. Indeed, the phrase has come to acquire a pejorative connotation in clinical medicine. Imagine that you are testing a new painkilling drug for back pain. Assume also that no one gets better spontaneously. To determine the efficacy of the drug, you give the pills to one hundred patients and find that, say, ninety patients get better. In a controlled clinical trial, it is customary for the comparison group of one hundred patients to receive a dummy pill—a placebo—(of course, the patient doesn't know this) to see what proportion of them, if any, get better simply as a result of the belief in the drug. If only 50 percent get better (instead of 90 percent), we are justified in concluding that the drug is indeed an effective painkiller.

But now let us turn to the mysterious 50 percent who got better as a result of the "placebo." Why did they get better? It was shown about a decade ago that these patients actually release painkilling chemicals, called endorphins, in their brains (indeed, in some cases the effect of the placebo can be counteracted by naloxone, a drug that blocks endorphins).

A fascinating but largely unexplored question concerns the specificity of the placebo response, and our laboratory has recently become very interested in this issue. Recall that only 50 percent got better from taking the placebo. Is this because there is something special about this group? What if the same one hundred patients (treated with a placebo for pain) went on to develop depression a few months later and you were to give a "new" placebo—telling them that it was a powerful new antidepressant? Would the same fifty patients get better, or would a new set of patients show improvement, overlapping only partially with the first set? In other words, is there such a thing as a "placebo responder"? Is the response specific to the malady, the pill, the person or all three? Indeed, consider what would happen if the same one hundred patients once again developed pain a year later and again you gave them the original placebo "painkiller." Would the same fifty get better or would it be a new group of patients? Dr. Eric Altschuler and I are presently conducting such a study.

Other aspects of placebo specificity also remain to be investigated. Imagine that a patient simultaneously develops a migraine and an ulcer—and you give him a placebo that you tell him is a new "antiulcer drug." Then would only the ulcer pain go away (assuming that he is a "placebo responder"), or would his brain become so flushed with endorphins that the migraine pain would also disappear as a bonus? This sounds unlikely, but if antipain neurotransmitters, such as endorphins, are released diffusely in his brain, then he may also get relief from his other aches and pains even though his belief pertains only to the ulcer. The question of how sophisticated beliefs are translated and understood by primitive brain mechanisms concerned with pain is a fascinating one.

9. For a review of multiple personality disorders, see Birnbaum and Thompson, 1996.

   For ocular changes, see Miller, 1989.

Chapter 12: Do Martians See Red?

1. For clear introductions to the problem of consciousness, see Humphrey, 1992; Searle, 1992; Dennett, 1991; P. Churchland, 1986; P.M. Churchland, 1993; Galin, 1992; Baars 1997; Block, Ramachandran and Hirstein, 1997; Penrose, 1989.

   The idea that consciousness—especially introspection—may have evolved mainly to allow you to simulate other minds (which inspired the currently popular notion of a "theory of other minds" module) was first proposed by Nick Humphrey at a conference that I had organized in Cambridge over twenty years ago.
2. Another very different type of translation problem also arises between the code or language of the left hemisphere and that of the right (see note 16, Chapter 7).
3. Some philosophers are utterly baffled by this possibility, but it's no more mysterious than striking your ulnar nerve at the elbow with a hammer to generate a totally novel electrical "tingling" qualia even though you may have never experienced anything quite like it before (or even the very first time a boy or girl experiences an orgasm).
4. Thus an ancient philosophical riddle going back to David Hume and William Molyneux can now be answered scientifically. Researchers at NIH have used magnets to stimulate the visual cortex of blind people to see whether visual pathways have degenerated or become reorganized, and we have also begun some experiments here at UCSD. But to my knowledge, the specific question of whether a person can experience a quale or subjective sensation totally novel to him or her has never been explored empirically.
5. The pioneering experiments in this field were performed by Singer, 1993, and Gray and Singer, 1989.

6. It is sometimes asserted—on grounds of parsimony—that one does not need qualia for a complete description of the way the brain works, but I disagree with this view. Occam's razor—the idea that the *simplest* of competing theories is preferable to more complex explanations of unknown phenomena—is a useful rule of thumb, but it can sometimes be an actual impediment to scientific discovery. Most science begins with a bold conjecture of what might be true. The discovery of relativity, for example, was not the product of applying Occam's razor to our knowledge of the universe at that time. The discovery resulted from rejecting Occam's razor and asking what if some deeper generalization were true, which was not required by the available data, but which made unexpected predictions (which later turned out to be parsimonious, after all). It's ironic that most scientific discoveries result not from brandishing or sharpening Occam's razor—despite the view to the contrary held by the great majority of scientists and philosophers—but from generating seemingly ad hoc and ontologically promiscuous conjectures that are not called for by the current data.

7. Please note that I am using the phrase "filling in" in a strictly metaphorical sense—simply for lack of a better one. I don't want to leave you with the impression that there is a pixel-by-pixel rendering of the visual image on some internal neural screen. But I disagree with Dennett's specific claim that there is no "neural machinery" corresponding to the blind spot. There is, in fact, a patch of cortex corresponding to each eye's blind spot that receives input from the other eye as well as the region surrounding the blind spot in the same eye. What we mean by "filling in" is simply this: that one quite literally sees visual stimuli (such as patterns and colors) as arising from a region of the visual field where there is actually no visual input. This is a purely descriptive, theory-neutral definition of filling in, and one does not have to invoke—or debunk—homunculi watching screens to accept it. We would argue that the visual system fills in not to benefit a homunculus but to make some aspects of the information explicit for the next level of processing.

8. Tovee, Rolls and Ramachandran, 1996. Kathleen Armel, Chris Foster and I have recently shown that if two completely different "views" of this dog are presented in rapid succession, naive subjects can see only chaotic, incoherent motion of the splotches, but once they see the dog, it is seen to jump or turn in the appropriate manner—emphasizing the role of the "top-down" object knowledge in motion perception (see Chapter 5).

9. Sometimes qualia become deranged, leading to a fascinating condition called synesthesia, in which a person quite literally tastes a shape or sees color in a sound. For example, one patient, a synesthete, claimed that chicken has a distinctly "pointy" flavor and told his physician, Dr. Richard Cytowic, "I wanted the taste of this chicken to be pointed, but it came out all round . . . well, I mean it's nearly spherical; I can't serve this if it doesn't have points." Another patient claimed to see the letter "U" as being yellow to light brown in color, whereas the letter "N" was a shiny varnished ebony hue. Some synesthetes see this union of the senses as a gift to inspire their art, not as brain pathology.

   Some cases of synesthesia tend to be a bit dubious. A person claims to see a sound or taste a color, but it turns out that she is merely being metaphorical—much the same way that you might speak of a sharp taste, a bitter memory or a dull sound (bear in mind, though, that the distinction between the metaphorical and the literal is extremely blurred in this curious condition). However, many other cases are quite genuine. A graduate student, Kathleen Armel, and I recently examined a patient named John Hamilton who had relatively normal vision up until the age of five, then suffered progressive deterioration in his sight as a result of retinitis pigmentosa, until finally at the age of forty he was completely blind. After about two or three years, John began to notice that whenever he touched objects or simply read Braille, his mind would conjure up vivid visual images, including flashes of light, pulsating hallucinations or sometimes the actual shape of the object he was touching. These images were highly intrusive and actually interfered with his Braille reading and ability to recognize objects through touch. Of course, if you or I close our eyes and touch a ruler, we don't hallucinate one, even though we may visualize it in our mind's eye. The difference, again, is that your visualization of the ruler is usually helpful to your brain since it is tentative and revocable—you have control over it—whereas John's hallucinations are often irrelevant and always irrevocable and intrusive. He can't do anything about them, and to him they are a spurious and distracting nuisance. It seems that the tactile signals evoked in John's somatosensory areas—his Penfield map—are being sent all the way back to his deprived visual areas, which are hungry for input. This is a radical idea, but it can be tested by using modern imaging techniques.

Interestingly, synesthesia is sometimes seen in temporal lobe epilepsy, suggesting that the merging of sense modalities occurs not only in the angular gyrus (as is often asserted) but also in certain limbic structures.

10. This question arose in a conversation I had with Mark Hauser.
11. Searle, 1992.
12. Jackendorf, 1987.
13. The patient may also say, "This is it; I finally see the truth. I have no doubts anymore." It seems ironic that our convictions about the absolute truth or falsehood of a thought should depend not so much on the propositional language system, which takes great pride in being logical and infallible, but on much more primitive limbic structures, which add a form of emotional qualia to thoughts, giving them a "ring of truth." (This might explain why the more dogmatic assertions of priests as well as scientists are so notoriously resistant to correction through intellectual reasoning!)
14. Damasio, 1994.
15. I am, of course, simply being metaphorical here. At some stage in science, one has to abandon or refine metaphors and get to the actual mechanism—the nitty-gritty of it. But in a science that is still in its infancy, metaphors are often useful pointers. (For example, seventeenth-century scientists often spoke of light as being made of waves or particles, and both metaphors were useful up to a point, until they became assimilated into the more mature physics of quantum theory. Even the gene—the independent particle of beanbag genetics—continues to be a useful word, although its actual meaning has changed radically over the years.)
16. For an insightful discussion of akinetic mutism, see Bogen, 1995, and Plum, 1982.
17. Dennett, 1991.
18. Trivers, 1985.

Bibliography and Suggested Reading

Adamec, R.E. 1989. "Kindling, Anxiety, and Personality." In T.G. Bowlig and M.R. Trimble (eds.), *The Clinical Relevance of Kindling*. Chichester: Wiley, 117–135.

Ader, R., ed. 1981. *Psychoneuroimmunology*. New York: Academic Press.

Aglioti, S.A., A. Bonazzi, F. Cortese. 1994. "Phantom Lower Limb as a Perceptual Marker for Neural Plasticity in the Mature Human Brain." *Proceedings of the Royal Society* (London) [Biol], 255:273–278.

Aglioti, S.A., J. DeSouza, and M. Goodale. "Size Contrast Illusions Deceive the Eye but Not the Hand." *Curr Biol*, 5:679–685.

Aglioti, S.A., N. Smania, A. Atzei, and G. Berlucchi. 1997. "Spatio-Temporal Properties of the Pattern of Evoked Phantom Sensations in a Left Index Amputee Patient." *Behav Neuro*, 111(5):867–872.

Albright, T.D. 1995. "Visual Motion Perception." *Proc Natl Acad Sci USA*, 92(7): 2433–2440.

Alley, T.R., and K.A. Hildebrandt. 1988. In T.R. Alley (ed.), *Social and Applied Aspects of Perceiving Faces*. Hillsdale, NJ: Lawrence Erlbaum.

Allman, J.M., and J.H. Kass. 1971. "Representation of the Visual Field in Striate and Adjoining Cortex of the Owl Monkey." *Brain Res*, 35:89–106.

Avery, O.T., C.M. Macleod, and M. McCarty. 1944. "Studies on the Chemical Nature of the Substance Inducing Transformation of the Pneumococcal Types." *J Exp Med*, 79:137–158

Baars, B. 1988. *A Cognitive Theory of Consciousness*. New York: Cambridge University Press.

Baars, B. 1997. *In the Theater of Consciousness*. Oxford: Oxford University Press.

Babinski, M.J. 1914. "Contribution à l'étude des troubles mentaux dans l'hémiplegie organique cérébrale." *Rev Neurol* 1:845–848.

Bach-y-Rita, P. 1995. *Non-Synaptic Diffusion Neurotransmission and Late Brain Reorganization*. New York: Demos.

Baddeley, A.D. 1986. *Working Memory*. Oxford: Churchill Livingtone.

Baddeley, A.D. 1994. "When Implicit Learning Fails: Amnesia and the Problem of Error Elimination." *Neuropsychologia*, 32:53–69.

Baddeley, A.D. 1995. "The Psychology of Memory Disorders." In A.D. Baddeley, B.A. Wilson, and F.N. Watts (eds.), *Handbook of Memory Disorders*. Chichester: Wiley, 3–25.

Bancaud, J., F. Brunet-Bourgin, P. Chavel, and E. Halgren. 1994. "Anatomical Origin of Déjà Vu and Vivid 'Memories' in Human Temporal Lobe Epilepsy." *Brain*, 127:71–90.

Barkow, J.H., L. Cosmides, and J. Tooby. 1992. *The Adapted Mind*. New York: Oxford University Press.

Barlow, H.B. 1987. "The Biological Role of Consciousness." *Mindwaves*, 361–381. Oxford: Basil Blackwell.

Baron-Cohen, S. 1995. *Mindblindness*. Cambridge, MA: MIT Press.

Bartlett, F.C. 1932. *Remembering*. Cambridge: Cambridge University Press.

Basbaum, A.I. 1996. "Memories of Pain." *Sci Am Med,* 22–31.

Bates, E., and J. Elman. 1996. "Learning Rediscovered." *Science,* 274 (5294): 1849–1850.

Bauer, R.M. 1984. "Autonomic Recognition of Names and Faces in Prosopagnosia." In H.D. Ellis, M.A. Jeeves, F. Newcombe, and A.W. Young (eds.), *Aspects of Face Processing.* Dordrecht: Nijhoff.

Bear, D.M., and P. Fedio. 1977. "Quantitative Analysis of Interictal Behavior in Temporal Lobe Epilepsy." *Arch Neuro,* 34:454–467.

Benson, F. 1997. In T. Feinberg and M. Farah (eds.), *Behavioral Neurology and Neuropsychology.* New York: McGraw-Hill.

Bever, T.G., and R.S. Chiarello. 1994. "Cerebral Dominance in Musicians and Nonmusicians." *Science,* 185:537–539.

Birnbaum, M.H., and K. Thompson. 1996. "Visual Function in Multiple Personality Disorder." *J Am Optom Assoc,* 67:327–334.

Bisiach, E., and C. Luzatti. 1978. "Unilateral Neglect of Representational Space." *Cortex,* 14:129–133.

Bisiach, E., M.L. Rusconi, and G. Vallar. 1992. "Remission of Somatophrenic Delusion Through Vestibular Stimulation." *Neuropsychologia,* 29:1029–1031.

Bivin, G.D., and M.P. Klinger. 1937. *Pseudocyesis.* Bloomington, IN: Principia Press.

Blakemore, C. 1977. *Mechanics of the Mind.* Cambridge: Cambridge University Press.

Block, N. 1995. "On a Confusion about a Function of Consciousness." *Behav Brain Sci,* 18:227–247.

Block, N. 1997. *The Nature of Consciousness: Philosophical Debates.* Cambridge, MA: MIT Press.

Bogen, J.E. 1975. "The Other Side of the Brain." *UCLA Educ,* 17:24–32.

Bogen, J.E. 1995. "On Neurophysiology of Consciousness. Part II. Constraining the Semantic Problem." *Consciousness Cognition,* 4:53–62.

Bonnet, C. 1760. *Essai Analyttique sur les facultés de l'âme.* Geneve: Philbert.

Borsook, B., S. Fishman, L. Becerra, A. Edwards, M. Stojanovic, H. Breiter, V.S. Ramachandran, et al. 1997. "Acute Plasticity in Human Somatosensory Cortex Following Amputation." *Soc Neurosci Abstr,* 1(173.1):438.

Botvinik, M., and J. Cohen. 1988. "Rubber Hands Feel Touch That Eyes See." *Nature,* 391:756.

Brain, W.R. 1941. "Visual Distortion with Special Reference to the Regions of the Right Hemisphere." *Brain,* 64:244–272

Brothers, L. 1997. *Friday's Footprint.* New York: Oxford University Press.

Brown, E., and P. Barglow. 1971. "Pseudocyesis." *Arch Gen Psych,* 24:221–229.

Bruens, J.H. 1971. "Psychosis in Epilepsy." *Psychiatr Neurol Neurochir,* 74: 175–192.

Caccace, A.T., T.J. Lovely, D.R. Winetr, S.M. Parnes, and D.J. McFarland. 1994. "Auditory Perceptual and Visual-Spatial Characteristics of Gaze Evoked Tinnitus." *Audiology,* 33:291–303.

Calford, M. 1991. "Curious Cortical Change." *Nature,* 352:759–760.

Capgras, J., and J. Reboul-Lachaux. "L'illusion des 'sosies' dans un délire systématise chronique." *Bull Soc Clin Med Mentale,* 2:6–16.

Cappa, S., R. Sterzi, G. Vallar, and E. Bisiach. 1987. "Remission of Hemineglect and Anosognosia after Vestibular Stimulation." *Neuropsychologia,* 25:755–782.

Chafe, W. 1987. "Humor as a Disabling Mechanism." *Am Behav Sci*, 30:16–26.

Churchland, P.S. 1986. *Neurophilosophy*. Cambridge, MA: MIT Press.

Churchland, P.M. 1993. *Matter and Consciousness*. Cambridge, MA: MIT Press.

Churchland, P.M. 1996. *The Engine of Reason, the Seat of the Soul*. Cambridge, MA: MIT Press.

Churchland, P.S., V.S. Ramachandran, and T. Sejnowski. 1994. In C. Koch and J.L. Davis (eds.), *A Critique of Pure Vision in Large Scale Neuronal Theories of the Brain*. Cambridge, MA: MIT Press.

Clarke, S., L. Regli, R.C. Janzer, G. Assal, and N. de Tribolet. 1996. "Phantom Face: Conscious Correlate of Neural Reorganization after Removal of Primary Sensory Neurons." *Neuroreport*, 7:2853–2857.

Cohen, L., S. Bandinell, T. Findlay, M. Hallet. 1991. "Motor Reorganization after Upper Limb Amputation in Man." *Brain*, 114:615–627.

Cohen, M.S., S.M. Kosslyn, and H.C. Breiter. 1996. "Changes in Cortical Activity during Mental Rotation: A Mapping Study Using Functional MRI." *Brain*, 119: 89–100.

Corballis, M. 1991. *The Lopsided Ape*. New York: Oxford University Press.

Corkin, S. 1968. "Acquisition of Motor Skill after Bilateral Medial Temporal Lobe Excision." *Neuropsychologia*, 6:255–265.

Cowey, A., and P. Stoerig. 1991. "The Neurobiology of Blindsight." *Trends Neurosci*, 29:65–80.

Cowey, A., and P. Stoerig. 1992. In D. Milner and M.D. Rugg (eds.), *Reflections on Blindsight: The Neuropsychology of Consciousness*. London: Academic Press, 11–37.

Crick, F.H.C. 1993. *The Astonishing Hypothesis*. New York: Charles Scribner.

Crick, F., and C. Koch. 1995. "Are We Aware of Neural Activity in Primary Visual Cortex?" *Nature*, 375:121–123.

Critchley, M. 1962. "Clinical Investigation of Disease of the Parietal Lobes of the Brain." *Med Clin North Am* 46:837–857.

Critchley, M. 1966. *The Parietal Lobes*. New York: Hafner.

Cronholm, B. 1951. "Phantom Limbs in Amputees: A Study of Changes in the Integration of Centripetal Impulses with Special Reference to Referred Sensations." *Acta Psychiatr Neurol Scand*, Suppl *72*:1–310.

Cutting, J. 1978. "Study of Anosognosia." *J Neurol Neurosurg Psychiatry*, 41: 548–555.

Cytowic, R. 1989. *Synaesthesia*. Heidelberg: Springer Verlag.

Cytowic, R. 1995. *The Neurological Side of Neuropsychology*. Cambridge, MA: Bradford Books.

Daly, M., and M. Wilson. 1983. *Sex, Evolution, and Behavior*. Boston: Willard Grant.

Damasio, A. 1994. *Descartes Error*. New York: G.P. Putnam.

Damasio, A.R., H. Damasio, and G.W. Van Hoesen. 1982. "Prosopagnosia: Anatomic Basis and Behavioral Mechanisms." *Neurology*, 32:331–341.

Damasio, A.R. 1985. "Prosopagnosia." *Trends Neurosci*, 8:132–135.

Darwin, C. 1871. *The Descent of Man*. London: John Murray.

Dawkins, R. 1976. *The Selfish Gene*. New York: Oxford University Press.

Dehaene, S. 1997. *The Number Sense*. New York: Oxford University Press.

Dennett, D. 1991. *Consciousness Explained*. Boston: Little, Brown.

Dennett, D. 1995. *Darwin's Dangerous Idea*. New York: Simon & Schuster.

DeWeerd, P., R. Gattass, R. Desimone, and L.G. Ungerleider. 1995. "Responses of Cells in Monkey Visual Cortex During Perceptual Filling-in of an Artificial Scotoma." *Nature*, 377:731–734.

Dewhurst, K., and A.W. Beard. 1970. "Sudden Religious Conversion in Temporal Lobe Epilepsy." *Br J Psychiatry*, 117:497–507.

DeYoe, E.A., and D.C. Van Essen. 1985. "Segregation of Efferent Connections and Receptive Fields in Visual Area V2 of the Macaque." *Nature*, 317:58–61.

Edelman, G.M. 1989. *The Remembered Present*. New York: Basic Books.

Eisley, L. 1958. *Darwin's Century*. New York: Doubleday.

Ekman, P. 1975. *Unmasking the Face: Guide to Recognizing Emotions from Facial Clues*. Englewood Cliffs, NJ: Prentice-Hall.

Ekman, P. 1992. "Are There Basic Emotions?" *Psychol Rev*, 99:550–553.

Erdelyi, M. 1985. *Psychoanalysis*. New York: W.H. Freeman.

Farah, M.J. 1989. "The Neural Basis of Visual Imagery." *Trends Neurosci*, 10: 395–399.

Farah, M. 1991. *Visual Agnosia*. Cambridge, MA: MIT Press.

Feinberg, T., and M. Farah. 1997. *Behavioral Neurology and Neuropsychology*. New York: McGraw-Hill.

Flanagan, O. 1991. *The Science of the Mind*. Cambridge, MA: Bradford Books.

Flor, H., T. Elbert, S. Knetch, C. Wienbruch, C. Pantev, N. Birbaumer, W. Larbig, and E. Taub. 1995. "Phantom Limb as a Perceptual Correlate of Cortical Reorganization Following Arm Amputation." *Nature*, 375:482–484.

Florence, S.L., and J.H. Kaas. 1995. "Large-Scale Reorganization at Multiple Levels of the Somatosensory Pathway Follows Therapeutic Amputation of the Hand in Monkeys." *J Neurosci*, 15:8083–8095.

Flor-Henry, P., L.T. Yeudall, Z.J. Koles, and B.G. Howarth. 1979. "Neuropsychological and Power Spectral EEG Investigations of the Obsessive-Compulsive Syndrome." *Biol Psychiatry*, 14:99–130.

Fodor, J. 1983. *Modularity of Mind*. Cambridge, MA: MIT Press.

Frackowiak, R.S.J., K.J. Friston, and C. Frith. 1997. *Human Brain Function*. New York: Academic Press.

Freud, A. 1946. *The Ego and the Mechanisms of Defense*. New York: International Universities Press.

Freud, S. 1996. *The Standard Edition of the Complete Works of Sigmund Freud*, Vol. 1–23. London: Hogarth Press.

Fried, I., C. Wilson, K. MacDonald, and E. Behnke. 1998. "Electric Current Stimulates Laughter." *Nature*, 391:850.

Friedman, H., T. Klein, and A. Friedman. 1996. *Psychoneuroimmunology, Stress and Infection*. Boca Raton, FL: CRC Press.

Frith, C.D., and R.J. Dolan. 1997. "Abnormal Beliefs: Delusions and Memory." Paper presented at the May 1997 Harvard Conference on Memory and Belief.

Fuster, J.M. 1980. *The Prefrontal Cortex: Anatomy, Physiology, and Neurophysiology of the Frontal Lobe*. New York: Raven Press.

Gabrieli, J.D.E., W. Milberg, M.M. Keane, and S. Corkin. 1990. "Intact Priming of Patterns Despite Impaired Memory." *Neuropsychologia*, 28:417–428.

Gainotti, G. 1972. "Emotional Behavior and Hemispheric Side of Tension." *Cortex*, 8:41–55.

Galin, D. 1974. "Implications for Psychiatry of Left and Right Cerebral Specialization." *Arch Gen Psychiatry,* 31:572–583.

Galin, D. 1976. "Two Modes of Consciousness in the Two Halves of the Brain." In P.R. Lee, R.E. Ornstein, and D. Galin (eds.), *Symposium on Consciousness.* New York: Viking Press.

Galin, D. 1992. "Theoretical Reflections of Awareness, Monitoring and Self in Relation to Anosognosia." *Consciousness Cognition,* 1:152–162.

Gallen, C.C., D.F. Sobel, T. Waltz, M. Aung, B. Copeland, B.J. Schwartz, E.C. Hirschkoff, and F.E. Bloom. 1993. "Noninvasive Neuromagnetic Mapping of Somatosensory Cortex." *Neurosurgery,* 33:260–268.

Gardner, H. 1993. In E. Perecman (ed.), *Cognitive Processing in the Right Hemisphere.* New York: Academic Press.

Gastaut, H. 1956. "Etude électroclinique des épisodes psychotiques survenant en dehors de crises cliniques: chez les épileptiques." *Rev Neurol,* 94:587–594.

Gazzaniga, M. 1992. *Nature's Mind.* New York: Basic Books.

Gazzaniga, M., J.E. Bogen, and R.W. Sperry. 1962. "Some Functional Effects of Sectioning the Cerebral Commisures in Man." *Proc Natl Acad of Sci USA,* U8: 1765–1769.

Gibbs, F.A. 1951. "Ictal and Non-Ictal Psychiatric Disorders in Temporal Lobe Epilepsy." *J Nerv Ment Dis,* 133:522–528.

Girgis, M. 1971. "The Orbital Surface of the Frontal Lobe of the Brain." *Acta Psychiatry Scand,* 222:1–58.

Gleick, J.L. 1987. *Chaos.* New York: Penguin.

Gloor, P. 1992. "Amygdala and Temporal Lobe Epilepsy." In J.P. Aggleton (ed.), *The Amygdala: Neurobiological Aspects of Emotion, Memory, Mental Dysfunction.* New York: Wiley-Liss.

Golberg, G. 1987. "From Intent to Action." In E. Perecman (ed.), *The Frontal Lobes Revised.* Hillsdale, NJ: Lawrence Erlbaum.

Goldberg, E., and R.M. Bilder, Jr. 1987. "The Frontal Lobes and Hierarchical Organization of Cognitive Control." In E. Perecman (ed.), *The Frontal Lobes Revisited.* Hillsdale, NJ: Lawrence Erlbaum.

Goldman-Rakic, P.S. 1987. "Circuitry of Primate Prefrontal Cortex and Regulation of Behavior by Representational Memory." *Handbook of Physiology: The Nervous System,* vol. 5., Bethesda, MD: American Psychological Society, 373–417.

Goldman-Rakic, P.S. 1988. "Topography of Cognition: Parallel Distributed Networks in Primate Association Cortex." *Annu Rev Neurosci,* 11:137–156.

Gould, S.J. 1981. *The Mismeasure of Man.* New York: W.W. Norton.

Gould, S.J. 1983. *Panda's Thumb.* New York: Penguin.

Gould, S.J. 1989. *Wonderful Life.* New York: W.W. Norton.

Gray, C.M., A.K. Engel, P. Konig, and W. Singer. 1992. "Synchronization of Oscillatory Neural Responses in Cat Striate Cortex: Temporal Properties." *Vis Neurosci,* 8(4):337–347.

Gray, C.M., and W. Singer. 1989. "Stimulus Specific Neural Oscillations." *Proc Natl Acad Sci USA,* 86:1689–1702.

Graziano, M.S.A., G.S. Yap, and C. Gross. 1994. "Coding of Visual Space by Premotor Neurons." *Science,* 266:1051–1054.

Gregory, R.L. 1966. *Eye and Brain.* London: Wiedenfeld and Nicolson.

Gregory, R.L. 1981. *Mind in Science.* Cambridge: Cambridge University Press.

Gregory, R.L. 1997. *Mirrors in Mind*. New York: Oxford University Press.

Gregory, R.L. 1991. *Odd Perceptions*. New York: Routledge, Chapman Hall.

Gross, C.G. 1992. "Representatives of Visual Stimuli in the Inferior Temporal Cortex." *Pro Roy Soc London* [Biol], 135:3–10.

Halligan, P.W., and J.C. Marshall, eds. 1994. *Spatial Neglect*. Hillsdale, NJ: Lawrence Erlbaum.

Halligan, P.W., J.C. Marshall, and V. S. Ramachandran. "Ghosts in the Machine: A Case Description of Visual and Haptic Hallucinations after Right Hemisphere Stroke." *Cog Neuropsychol*, 11:459–477.

Halligan, P.W., J.C. Marshall, D.T. Wade, J. Davey, and D. Morrison. 1993. "Thumb in Cheek? Sensory Reorganization and Perceptual Plasticity after Limb Amputation." *Neuroreport*, 4:233–236.

Hameroff, S., and R. Penrose. 1995. "Orchestrated Reduction of Quantum Coherence in Brain Molecules: A Model for Consciousness." In J. King and K.H. Pribram (eds.), *Conscious Experience: Is the Brain Too Important to Be Left to Specialists to Study?* Hillsdale, NJ: Lawrence Erlbaum, 241–274.

Hamilton, W.D. 1964. "The Genetical Evolution of Social Behavior." *J Theor Biol*, 7:1–52.

Hamilton, W.D., and M. Zuk. 1982. "Heritable True Fitness and Bright Birds: A Role for Parasites?" *Science*, 218:384–387.

Harrington, A. 1989. *Medicine, Mind, and the Double Brain*. Princeton, NJ: Princeton University Press.

Head, H. 1918. "Sensation and the Cerebral Cortex." *Brain*, 41:57–253.

Heilman, J. 1991. In G. Prigatano and D. Schacter (eds.), *Awareness of Deficits after Brain Injury*. New York: Oxford University Press.

Hermelin, B., and N. O'Connor. 1990. "Factors and Primes: A Specific Numerical Ability." *Psychol Med*, 20:163–189.

Hill, A.L. 1978. In N.R. Eller (ed.), *Mentally Retarded Individuals with Special Skills*, Vol. 9. New York: Academic Press.

Hirstein, W., and V.S. Ramachandran. 1997. "Capgras' Syndrome: A Novel Probe for Understanding the Neural Representation of Identity and Familiarity of Persons." *Proc R Soc London* [Biol], 264:437–444.

Hobson, J.A. 1988. *The Dreaming Brain*. New York: Basic Books.

Hochberg, J.E. 1964. *Perception*. Englewood Cliffs, NJ: Prentice-Hall.

Hoffman, J. 1955. "Facial Phantom Phenomena." *J Nerv Ment Dis*, 122:143.

Horgan, J. 1994. "Can Science Explain Consciusness?" *Sci Am*, 271:88–94.

Hubel, D.H., and T.N. Wiesel. 1979. "Brain Mechanisms of Vision." *Sci Am*, 241: 150–162.

Hubel, D.H., and M.S. Livingstone. 1985. "Complex Unoriented Cells in a Subregion of Primate Area 18." *Nature*, 315:325–327.

Humphrey, N. 1992. *A History of the Mind*. New York: Simon & Schuster.

Humphrey, N. 1993. *History of the Mind: Evolution and the Birth of Consciousness*. New York: HarperCollins.

Ironside, R. 1955. "Disorder of Laughter Due to Brain Lesions." Presidential Address, Neurological Section, Royal Society of Medicine, London.

Jackendorf, R. 1987. *Conciousness and the Computational Mind*. Cambridge, MA: MIT Press.

Jacobs, B. 1994. "Serotonin, Motor Activity and Depression-Related Disorders." *American Scientist*, 82:456–463.

James, W. 1887. "The Consciousness of Lost Limbs." *Proc Am Soc Psychic Res*, 1: 249–258.

James, W. 1890. *The Principles of Psychology*. New York: Henry Holt, 288–289.

Johanson, D., and B. Edward. 1996. *From Lucy to Language*. New York: Simon & Schuster.

Johnson, G. 1995. *Fire in the Mind*. New York: Random House.

Jones, E. 1982. "Thalamic Basis of Place- and Modality-Specific Columns in Monkey Somatosensory Cortex: A Correlative Anatomical and Physiological Study." *J Neurophysiol*, 48:546–568.

Joseph, R. 1990. *Neuropsychology, Neuropsychiatry, and Behavioral Neurology*. New York: Plenum Press.

Joseph, R. 1992. *The Right Brain in the Unconscious*. New York: Plenum Press.

Joseph, R. 1993. *The Naked Neuron*. New York: Plenum Press.

Juba, A. 1949. "Beitrag zur Strukdur der ein und doppelsietgen Korshemastorungen." *Monatsschr Psychiatr Neurol*, 118:11–29.

Kaas, J.H., R.J. Nelson, M. Sur, and M.M. Merzenich. 1981. *The Organization of the Cerebral Cortex*. Cambridge, MA: MIT Press, 237–261.

Kaas, J.H., and S.L. Florence. 1996. "Brain Reorganization and Experience." *Peabody J Educ*, 71:152–167.

Kallio, K.E. 1950. "Phantom Limb of Forearm Stump Cleft by Kineplastic Surgery." *Acta Chir Scand*, 99:121–132.

Kandel, E.R., J.H. Schwartz, and T.M. Jessell. 1991. *Principles of Neural Science*. New York: Elsevier.

Kaufmann, S. 1993. *The Origins of Order*. New York: Oxford University Press.

Kaufmann, S. 1995. *At Home in the Universe*. New York: Oxford University Press.

Kew, J.J.M., P.W. Halligan, J.C. Marshall, R.E. Passingham, J.C. Rothwell, M.C. Ridding, et al. 1997. "Abnormal Access of Axial Vibrotactile Input to Deafferented Somatosensory Cortex in Human Upper Limb Amputees." *J Neurophysiol*, 77:2753–2764.

Kinney, H. 1995. *James Thurber, His Life and Times*. New York: Henry Holt.

Kinsbourne, M. 1989. "A Model of Adaptive Behavior As It Relates to Cerebral Participation in Emotional Control." In G. Gainnotti and C. Caltagrione (eds.), *Emotions and the Dual Brain*. Heidelberg: Springer Verlag.

Kinsbourne, M. 1995. "The Intralaminar Thalamic Nuclei." *Consciousness Cognition*, 4:167–171.

Kleffner, D.A., and V.S. Ramachandran, 1992. "On the Perception of Shape from Shading." *Perception Psychophysics*, 52:18–36.

Kosslyn, S. 1996. *Image and Brain*. Cambridge, MA: MIT Press.

Lackner, J.R. 1988. "Some Proprioceptive Influences on Perceptual Representation." *Brain*, III:281–297.

LaCroix, R., R. Melzack, D. Smith, and N. Mitchell. 1992. "Multiple Phantom Limbs in a Child." *Cortex*, 28:503–507.

Leakey, R. 1993. *The Origin of Humankind*. New York: Basic Books.

LeDoux, J. 1996. *The Emotional Brain*. New York: Simon & Schuster.

Lettvin, J. 1976. "A Sidelong Glance at Seeing." *Sciences,* 16:1–20.

Levine, D.N. 1990. "Unawareness of Visual and Sensorimoter Defects: A Hypothesis." *Brain Cognition,* 13:233–281.

Livingstone, M.S., and D.H. Hubel. 1987. "Psychophysical Evidence for Separate Channels for the Perception of Form, Colour, Movement, and Depth." *J Neurosci,* 7:3416–3468.

Luria, A. 1968. *The Mind of a Mnemonist.* New York: Basic Books.

Luria, A. 1976. *Working Brain: An Introduction to Neuropsychology.* New York: Basic Books.

Maclean, P. 1973. *A Triune Concept of the Brain and Behavior.* Toronto, Can.: University of Toronto Press.

Marcel, A.J. 1983. "Conscious and Unconscious Perception: Experiments on Visual Masking and Word Recognition." *Cognit Psychol,* 15:197–237.

Marcel, A.J. 1993. "Slippage in the Unity of Consciousness in Experimental and Theoretical Studies on Consciousness." *CIBA Foundation Symposium,* no. 174. Chichester: Wiley.

Marcel, A.J., and E. Bisiach. 1988. *Consciousness in Contemporary Science.* Oxford: Clarendon Press.

Marr, D. 1981. *Vision.* San Francisco: W.H. Freeman.

Marshall, J., and P.W. Halligan. 1988. "Blindsight and Insight in the Visuospatial Neglect." *Nature,* 336:766–767.

Martin, J.P. 1950."Fits of Laughter in Organic Cerebral Disease." *Brain,* 73:453–464.

Maynard-Smith, J. 1978. *The Evolution of Sex.* Cambridge: Cambridge University Press.

McGlynn, S.M., and D.L. Schacter. 1989. "Unawareness of Deficits in Neuropsychological Syndromes." *J Clin Exp Neuropsychol,* 11:143–295.

McNaughton, B., J. McClelland, and R. O'Reilly. (1995). "Why There Are Complementary Learning Systems in the Hippocampus and Neocortex? Insights from the Successes and Failures of Connectionist Models of Learning and Memory." *Psychol Rev,* 102(3):419–457.

Melzack, R. 1990. "Phantom Limbs and the Concept of a Neuromatrix." *Trends Neurosci,* 13:88–92.

Melzack, R. 1992. "Phantom Limbs." *Sci Am,* 266:90–96.

Melzack, R., R. Israel, R. Lacroix, and G. Schultz. 1997. "Phantom Limbs in People with Congenital Limb Deficiency or Amputation in Early Childhood," part 9. *Brain,* 120:1603–1620.

Merzenich, M.M., and J.H. Kaas. 1980. "Reorganization of Mammalian Somatosensory Cortex Following Peripheral Nerve Injury." *Trends Neurosci,* 5:434–436.

Merzenich, M.M., R.J. Nelson, M.S. Stryker, M.S. Cyander, A. Schoppmann, and J.M. Zook. 1984. "Somatosensory Cortical Map Changes Following Digit Amputation in Adult Monkeys." *J Comp Neurol,* 224:591–605.

Miller, S.O. 1989. "Optical Differences in Cases of Multiple Personality Disorders." *J Nerv Ment Disord,* 177:480–486.

Milner, B. 1966. "Amnesia Following Operation on Temporal Lobes." In C.W.M. Whitty and O.L. Zangwill (eds.), *Amnesia.* London: Butterworths.

Milner, B., S. Corkin, and H.L. Teuber. 1968. "Further Analysis of the Hippocampal Amnesic Syndrome: Fourteen Year Follow-up Study of HM." *Neuropsychologia,* 6:215–234.

Milner, D., and M. Goodale. 1995. *The Visual Brain in Action.* New York: Oxford University Press.

Mishkin, M. 1978. "Memory in Monkeys Severely Impaired by Combined but Not Separate Removal of the Amygdala and Hippocampus." *Nature,* 273:297–298.

Mitchell, S.W. 1871. "Phantom Limbs." *Lippincott's Magazine for Popular Literature and Science,* 8:563–569.

Morsier, G. 1967. "Le syndrome de Charles Bonnet, hallucinations visuale sans déficience mentale." *Ann Medico-Psychol,* 2(5):677–702.

Moscovitch, M. 1992. "Memory and Working-with-Memory: A Component Process Model Based on Modules and Central Systems." *Journal of Cognitive Neuroscience,* vol. 4, no. 3:257–267.

Mountcastle, V.B. 1957. "Modality and Topographic Properties of Single Neurons of Cat's Somatic Sensory Cortex." *J Neurophysiol,* 5:377–390.

Mountcastle, V. 1995. "The Evolution of Ideas Concerning the Function of the Neocortex." *Cerebral Cortex,* 5:289–295; 1047–3211.

Mountcastle, V. 1995. "The Parietal System and Some Higher Brain Functions." *Cerebral Cortex,* 5:377–390; 1047–3211.

Nadel, L., and M. Moscovitch. 1997. "Memory Consolidation: Retrograde Amnesia and the Hippocampal Complex." *Cur Opin Neurobiol,* 7:217–227.

Nakamura, R.K., and M. Mishkin. 1980. "Blindness in Monkeys Following Non-Visual Cortical Lesions." *Brain Res,* 188:572–577.

Nathanson, M., P. Bergman, and G. Gordon. 1952. "Denial of Illness." *A.M.A. Archives of Neurology and Psychiatry,* 68:380–387.

Newsome, W.T., A. Mikami, and R.H. Wurtz. 1986. "Motion Selectivity in Macaque Visual Cortex. III: Psychophysics and Physiology of Apparent Motion." *J Neurophysiol,* 55:1340–1351.

Nielsen, H., and O. Kristensen. 1981. "Personality Correlates of Sphenoidal EEG Foci in Temporal Lobe Epilepsy." *Acta Neurol Scand,* 64:289–300.

Nudo, R.J., B.M. Wise, F. SiFuentes, and G. Milliken. 1996. "Neural Substrates for the Effects of Rehabilitative Training on Motor Recovery after Ischemic Infarct." *Science,* 272:1791–1794.

Ornstein, R. 1997. *The Right Mind.* New York: Harcourt Brace.

Papez, J.W. 1937. "A Proposed Mechanism of Emotion." *Arch Neurol Psychiatry,* 38:725–739.

Pascual-Leone, A., M. Peris, J.M. Tormos, A.P. Pascual, and M.D. Catala. 1995. "Reorganization of Human Cortical Motor Output Maps Following Traumatic Forearm Amputation." *Neuroreport,* 7:2068–2070.

Penfield, W., and T. Rasmussen. 1950. *The Cerebral Cortex of Man: A Clinical Study of Localization of Function.* New York: MacMillan.

Penrose, R. 1989. *The Emperor's New Mind.* Oxford: Oxford University Press.

Phelps, M.E., D.E. Kuhl, and J.C. Mazziota. 1981. "Metabolic Mapping of the Brain's Response to Visual Stimulation: Studies in Humans." *Science,* 211(4489): 1445–1448.

Pinker, S. 1997. *How the Mind Works.* New York: W.W. Norton.

Plum, F. 1982. *The Diagnosis of Stupor and Coma.* Philadelphia: F.A. Davis.

Poeck, K. 1969. "Phantom Limbs After Amputation and in Congenital Missing Limbs." *Deutsch Med Woch,* 94:2367–2374.

Pons, T.P., E. Preston, and A. K. Garraghty. 1991. "Massive Cortical Reorganization after Sensory Deafferentation in Adult Macaques:" *Science,* 252:1857–1860.

Poppel, E., R. Held, and D. Frost. 1973. "Residual Vision Function after Brain Wounds Involving the Central Visual Pathways in Man." *Nature,* 243:295–296.

Posner, M., and M. Raichle. 1997. *Images of Mind.* New York: W.H. Freeman.

Pribram, K. "The Role of Analogy in Transcending Limits in the Brain Sciences." *Daedalus,* 109(2):19–38.

Profet, M. 1997. *Pregnancy Sickness.* Reading, MA: Addison-Wesley.

Ramachandran, V.S. 1988a. "Perception of Depth from Shading." *Sci Am,* 269: 76–83.

Ramachandran, V.S. 1988b. "Perception of Shape from Shading." *Nature,* 331: 163–166.

Ramachandran, V.S. 1988c. "Interactions Between Motion, Depth, Color and Form: The Utilitarian Theory of Perception." In C. Blakemore (ed.), *Vision: Coding and Efficiency (Essays in Honour of H.B. Barlow).* Cambridge: Cambridge University Press.

Ramachandran, V.S. 1989a. Vision: A Biological Perspective. Presidential Lecture Given at the Annual Meeting of the Society for Neuroscience, Phoenix, AZ.

Ramachandran, V.S. 1989b. "The Neurobiology of Perception." Presidential Lecture at the Annual Meeting of the Society for Neuroscience, Phoenix, AZ.

Ramachandran, V.S. 1990. "Visual Perception in People and Machines." In A. Blake and T. Troscianko (eds.), *AI and the Eye.* Sussex, Eng.: John Wiley and Sons, 21–77.

Ramachandran, V.S. 1991. "Form, Motion, and Binocular Rivalry." *Science,* 251: 950–951.

Ramachandran, V.S. 1992. "Blind Spots." *Sci Am,* 266:85–91.

Ramachandran, V.S. 1993a. "Behavioral and MEG Correlates of Neural Plasticity in the Adult Human Brain." *Proc Natl Acad Sci USA,* 90:10413–10420.

Ramachandran, V.S. 1993b. "Filling in Gaps in Perception: Part II. Scotomas and Phantom Limbs." *Curr Directions Psychol Sci,* 2:56–65.

Ramachandran, V.S. 1994. "Phantom Limbs, Neglect Syndromes, Repressed Memories and Freudian Psychology." *Int Rev Neurobiol,* 37:291–333.

Ramachandran, V.S. 1995a. "Anosognosia in Parietal Lobe Syndrome." *Consciousness Cognition,* 4:22–51.

Ramachandran, V.S. 1995b. "2-D or Not 2-D: That Is the Question." In R.L. Gregory, J. Harris, P. Heard, and D. Rose (eds.), *The Artful Eye.* Oxford: Oxford University Press, 249–267.

Ramachandran, V.S. 1995c. Editor-in-Chief, *Encyclopedia of Human Behavior,* Vol. 1 to 4. New York: Academic Press.

Ramachandran, V.S. 1995d. "Plasticity in the Adult Human Brain: Is There Reason for Optimism?" In B. Julesz and I. Kovacs (eds.), *Santa Fe Institute for Studies in the Sciences on Complexity,* Vol. XXIII. Reading, MA: Addison-Wesley, 179–197.

Ramachandran, V.S. 1996. "What Neurological Syndromes Can Tell Us about Human Nature: Some Lessons from Phantom Limbs, Capgras' Syndrome, and Anosognosia." *Cold Spring Harbor Symposia,* LXI:115–134.

Ramachandran, V.S. 1997. "Why Do Gentleman Prefer Blondes?" *Med Hypotheses,* 48:19–20.

Ramachandran, V.S. 1998. "Evolution and Neurology of Laughter and Humor." *Med Hypotheses.* In press.

Ramachandran, V.S., E.L. Altschuler, and S. Hillyer. 1997. "Mirror Agnosia." *Proc R Soc London,* 264:645–647.

Ramachandran, V.S., S. Cobb, and L. Levi. 1994a. "Monocular Double Vision in Strabismus." *Neuroreport,* 5:1418.

Ramachandran, V.S., S. Cobb, and L. Levi. 1994b. "The Neural Locus of Binocular Rivalry and Monocular Diplopia in Intermittent Exotropes." *Neuroreport,* 5: 1141–1144.

Ramachandran, V.S., and R.L. Gregory. 1991. "Perceptual Filling In of Artificially Induced Scotomas in Human Vision." *Nature,* 350:699–702.

Ramachandran, V.S., R.L. Gregory, and W. Aiken. 1993. "Perceptual Fading of Visual Texture Borders." *Vision Res,* 33:717–721.

Ramachandran, V.S., and W. Hirstein. 1997. "Three Laws of Qualia." *J Consciousness Studies,* 4(5–6):429–457.

Ramachandran, V.S., W. Hirstein, K.C. Armel, E. Tecoma, and V. Iragui. 1998. "The Neural Basis of Religious Experience." *Soc Neurosci Abst,* 23:519.1.

Ramachandran, V.S., W. Hirstein, and D. Rogers-Ramachandran. 1998. "Phantom Limbs, Body Image, and Neural Plasticity." *IBRO News,* 26(1):10–11.

Ramachandran, V.S., L. Levi, L. Stone, D. Rogers-Ramachandran, R. McKinney, M. Stalcup, G. Arcilla, R. Zweifler, A. Schatz, and A. Flippin. 1996. "Illusions of Body Image: What They Reveal about Human Nature." In R. Llinas and P.S. Churchland (eds.), *The Mind-Brain Continuum.* Cambridge, MA: MIT Press, 29–60.

Ramachandran, V.S. and D. Rogers-Ramachandran. 1996a. "Denial of Disabilities in Anosognosia." *Nature,* 382:501.

Ramachandran, V.S., and D. Rogers-Ramachandran. 1996b. "Synaesthesia in Phantom Limbs Induced with Mirrors." *Proc R Soc London,* 263:377–386.

Ramachandran, V.S., D. Rogers-Ramachandran, and S. Cobb. 1995. "Touching the Phantom Limb." *Nature,* 377:489–490.

Ramachandran, V.S., D. Rogers-Ramachandran, and M. Stewart. 1992. "Perceptual Correlates of Massive Cortical Reorganization." *Science,* 258:1159–1160.

Ramachandran, V.S., M. Stewart, and D. Rogers-Ramachandran. 1992. "Perceptual Correlates of Massive Cortical Reorganization." *Neuroreport,* 3:583–586.

Riddoch, G. 1941. "Phantom Limbs and Body Shape." *Brain,* 64:197.

Ridley, M. 1997. *The Origins of Virtue.* New York: Viking Penguin.

Robinson, R.G., K.L. Kubos, L.B. Starr, K. Rao, and T.R. Price. 1983. "Mood Changes in Stroke Patients." *Comp Psychiatry,* 24:555–566.

Robinson, R.G., K.L. Kubos, and L.B. Starr. 1984. "Mood Disorders in Stroke Patients." *Brain,* 107:81–93.

Rock, I. 1985. *The Logic of Perception.* Cambridge, MA: MIT Press.

Rodin, E., and S. Schmaltz. 1984. "The Bear-Fedio Personality Inventory." *Neurology,* 34:591–596.

Rolls, E.T. 1995. "A Theory of Emotion and Consciousness, and Its Application to Understanding the Neural Basis of Emotion." In M.S. Gazzinga (ed.), *The Cognitive Neurosciences*. Cambridge, MA: MIT Press.

Rossetti, Y. 1996. "Implicit Perception in Action: Short-Lived Motor Representations of Space Evidenced by Brain-Damaged and Healthy Subjects." In P.G. Grossenbacher (ed.), *Consciousness and Brain Circuitry: Neurocognitive Systems Which Mediate Subjective Experience*. Advances in Consciousness Research. Philadelphia: J. Benjamins Publ.

Saadeh, E.S., and R. Melzack. 1994. "Phantom Limb Experiences in Congenital Limb-Deficient Adults." *Cortex*, 30:479–485.

Sacks, O. 1984. *A Leg to Stand On*. New York: Harper and Row.

Sacks, O. 1985. *The Man Who Mistook His Wife for a Hat*. New York: HarperCollins.

Sacks, O. 1990. *Awakenings*. New York: HarperPerennial Library.

Sacks, O. 1990. *Seeing Voices*. New York: HarperCollins.

Sacks, O. 1995. *An Anthropologist on Mars*. New York: Alfred A. Knopf.

Schacter, D.L. 1992. "Consciousness and Awareness in Memory and Amnesia: Critical Issues." In A.D. Milner and M.D. Rugg (eds.), *Neuropsychology of Consciousness*. London: Academic Press, 179–200.

Schacter, D.L. 1996. *Searching for Memory*. New York: Basic Books.

Schopenhauer, A. 1819. *Die welt als wille und virstellung*. Leipzig.

Searle, J. 1992. "Minds, Brains, and Programs." *Behav Brain Sci*, 3:417–458.

Searle, J. 1994. *The Rediscovery of the Mind*. Cambridge, MA: MIT Press.

Sereno, M.I., A.M. Dale, J.B. Reppas, K.K. Kwong, J.W. Belliveau, T.J. Brady, B.R. Rosen, R.B. Tootell, et al. 1995. "Borders of Multiple Visual Areas in Humans Revealed by Functional Magnetic Resonance Imaging." *Science*, 268: 889–893.

Sergent, J. 1988. "An Investigation into Perceptual Completion in Blind Areas of the Visual Field." *Brain*, 111:347–373.

Shallice, T. 1988. *From Neuropsychology to Mental Structure*. Cambridge: Cambridge University Press.

Simmel, M. 1962. "The Reality of Phantom Sensations." *Soc Res*, 29:337–356.

Sinclair-Gieben, A.H.C., and D. Chalmers. 1959. "Evaluation of Treatment of Warts by Hypnosis." *Lancet*, 2: 480–482.

Singer, W. 1993. "Synchronization of Cortical Activity and Its Putative Role in Information Processing and Learning." *Ann Rev Physiol*, 55:349–374.

Slater, E., and A.W. Beard. 1963. "The Schizophrenia-like Psychoses of Epilepsy. V. Discussion and Conclusions." *Br J Psychiatry*, 109:95–150.

Snyder, A., and M. Thomas. 1997 "Autistic Savants Give Clues to Cognition." *Perception*, 26:93–96.

Spanos, N.P., R.S. Stenstrom, and M.A. Johnston. 1988. "Hypnosis, Placebo, and Suggestion in the Treatment of Warts." *Psychosom Med*, 50:245–260.

Springer, S., and G. Deutsch. 1998. *Left Brain, Right Brain*. San Francisco: W.H. Freeman.

Squire, L. 1987. *Memory and the Brain*. New York: Oxford Press.

Squire, L.R., and S. Zola-Morgan. 1983. "The Neurology of Memory: The Case for Correspondence Between the Findings for Human and Nonhuman Primates." In

J.A. Deutsch (ed.) *The Physiological Basis of Memory,* 2nd ed. New York: Academic Press.

Starkman, M., J. Marshall, J. La Ferla, and R.P. Kelch. 1985. "Pseudocyesis." *Psychosom Med,* 47:46–57.

Starr, A., and L. Phillips. 1970. "Verbal and Motor Memory in the Amnesic Syndrome." *Neuropsychologia,* 8:75–88.

Stoerig, P., and A. Cowey. 1989. "Wavelength Sensitivity in Blindsight." *Nature,* 342:916–918.

Sunderland, S. 1972. *Nerves and Nerve Injuries.* Edinburgh: Churchill Livingstone.

Sur. M., P.E. Garraghty, and C.J. Bruce. 1985. "Somatosensory Cortex in Macaque Monkeys: Laminar Differences in Receptive Field Size." *Brain Res,* 342: 391–395.

Surman. O.S., K. Sheldon, and T.P. Hackett. 1973. "Hypnosis in the Treatment of Warts." *Arch Gen Psychiatry,* 28:438–441.

Symons, D. 1979. *The Evolution of Human Sexuality.* New York: Oxford University Press.

Symons, D. 1995. In P. Abramson and S.D. Pinkerton (eds.), *Sexual Nature and Sexual Culture.* Chicago and London: University of Chicago Press.

Taub, E., N.E. Miller, T.A. Novack, E.W. Cook, W.C. Fleming, C.S. Neomuceno, J.S. Connell, and J.E. Crago. 1993. "Technique to Improve Chronic Motor Deficit After Stroke." *Arch Phys Med Rehabil,* 74:347–354.

Toga, A.W., and J.C. Mazziotta. 1996. *Brain Mapping: The Methods.* New York: Academic Press.

Tovee, M.J., E. Rolls, and V.S. Ramachandran. 1996. "Rapid Visual Learning in Neurons in the Primate Visual Cortex." *Neuroreport,* 7:2757–2760.

Tranel, D., and A.R. Damsio. 1985. "Knowledge Without Awareness: An Automatic Index of Facial Recognition by Prosopagnosics." *Science,* 228:235–249.

Treisman, A. 1986. "Features and Objects in Visual Processing." *Sci Am,* 225:114–126.

Trevarthen, C.B. 1968. "Two Mechanisms of Vision in Primates." *Psychol Forsch,* 31:299–337.

Trimble, M.R. 1992. "The Gastaut-Geschwind Syndrome." In M.R. Trimble and T.G. Bolwig (eds.), *The Temporal Lobes and the Limbic System.* Petersfield, Eng.: Wrightson Biomedical.

Trivers, R. 1985. *Social Evolution.* Menlo Park, CA: Benjamin-Cummings.

Tucker, D.M. 1981. "Lateral Brain, Function, Mood, and Conceptualization." *Psychological Bulletin,* 89:19–46.

Turnbull, O.H. 1997. "Mirror, Mirror on the Wall—Is the Left Side There at All?" *Current Biology,* 7R:709–711.

Turnbull, O.H., D. Carey, and R. McCarthy. 1997. "The Neuropsychology of Object Constancy." *Journal of the International Neuropsychological Society,* 3: 288–298.

Van der Berghe, L., and P. Frost. 1986. "Skin Color Preference, Sexual Dimorphism and Sexual Selection: A Case of Gene Co-evolution." *Ethnic Racial Studies,* 9: 87–113.

Van Essen, D.C. 1979. "Visual Cortical Areas." In W.M. Cowan (ed.), *Annual Reviews in Neuroscience,* Vol. 2. Palo Alto, CA: Palo Alto Annual Reviews, 227–263.

Wall, P.D. 1977. "The Presence of Inaffective Synapses and the Circumstances Which Unmask Them." *Philos Trans R Soc Lond* [Biol], 278:361–372.

Wall, P.D. 1984. "The Painful Consequences of Peripheral Injury." *J Hand Surg Br*, 9:37–39.

Walker, R., and J.B. Mattingley. 1997. "Ghosts in the Machine? Pathological Visual Completion Phenomena in the Damaged Brain." *Neurocase*, 3:313–335.

Warrington, E.K., and L. Weiskrantz. 1970. "Amnesic Syndrome: Consolidation or Retrieval?" *Nature*, 228:628–630.

Warrington, E.K., and L. Weiskrantz. 1971. "Organizational Aspects of Memory in Amnesic Patients." *Neuropsychologia*, 9:67–73.

Warrington, E.K., and L.W. Duchen. 1992. "A Reappraisal of a Case of Persistent Global Amnesia Following Right Temporal Lobectomy—A Clinicopathological Study." *Neuropsychologia*, 30:437–450.

Waxman, S.G., and N. Geschwind. 1975. "The Interictal Behavior Syndrome of Temporal Lobe Epilepsy." *Arch Gen Psychiatry*, 32:1580–1586.

Weinberger, N.M., J.L. McGaugh, and G. Lynch. 1985. *Memory Systems of the Brain*. New York: Guilford Press.

Weinstein, E.A., and R.L. Kahn. 1950. "The Syndrome of Anosognosia." *Arch Neurol Psychiatry*, 64:772–791.

Weir Mitchell, S. 1872. *Injuries of Nerves and Their Consequences*. Philadelphia: Lippincott.

Weir Mitchell, S. 1871. "Phantom Limbs." *Lippincott's Magazine*, 8:563–569.

Weiskrantz, L. 1985. "Issues and Theories in the Study of the Amnesic Syndrome." In N.M. Weinberger, J.L. McGaugh, and G. Lynch (eds.), *Memory Systems of the Brain: Animal and Human Cognitive Processes*. New York: Guilford Press, 380–415.

Weiskrantz, L. 1986. *Blindsight*. Oxford: Oxford University Press.

Weiskrantz, L. 1987. "Neuroanatomy of Memory and Amnesia: A Case for Multiple Memory Systems." *Hum Neurobiol*, 6:93–105.

Weiskrantz, L. 1997. *Consciousness Lost and Regained*. New York: Oxford University Press.

Wieser, H.G. 1983. "Depth Recorded Limbic Seizures and Psychopathy." *Neurosci Behav Rev*, 7:427–440.

Williams, G. 1966. *Adaptation and Natural Selection*. Princeton, NJ: Princeton University Press.

Wills, C. 1993. *The Runaway Brain*. New York: Basic Books.

Wilson, E.O. 1978. *On Human Nature*. Cambridge, MA: Harvard University Press.

Winson, J. 1986. *Brain and Psyche*. New York: Vintage Books, Random House.

Wright, R. 1994. *The Moral Animal*. New York: Random House.

Yang, T., C. Gallen, B. Schwartz, F. Bloom, V.S. Ramachandran, and S. Cobb. 1994. "Sensory Maps in the Human Brain." *Nature*, 368:592–593.

Yang, T., C. Gallen, V.S. Ramachandran, B.J. Schwartz, and F.E. Bloom. 1994b. "Noninvasive Detection of Cerebral Plasticity in Adult Human Somatosensory Cortex." *Neuroreport*, 5:701–704.

Young, A.W., and E.H.F. De Haan. 1992. "Face Recognition and Awareness after Brain Injury." In A.D. Milner and M.D. Rugg (eds.), *The Neuropsychology of Consciousness*. London: Academic Press, 69–90.

Young, A.W., H.D. Ellis, A.H. Quayle, and K.W. De Pauw. 1993. "Face Processing

Impairments and the Capgras Delusion." *Br J Psychiatry,* 162: 695–698.

Zaidel, E. 1985. "Academic Implications of Dual Brain Theory." In D. Benson and E. Zaidel (eds.), *The Dual Brain*. New York: Guilford Press.

Zeki, S. 1980. "The Representation of Colours in the Cerebral Cortex." *Nature,* 284:412–418.

Zeki, S.M. 1978. "Functional Specialisation in the Visual Cortex of the Rhesus Monkey." Nature 274:423–428.

Zeki, S.M. 1993. *A Vision of the Brain*. Oxford: Oxford University Press.

Zihl, J., D. von Cramon, and N. Mai. 1983. "Selective Disturbance of Movement Vision after Bilateral Brain Damage." *Brain,* 106:313–340.

Zuk, M., K. Johnson, R. Thornhill, and D.J. Ligon. 1990. "Mechanisms of Female Choice in Red Jungle Fowl." *Evolution,* 44:477–485.

Index

Page numbers in *italics* refer to illustrations.